T0195421

Renal Cancer: Old and New Paradigms

Editors

STEVEN L. CHANG
MICHAEL L. BLUTE Sr.

UROLOGIC CLINICS
OF NORTH AMERICA

www.urologic.theclinics.com

Consulting Editor
KEVIN R. LOUGHLIN

May 2023 • Volume 50 • Number 2

ELSEVIER

1600 John F. Kennedy Boulevard • Suite 1800 • Philadelphia, Pennsylvania, 19103-2899

http://www.theclinics.com

UROLOGIC CLINICS OF NORTH AMERICA Volume 50, Number 2
May 2023 ISSN 0094-0143, ISBN-13: 978-0-443-18286-0

Editor: Kerry Holland
Developmental Editor: Diana Ang

Urologic Clinics of North America (ISSN 0094-0143) is published quarterly by Elsevier Inc., 360 Park Avenue South, New York, NY 10010-1710. Months of issue are February, May, August, and November. Business and Editorial Offices: 1600 John F. Kennedy Blvd., Suite 1800, Philadelphia, PA 19103-2899. Periodicals postage paid at New York, NY and additional mailing offices. Subscription prices are $415.00 per year (US individuals), $832.00 per year (US institutions), $100.00 per year (US students and residents), $473.00 per year (Canadian individuals), $1040.00 per year (Canadian institutions), $100.00 per year (Canadian students/residents), $546.00 per year (foreign individuals), $1040.00 per year (foreign institutions), and $240.00 per year (foreign students/residents). Foreign air speed delivery is included in all *Clinics* subscription prices. All prices are subject to change without notice. **POSTMASTER:** Send address changes to *Urologic Clinics of North America*, Elsevier Health Sciences Division, Subscription Customer Service, 3251 Riverport Lane, Maryland Heights, MO 63043. **Customer Service: 1-800-654-2452 (US). From outside the United States, call 1-314-447-8871. Fax: 1-314-447-8029. E-mail: JournalsCustomerServiceusa@elsevier.com (for print support)** and **JournalsOnlineSupport-usa@elsevier.com (for online support)**.

Reprints. For copies of 100 or more, of articles in this publication, please contact the Commercial Reprints Department, Elsevier Inc., 360 Park Avenue South, New York, New York 10010-1710. Tel.: 212-633-3874; Fax: 212-633-3820; E-mail: reprints@elsevier.com.

Urologic Clinics of North America is covered in MEDLINE/PubMed (*Index Medicus*), *Excerpta Medica, Current Contents/Clinical Medicine, Science Citation Index,* and *ISI/BIOMED*.

Contributors

CONSULTING EDITOR

KEVIN R. LOUGHLIN, MD, MBA
Emeritus Professor of Surgery (Urology),
Harvard Medical School, Visiting Scientist,
Vascular Biology Research Program at Boston
Children's Hospital, Boston, Massachusetts

EDITORS

STEVEN L. CHANG, MD, MS
Associate Professor of Surgery, Harvard
Medical School Co-Director of the Kidney
Cancer Center, Dana-Farber Cancer Institute
Section Chief of Urologic Oncology, Division of
Urology, Brigham and Women's Hospital
Boston, Massachusetts, USA

MICHAEL L. BLUTE Sr., MD
Walter S. Kerr Jr Professor of Surgery, Harvard
Medical School, Chief, Department of Urology,
Massachusetts General Hospital, Boston,
Massachusetts, USA

AUTHORS

ROBERT ABOUASSALY, MD
Staff Urologist, Glickman Urological and
Kidney Institute, Cleveland Clinic Foundation,
Cleveland, Ohio, USA

REZA ALAGHEHBANDAN, MD
Department of Pathology, Robert J. Tomsich
Pathology and Laboratory Medicine Institute,
Cleveland Clinic, Cleveland, Ohio, USA

SOHRAB NAUSHAD ALI, MD, MSc, FRCSC
Assistant Clinical Professor, Department of
Urology, University of California, Irvine, Irvine,
California, USA

MAJED ALRUMAYYAN, MD
Division of Urology, Department of Surgery,
Princess Margaret Cancer Centre, University
Health Network, Toronto, Ontario, Canada

TARIK BENIDIR, MD, MSc
Urologic Oncology Fellow, Glickman
Urological and Kidney Institute, Cleveland
Clinic Foundation, Cleveland, Ohio, USA

MICHAEL L. BLUTE Sr., MD
Walter S. Kerr Jr Professor of Surgery, Harvard
Medical School, Chief, Department of Urology,
Massachusetts General Hospital, Boston,
Massachusetts, USA

DAVID A. BRAUN, MD, PhD
Center of Molecular and Cellular Oncology,
Yale Cancer Center, Yale School of Medicine,
New Haven, Connecticut, USA

REBECCA A. CAMPBELL, MD
Chief Resident - Urology, Glickman
Urological and Kidney Institute, Cleveland
Clinic Foundation, Cleveland, Ohio,
USA

STEVEN C. CAMPBELL, MD, PhD
Professor of Surgery, Residency Program
Director, Vice Chair, Department of Urology,
Glickman Urological and Kidney Institute,
Cleveland Clinic Foundation, Cleveland, Ohio,
USA

ALEX CHUNG, MD
Assistant Professor, Department of Radiology, David Geffen School of Medicine at UCLA, Los Angeles, California, USA

STEVEN L. CHANG, MD, MS, FACS
Division of Urology, Brigham and Women's Hospital, Boston, Massachusetts, USA

BENJAMIN I. CHUNG, MD, MS
Department of Urology, Stanford University School of Medicine, Stanford, California, USA

SHAWN DASON, MD
Division of Urologic Oncology, The Ohio State University Comprehensive Cancer Center, Columbus, Ohio, USA

ANTONIO FINELLI, MD, MSc
Division of Urology, Department of Surgery, Princess Margaret Cancer Centre, University Health Network, Toronto, Ontario, Canada

OTHON ILIOPOULOS, MD
VHL Comprehensive Clinical Care Center and Hemangioblastoma Center, Division of Hematology-Oncology, Department of Medicine, Massachusetts General Hospital, Center for Cancer Research, Massachusetts General Hospital Cancer Center, Charlestown, Massachusetts, USA; Associate Professor of Medicine, Harvard Medical School, Boston, Massachusetts, USA

SOKI KASHIMA, MD, PhD
Center of Molecular and Cellular Oncology, Yale Cancer Center, Yale School of Medicine, New Haven, Connecticut, USA; Department of Urology, Akita University, Graduate School of Medicine, Akita, Japan

JAIME LANDMAN, MD
Professor and Chair, Department of Urology, University of California, Irvine, Irvine, California, USA

KEITH A. LAWSON, MD, PhD
Division of Urology, Department of Surgery, Princess Margaret Cancer Centre, University Health Network, Toronto, Ontario, Canada

JONATHAN E. LEEMAN, MD
Department of Radiation Oncology, Dana-Farber Cancer Institute, Brigham and Women's Hospital, Boston, Massachusetts, USA

JEFFREY J. LEOW, MBBS, MPH, MRCS, FAMS(Urology)
Department of Urology, Tan Tock Seng Hospital, Singapore, Singapore

KEVIN R. LOUGHLIN, MD, MBA
Emeritus Professor of Surgery (Urology), Harvard Medical School, Visiting Scientist, Vascular Biology Research Program, Boston Children's Hospital, Karp Family Research Laboratories, Boston, Massachusetts, USA

JESSE K. McKENNEY, MD
Department of Pathology, Robert J. Tomsich Pathology and Laboratory Medicine Institute, Cleveland Clinic, Cleveland, Ohio, USA

JAHAN MOHEBALI, MD, MPH
Division of Vascular and Endovascular Surgery, Massachusetts General Hospital, Harvard Medical School, Boston, Massachusetts, USA

JOSÉ IGNACIO NOLAZCO, MD
Division of Urological Surgery, Brigham and Women's Hospital, Harvard Medical School, Boston, Massachusetts, USA; Servicio de Urología, Hospital Universitario Austral, Universidad Austral, Pilar, Argentina

STEVEN S. RAMAN, MD, FSAR, FSIR
Professor of Radiology, Urology and Surgery, David Geffen School of Medicine at UCLA, Los Angeles, California, USA

NITYAM RATHI, BS
Medical Student, Glickman Urological and Kidney Institute, Cleveland Clinic Foundation, Cleveland, Ohio, USA

LUCSHMAN RAVEENDRAN, MD, MSc
Division of Urology, Department of Surgery, Princess Margaret Cancer Centre, University Health Network, Toronto, Ontario, Canada

SHAGNIK RAY, MD
Division of Urologic Oncology, The Ohio State University Comprehensive Cancer Center, Columbus, Ohio, USA

KEYAN SALARI, MD, PhD
Department of Urology, Massachusetts General Hospital, Harvard Medical School, Boston, Massachusetts, USA; Broad Institute of MIT and Harvard, Cambridge, Massachusetts, USA

ERIC A. SINGER, MD, MA, MS, FACS, FASCO
Division of Urologic Oncology, The Ohio State University Comprehensive Cancer Center, Columbus, Ohio, USA

SIMON JOHN CHRISTOPH SOERENSEN, MD
Department of Urology, Stanford, California, USA; Department of Epidemiology and Population Health, Stanford University School of Medicine, Stanford, USA

ZACHARY TANO, MD
Department of Urology, University of California, Irvine, Irvine, California, USA

CHRISTOPHER J. WEIGHT, MD
Center Director Urologic Oncology, Fellowship Director, Society of Urologic Oncology Fellowship, Glickman Urological and Kidney Institute, Cleveland Clinic Foundation, Cleveland, Ohio, USA

ANDREW M. WOOD, MD, MS
Urologic Oncology Fellow, Glickman Urological and Kidney Institute, Cleveland Clinic Foundation, Cleveland, Ohio, USA

KENDRICK YIM, MD
Division of Urology, Brigham and Women's Hospital, Boston, Massachusetts, USA

Contents

There is a clear benefit of imaging-based differentiation of small indeterminate renal masses to its possible subtypes of clear cell renal cell carcinoma (RCC), chromophobe RCC, papillary RCC, fat poor angiomyolipoma and oncocytoma because it helps guide the next step options for the patients. Different parameters in computed tomography, MRI, and contrast-enhanced ultrasound demonstrate many reliable imaging features that can suggest certain tissue subtypes. Likert score-based risk stratification systems can help determine management, and new techniques such as perfusion, radiogenomics, single-photon emission tomography, and artificial intelligence can add to the imaging-based evaluation of indeterminate renal masses.

The pathologic classification of renal tumors is a dynamic and complex process, which has evolved to a "histomolecular" driven system. Despite advances in molecular characterization, most renal tumors can be diagnosed by morphology with or without using a limited set of immunohistochemical stains. If access to molecular resources and specific immunohistochemical markers is limited, pathologists may face difficulties in following an optimal algorithm to classify renal tumors. In this article, we detail the historical evolution of renal tumor classification, including a synopsis of major changes introduced by the current fifth edition World Health Organization 2022 classification of renal epithelial tumors.

Renal cell carcinoma (RCC) is a heterogeneous disease characterized by a broad spectrum of disorders in terms of genetics, molecular and clinical characteristics. There is an urgent need for noninvasive tools to stratify and select patients for treatment accurately. In this review, we analyze serum, urinary, and imaging biomarkers that have the potential to detect malignant tumors in patients with RCC. We discuss the characteristics of these numerous biomarkers and their ability to be used routinely in clinical practice. The development of biomarkers continues to evolve with promising prospects.

venous tumor thrombus. Surgical resection is indicated for most patients with RCC and an inferior vena cava (IVC) thrombus in the absence of metastatic disease. Resection also has an important role in selected patients with metastatic disease. In this review, we discuss the comprehensive management of the patient with RCC with IVC tumor thrombus, emphasizing a multidisciplinary approach to the surgical techniques and perioperative management.

Because metachronous metastatic disease will develop in 20% to 40% of patients with presumed localized renal cell carcinoma (RCC) treated surgically, research is focused on neoadjuvant and adjuvant systemic therapy, to improve disease-free and overall survival. Neoadjuvant therapies trialed include anti–vascular endothelial growth factor (VEGF) tyrosine kinase inhibitor (TKI) agents, or combination therapies (immunotherapy with TKI), and aim to improve resectability of locoregional RCC. Adjuvant therapies trialed include cytokines, anti-VEGF TKI agents, or immunotherapy. These therapeutics can facilitate the surgical extirpation of the primary kidney tumor in the neoadjuvant setting and improve disease-free survival in the adjuvant setting.

Paraneoplastic syndromes can occur in 8% to 20% of individuals with malignancies. They can occur in a variety of cancers that include breast, gastric, leukemia, lung, ovarian, pancreatic, prostate, testicular, as well as kidney. The classic presentation of the triad of mass, hematuria, and flank pain occurs in less than 15% of patients with renal cancer. Because of the protean presentations of renal cell cancer, it has been referred to as the internist's tumor or the great masquerader. This article will provide a review of the causes of these symptoms.

The role of surgery for patients with locally advanced and metastatic renal cell carcinoma (RCC) is not precisely defined in our contemporary era of systemic therapies. Research in this field is focused on the role of regional lymphadenectomy, along with indications and timing of cytoreductive nephrectomy and metastasectomy. As our understanding of the molecular and immunological basis of RCC continues to develop along with the advent of novel systemic therapies, prospective clinical trials will be critical in defining how surgery should be integrated into the treatment paradigm of advanced RCC.

Renal cell carcinoma (RCC) has historically been considered resistant to radiotherapy. However, advances in the field of radiation oncology have led to safe delivery of higher radiation doses through the use of stereotactic body radiotherapy (SBRT) that have shown significant activity against RCC. SBRT has now been shown to be a highly effective modality for management of localized RCC for nonsurgical candidates. Increasing evidence also points to a role for SBRT in the management of oligometastatic RCC as a means for not only providing palliation but prolonging time to progression and potentially improving survival.

The management of advanced renal cell carcinoma has advanced tremendously over the past decade, but most patients still do not receive durable clinical benefit from current therapies. Renal cellcarcinoma is an immunogenic tumor, historically with conventional cytokine therapies, such as interleukin-2 and interferon-α, and contemporarily with the introduction of immune checkpoint inhibitors. Now the central therapeutic strategy in renal cell carcinoma is combination therapies including immunecheckpoint inhibitors. In this Review, we look back on the historical changes in systemic therapy for advanced renal cell carcinoma, and focus on the latest developments and prospects in this field.

UROLOGIC CLINICS OF NORTH AMERICA

SERIES OF RELATED INTEREST
Surgical Clinics of North America
https://www.surgical.theclinics.com/

Foreword

When You Hear Hoofbeats, Sometimes Think of Zebras

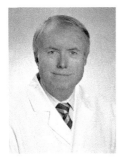

Kevin R. Loughlin, MD, MBA
Consulting Editor

Theodore Woodward, MD, a professor at the University of Maryland, is credited with telling his medical interns in the 1940s, "When you hear hoofbeats behind you, don't expect to see a zebra."[1] By 1960, it was widely quoted throughout the medical profession. The phrase delivered the message that, "Common things occur commonly," and has been part of medical dogma for decades.[2]

However, renal cancers have traditionally been recognized as exceptions to that rule. Renal cancers have been referred to as "The Great Masquerader" or "The Internist's Tumor" and can be elusive to diagnose. At the same time that we recognize the challenges of diagnosing renal cancers, Drs Blute and Chang have provided us with a wonderful resource of the latest recommendations by recognized experts on the diagnosis, management, and prognosis of renal cell carcinoma.

The topics covered in this issue of *Urologic Clinics of North America* include imaging, pathologic classification, biomarkers, the role of renal mass biopsy, surgery, adjuvant and neoadjuvant therapy, and immunotherapy as part of the treatment armamentarium for renal malignancy.

Renal cancer remains a significant challenge to treating physicians. The good news is when a zebra is discovered, we can rely on the information contained in this excellent issue to guide treatment.

Kevin R. Loughlin, MD, MBA
Vascular Biology Research Program at
Boston Children's Hospital
300 Longwood Avenue
Boston, MA 02115, USA

E-mail address:
KLOUGHLIN@PARTNERS.ORG

REFERENCES

1. Available at: en.wikipedia.org/wiki/Zebra_(medicine). Accessed December 13, 2022.
2. Harvey AM. Differential diagnosis. 3rd edition. Philadelphia: W.B. Saunders; 1979. p. 15.

Preface

The Progession Landscape of Diagnostic and Treatment Options for Kidney Cancer

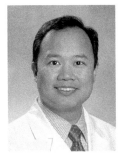 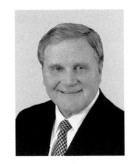

Steven L. Chang, MD, MS   Michael L. Blute Sr., MD
Editors

The management approaches for kidney cancer have undergone a dramatic transformation over the past 20 years. While recent developments in systemic therapeutic options for advanced disease have received a great deal of attention, in truth it is but one of a multitude of notable breakthroughs in the care of patients with kidney cancer, all of which have served to improve patient outcomes.

Arguably, the most important development for kidney cancer has been the shift to an integrated multimodal approach. This issue of *Urologic Clinics of North America* takes the reader on a comprehensive journey demonstrating the innumerable improvements in the various disciplines critical in the treatment of kidney cancer. There have been enhancements in the assessment of renal masses and renal cysts from advancements in imaging to the increasing utilization of renal mass biopsy—with biomarkers on the horizon to achieve greater diagnostic precision. Both the recent refinements in the pathologic classification of kidney cancer and better understanding of hereditary syndromes have established the underlying molecular and genetic alterations of kidney cancer, which in turn laid the groundwork for game-changing pharmacotherapies. The advent of these systemic therapies, including tyrosine kinase inhibitors and more recently immuno-oncology, as well as the simultaneous shift to lower stages of disease at presentation has

consequently impacted the role of surgery. Historically, expeditious surgery was the only option. Now, for low-stage disease (eg, small renal masses and renal cysts), surgery is weighed against nonsurgical options, such as active surveillance and thermal ablation, with strong consideration for patient comorbidities and treatment consequences (eg, chronic kidney disease). For high-stage disease, multidisciplinary management with a focus on quality of life, by addressing paraneoplastic syndrome and other presenting symptoms, along with oncologic outcomes requires a careful coordination between urology, medical oncology, and other specialties. Even radiation therapy, previously not considered an option because kidney cancer was thought to be radioresistant, is now showing promise as a curative treatment for low-stage disease and an effective modality for palliation and consolidation for high-stage disease. Future developments will undoubtedly lead to further evolution in the multimodal treatment of kidney cancer.

The advancements described in this issue were the culmination of an amazing international network of clinicians and researchers collaborating across clinics, academia, and industry. The determined efforts of patients, family members, and patient advocates impacted by kidney cancer are at the core of the progress. While there remains much work ahead, the rapid pace of the advancements in recent years fuels the optimism

Urol Clin N Am 50 (2023) xv–xvi
https://doi.org/10.1016/j.ucl.2023.02.002
0094-0143/23/© 2023 Published by Elsevier Inc.

for further paradigm shifts in the treatment of kidney cancer in the next 20 years.

Steven L. Chang, MD, MS
Harvard Medical School
Dana-Farber Cancer Institute
Brigham and Women's Hospital
Division of Urology
45 Francis Street
Boston, MA 02115, USA

Michael L. Blute Sr., MD
Harvard Medical School
Department of Urology
Massachusetts General Hospital
55 Fruit Street
Boston, MA 02114, USA

E-mail addresses:
slchang@bwh.harvard.edu (S.L. Chang)
mblute@mgh.harvard.edu (M.L. Blute)

Radiologist's Disease
Imaging for Renal Cancer

Alex Chung, MD[a], Steven S. Raman, MD, FSAR, FSIR[b],*

KEYWORDS

- CT • MRI • Ultrasound • Multiphasic contrast imaging

KEY POINTS

- US, CT and MRI imaging can be used to detect and characterize the majority of incidentally detected renal masses.
- A renal mass characterization protocol includes unenhanced, and multiphasic contrast enhanced phases in the corticomedullary (40-70sec), nephrographic (90-180 sec) and excretory (300-480sec) after intravenous contrast injection.
- MRI enables characterization with additonal sequences including T2, in and opposed phase gradient T1 and T1 fat saturated images.
- Contrast enhanced Ultrasound enables detection and characterization with no nephrotoxicity or nephrogenic systemic fibrosis risk.

INTRODUCTION

In part due to the increasing volume of abdominal imaging, there is a corresponding increase in the number of incidentally discovered nonfatty solid and cystic renal masses, most of which are low-grade renal cancers but some which are also benign lesions like fat poor angiomyolipoma (AML) or oncocytoma.[1] Size is one of the most important parameters for triaging indeterminate solid renal masses, where approximately 40% of lesions under 1 cm are benign but under 20% of lesions over 3 to 4 cm are benign.[2] Traditionally, solid nonfatty renal lesions were often surgically resected with up to 20% to 30% yielding a benign diagnosis on final pathologic analysis.[3] The approach to managing incidentally detected small renal masses under 3 cm has evolved with new tools including greyscale ultrasound (US), contrast-enhanced US (CEUS), computed tomography (CT) or MRI imaging-based characterization protocols and schemes, recognition of imaging as a biomarker for aggressive disease, improved availability and accuracy of percutaneous renal mass biopsy, and the adoption of active surveillance or percutaneous thermal ablation due to

the recognition that most solid renal masses grow slowly and tend to be of low histologic grade[4] instead of the traditional presumption of malignancy and partial nephrectomy.[5] Accurate imaging characterization of the small indeterminate renal masses is important because it allows for optimal triage of these lesions based on the level of risk to active surveillance only, biopsy, or ablation/surgical treatment. This article highlights recent advances in imaging-based methods of lesion characterization on multiphasic imaging and summarize the various fields of forthcoming advancements in radiology for characterizing indeterminate renal masses (see **Fig. 13**).

Normal Anatomy and Conventional Imaging Technique

The Society of Abdominal Radiology (SAR) guidelines for renal mass imaging recommend at minimum a two-phase CT protocol consisting of both an unenhanced and post intravenous iodinated contrast-enhanced nephrographic (120 s) phase imaging on CT to assess for enhancement to confirm the detection of a solid renal mass (**Table 1**) (**Fig. 1**).[7] Unenhanced images serve as a baseline

[a] Department of Radiology, David Geffen School of Medicine at UCLA, Los Angeles, CA 90095, USA; [b] David Geffen School of Medicine at UCLA, 757 Westwood Bl, RRMC, Los Angeles, CA, USA
* Corresponding author. 1621H RRH, 757 Westwood Boulevard RRMC, Los Angeles, CA 90095, USA
E-mail address: sraman@mednet.ucla.edu

Urol Clin N Am 50 (2023) 161–180
https://doi.org/10.1016/j.ucl.2023.01.006

Table 1
Imaging on computed tomography

Imaging Protocols				
CT (6)				
Contrast: Low or iso-osmolar, 35 to 52.5 g iodine (appx. 100 to 150 mL of 350 mg iodine/mL), rate: 2 to 5 cc/s				
Phase	*Anatomic Coverage*	*Acquisition*	*Reconstructions*	*Additional Reformats*
Pre-contrast	Kidneys only	Axial	3 mm slices, with or without 50% overlap	
Corticomedullary	Kidneys only	Axial, 40 to 70 s delay	3 mm slices, with or without 50% overlap	Coronal/sagittal, 3 mm slices without overlap
Nephrographic	Kidneys only	Axial, 100 to 120 s delay	3 mm slices, with or without 50% overlap	Coronal/sagittal, 3 mm slices without overlap
Excretory	Diaphragm to iliac crests	Axial, 7 to 10 min delay	3 mm slices, with or without 50% overlap	Coronal/sagittal, 3 mm slices without overlap
MRI (9)				
Contrast: Extracellular gadolinium-based, 0.1 mL/kg, rate: 1 to 2 mL/s followed by 10 to 20 mL saline				
Sequence	*Planes/Thickness/Gap*		*Details/Alternatives*	
2D T2 SSFSE	Axial/4 to 5 mm/no gap Coronal/5 to 6 mm/no gap		2D T2 FSE/4 to 5 mm slice thickness/no gap	
2D T1 GRE in/out of phase	Axial/5 to 6 mm/0.5 to 1 mm		3D Dixon/3 to 4 mm slice thickness/no gap	
3D T1 SPGR fat saturation, pre-contrast	Axial/3 to 4 mm/no gap Coronal/3 to 4 mm/no gap			
3D T1 dynamic SPGR fat saturation, post-contrast	Axial/3 to 4 mm/no gap Coronal/3 to 4 mm/no gap		Post-contrast timing: 30, 90 to 100, 180 to 210 s, and 5 to 7 min Obtain subtraction images as well	
Diffusion-weighted imaging	Axial/5 to 6 mm/no gap		B-values: 0 to 50, 400 to 500, and 800 to 1000 s/mm^2	

for further characterization of enhancement patterns and allow for characterization of calcifications, macroscopic fat, and lesion homogeneity.[8] Nephrographic phase is important for most hypo and hypervascular lesion detection but is insufficient for contemporary schemes relying on multiple phases for lesion characterization.[8]

For solid renal lesion characterization and optimal lesion detection of hypervascular lesions, the SAR guidelines also recommend the addition of corticomedullary and excretory phases, which help delineate renal vasculature, cortical enhancement, lesion enhancement and de-enhancement relative to cortex and assessment of the renal collecting system anatomy before potential interventions. Contemporary imaging schemes such as the clear cell score and others provide a preoperative imaging-based qualitative and quantitative renal mass characterization scheme to distinguish clear cell renal cell carcinoma (RCC) from other renal cancer subtypes and other benign lesions such as oncocytoma and fat-poor AML.[7]

Active surveillance schemes may rely on serial imaging with US, CEUS, CT or MRI. Using a CT only based imaging surveillance increases radiation exposure to patients and while care is taken to minimize dose for all patients, it is particularly important for younger patients whose risk of lifetime cancer risk can theoretically increase from 1/1000 to 1/82 with the equivalent of 8 lifetime CT scans although no known secondary cancer cases have been documented from medical dose radiation from CT scans.[9]

Dynamic contrast-enhanced MRI (DCE MRI) relies on intravenous gadolinium and provides several advantages over CT including unenhanced lesion imaging characteristics such as T2 weighted signal, fat- and water-specific T1-weighted Dixon sequences, and diffusion-weighted imaging (see **Table 1**) (see **Fig. 1**).[10] Even though it has the

MRI   CT

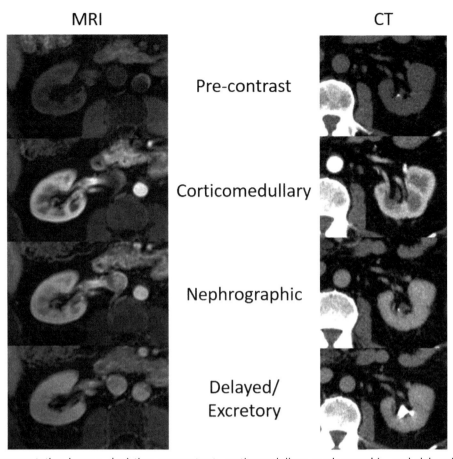

Pre-contrast

Corticomedullary

Nephrographic

Delayed/
Excretory

Fig. 1. Representative images depicting pre-contrast, corticomedullary, nephrographic, and delayed/excretory phases on both CT and MRI.[6] (*From* Allgood E, Raman SS. Image Interpretation: Practical Triage of Benign from Malignant Renal Masses. Radiol Clin North Am. Sep 2020;58(5):875-884. https://doi.org/10.1016/j.rcl.2020.06.002.)

benefit of lack of ionizing radiation compared with CT, MRI may have its own limitations related to longer imaging times, poor detection of lesion calcifications, variable imaging quality due to patient factors such as body habitus, claustrophobia, motion, and pacemakers or other metallic implanted devices or foreign bodies causing signal loss as well as longer time for image acquisition.

CEUS is an alternative emerging imaging modality with its own unique benefits over CT or MRI, such as minimal risk of contrast-related morbidity, lack of nephrotoxicity and ionizing radiation exposure, real-time scanning, and the ability to give contrast multiple times during image acquisition.[10] Limitations of CEUS are operator dependence with limited availability, higher inter-operator variability, the difficulty of reproducibility, and limited imaging in patients with large-body habitus.[11]

In general, multiphasic CT is widely available with well-defined protocols for imaging renal masses while DCE MRI is best performed on a 3 T system with high-performance gradients and

CEUS requires special software and training in the use of microbubbles. The combination of all of these modalities can be used for the diagnosis of indeterminate renal masses and can be used in a serial fashion for active surveillance, especially in elderly patients or patients with multiple comorbidities precluding surgery or ablation.

Imaging Findings/Pathology

After the detection of any given incidental renal lesion, the first step is to determine if it is solid or cystic. Cystic lesions are very common and may be categorized according to the Bosniak classification initially published in 1986 and most recently updated in 2019.[12] Cystic lesions are more commonly exophytic and are at least 70% fluid filled with relatively thin walls. Solid-enhancing lesions are less common than cystic lesions although most renal benign and malignant tumors are solid. Bosniak I cysts are lesions that have uniformly low attenuation (<15 HU) on unenhanced

CT, uniformly high T2 signal on MRI, and anechoic on US without any perceptible wall or mural enhancement. More complex cystic lesions are categorized according to the higher attenuation of the cyst contents, decreasing T2 signal and increasing T1 signal on MRI and echogenicity on US reflecting proteinaceous or hemorrhagic contents. Further cyst complexity is categorized by the number, size, and enhancement of septations as well as presence of enhancing nodules in the wall or in septations to provide increased confidence for a low-grade cystic malignancy.

Solid lesions with macroscopic fat (<−25 HU on CT, T1 hypointense on MRI with fat saturation, and hyperechoic on US) and absence of calcifications, especially if lobular and exophytic with a contour that conforms to the surrounding renal tissue, can be confidently diagnosed as benign AML.[1] In other solid lesions, more aggressive features such as, poor lesion margins, contour irregularity, lesion heterogeneity, local invasion, and infiltrative spread pattern can be used to distinguish sarcomatoid RCC and collecting duct carcinoma from more common and indolent subtypes of RCC or benign lesions.[13] If a renal lesion does not satisfy these criteria, it is considered indeterminate renal mass with most likely differential diagnosis of clear cell (ccRCC), papillary (pRCC), or chromophobe RCC (chrRCC), or common benign entities such as oncocytoma or fat-poor AML (FP-AML).

Most of these incidentally detected solid renal lesions can be categorized using a multiphasic contrast-enhanced CT or MRI with unenhanced, cortical, nephrographic phase, and excretory phase imaging, and the remainder can be characterized by percutaneous biopsy. Classifying solid lesions into one of the five most common benign and malignant renal lesions enables triage of these lesions to clinical options of active surveillance, biopsy, ablation, surgical treatment or no further follow-up. For lesion characterization, measuring the peak enhancement in the corticomedullary and de-enhancement in the nephrographic and excretory phases has been shown to be of value because most of these lesions had different shape and timing of peak enhancement curves over the four phases on both CT and MRI (absolute enhancement).[14,15] In follow-up studies, by Lee-Felker and colleagues and Young and colleagues on both CT and MRI, most of the clear cell renal cell cancers enhance rapidly above background renal cortex in the corticomedullary phase (relative enhancement) with rapid washout. Other lesions have their own characteristic patterns of enhancement in these post-contrast phases as described below (**Fig. 2**).[15,16] Similar observations and patterns of enhancement have also been shown on CEUS.[11] Further refinement of these methods and greater sample sizes show higher reliability and accuracy in differentiating the enhancing

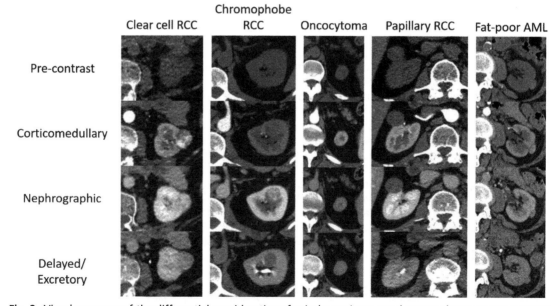

Fig. 2. Visual summary of the differential considerations for indeterminate renal masses shown at pre-contrast, corticomedullary, nephrographic, and excretory/delayed phases. Although there are some characteristics that allow for differentiation between these lesions, there is significant overlap in the subjective appearances of oncocytoma, fat-poor AML, clear cell, papillary, and chromophobe renal cell carcinoma.[6] (*From* Allgood E, Raman SS. Image Interpretation: Practical Triage of Benign from Malignant Renal Masses. Radiol Clin North Am. Sep 2020;58(5):875-884. https://doi.org/10.1016/j.rcl.2020.06.002.)

indeterminate renal masses via imaging with further details summarized below.

Clear cell RCC tend to be round, oval or lobular in shape with obtuse angles to the renal cortex with a claw sign heterogeneous enhancement with unenhanced hounsfield units (HU); between 25 and 40, corticomedullary phase peak absolute HU above 160, nephrographic phase HU of 120 and excretory HU of 100.

Papillary RCC is the second most common malignant histology after clear cell RCC and tends to have slightly higher unenhanced CT attenuation (35 to 45 HU), relatively poor and progressive enhancement in the corticomedullary phase (60 to 80 HU), with peak enhancement in the nephrographic phase (<100 HU) and de-enhancement on the excretory phase.

Chromophobe RCC is the third most common malignant histology and tends to be larger in size larger size, is heterogeneous, and shows peak absolute HU of 60 to 80 in the nephrographic and excretory phase, which is in contrast to above three lesions. Although these enhancement patterns are distinct for the majority of lesions, there is overlap in up to 20% of several characteristics among the five different renal masses that pose a challenge to a high-confidence differentiation (see **Fig. 2**).

The most common benign mimic of clear cell RCC is oncocytoma, which has a similar shape and tends to have a more homogeneous enhancement with unenhanced HU between 25 and 40, corticomedullary phase peak absolute HU below 120 and slower washout with nephrographic phase HU and excretory phase enhancement below 100. A subset of both oncocytomas and clear cell RCC have a central scar with delayed enhancement. Another mimic of clear cell RCC is fat-poor AML, which tends to have a lobular, mushroom or ovoid shape lesion often with acute angles to the renal cortex. However, it tends to occur in the younger population and has slightly different enhancement characteristics with homogeneous enhancement pattern with high unenhanced HU between 45 and 55, corticomedullary phase peak absolute HU of 140, with washout nephrographic phase HU of 100 to 120, and excretory HU of 80 to 100.

DCE-MRI replicates these lesional enhancement patterns with added information on T2 weighted imaging, T1 gradient echo opposed phase imaging and diffusion-weighted imaging. T2 signal tends to be hypointense in fat-poor AML (**Fig. 3**) and papillary RCC and mildly hyperintense in clear cell RCC, chromophobe RCC, and oncocytoma (**Fig. 4**). Loss of signal on T1 in-phase to opposed-phase imaging suggests microscopic fat mostly in clear cell RCC and sometimes in fat poor AML. Conversely, a gain of signal from in-phase to opposed-phase suggests

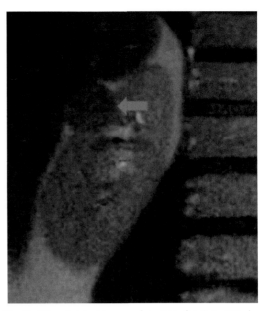

Fig. 3. T2-weighted image showing characteristic hypointensity of a papillary renal cell carcinoma (*red arrow*).[6] (*From* Allgood E, Raman SS. Image Interpretation: Practical Triage of Benign from Malignant Renal Masses. Radiol Clin North Am. Sep 2020;58(5):875-884. https://doi.org/10.1016/j.rcl.2020.06.002.)

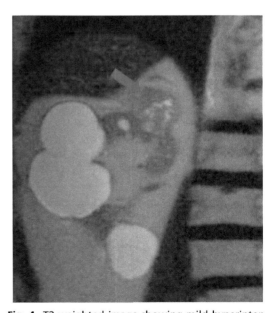

Fig. 4. T2-weighted image showing mild hyperintensity within a clear cell renal cell carcinoma (*red arrow*). Additional homogeneous T2 hyperintense simple cysts are also seen within the right kidney.[6] (*From* Allgood E, Raman SS. Image Interpretation: Practical Triage of Benign from Malignant Renal Masses. Radiol Clin North Am. Sep 2020;58(5):875-884. https://doi.org/10.1016/j.rcl.2020.06.002.)

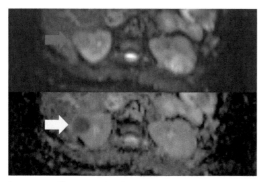

Fig. 5. Papillary renal cell carcinoma showing restriction of diffusion with the diminished signal on ADC (*yellow arrow*) compared with DWI (*red arrow*).[6] (*From* Allgood E, Raman SS. Image Interpretation: Practical Triage of Benign from Malignant Renal Masses. Radiol Clin North Am. Sep 2020;58(5):875-884. https://doi.org/10.1016/j.rcl.2020.06.002.)

hemosiderin presence in papillary RCC and sometimes in clear cell RCC. Restricted diffusion in renal lesions by an increased signal on high b-value diffusion weight imaging and decreased signal on apparent diffusion coefficient (ADC) is most robust in papillary RCC[17] (**Fig. 5**).

Mean Enhancement

Mean enhancement, which measures the enhancement of the whole lesion including the areas of hypoenhancing scar and necrosis, tends to average high and low enhancing areas and showed statistically significant difference between oncocytoma and all other types of RCC.[18] However, there is substantial overlap between oncocytoma and clear cell RCC using mean enhancement in the nephrographic phase alone. Further, there is high variability within RCC as RCC has a higher propensity for necrosis than oncocytoma, there was underestimation of peak enhancement of the lesions and limited ability to differentiate the subtypes of RCC.

Absolute Enhancement

Absolute enhancement measures peak HU of small region of interest (ROI) located on the most enhancing portion of a lesion, which is done on corticomedullary phase and replicated in the same location on other phases. There is statistically significant higher absolute enhancement of ccRCC versus other RCC and benign lesions in the corticomedullary phase[16,17] (**Fig. 6**).

In the nephrographic phase, peak HU is suboptimal for use in differentiation because almost all lesions except pRCC were observed to enhance similarly in a small range between 70 and 90 HU. pRCC shows peak enhancement during nephrographic phase around 70 to 80HU, which is different phase at which there is peak enhancement compared with ccRCC. chrRCC shows peak enhancement in either corticomedullary or nephrographic phases[17] (**Fig. 7**).

An additional value of nephrographic phase absolute enhancement for ccRCC is its correlation to higher Fuhrman grade with lower enhancement,[19] with less than 52.1HU in enhancement in nephrographic phase as a predictor of higher Fuhrman grade in ccRCC.[20]

Excretory phase absolute enhancement was shown to have a higher enhancement in ccRCC versus pRCC, chrRCC, or oncocytoma with non-overlapping confidence intervals.[17] Like nephrographic phase, excretory phase absolute enhancement for ccRCC is its correlation to higher Fuhrman grade with lower enhancement.[19]

MRI has also shown similar dynamic contrast enhancement, with ccRCC showing greatest peak enhancement and de-enhancement from the peak compared with oncocytoma, FP-AML, and chrRCC, with the least absolute enhancement seen in pRCC.[15,21]

Radiocytogenetics also correlates with differences in absolute enhancement, with gain of chromosome 12 in ccRCC associated with higher nephrographic and excretory phase enhancement compared with ccRCC without gain of chromosome 12, where the gain of chromosome 12 is associated with higher tumor grade and worse prognosis.[22]

Relative Enhancement

Relative enhancement is calculated from peak absolute enhancement subtracted against peak

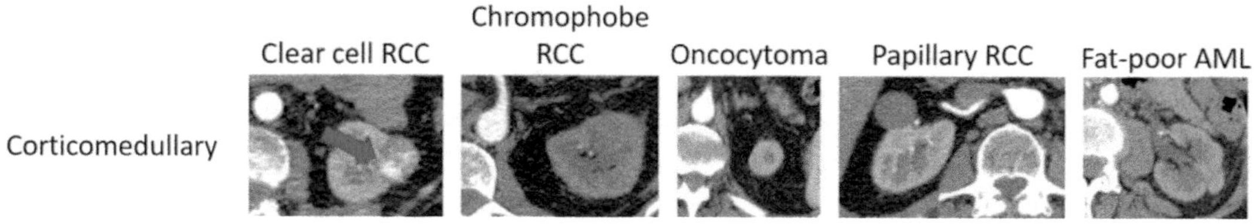

	Clear cell RCC	Chromophobe RCC	Oncocytoma	Papillary RCC	Fat-poor AML
Corticomedullary					

Fig. 6. Corticomedullary phase of oncocytoma, fat-poor AML, clear cell, papillary, and chromophobe RCC with clear cell RCC subjectively depicting the highest level of absolute enhancement (red arrow).[6] (*From* Allgood E, Raman SS. Image Interpretation: Practical Triage of Benign from Malignant Renal Masses. Radiol Clin North Am. Sep 2020;58(5):875-884. https://doi.org/10.1016/j.rcl.2020.06.002.)

Chromophobe RCC   Papillary RCC

Pre-contrast

Corticomedullary

Nephrographic

Delayed/
Excretory

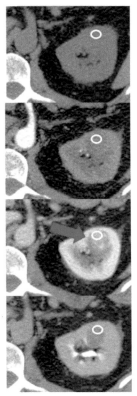
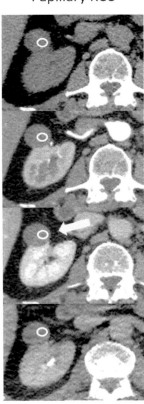

Fig. 7. Pre- and post-contrast phases of chromophobe and papillary RCC showing subtle absolute peak enhancement in the nephrographic phase (*red and yellow arrows*, respectively). ROIs placed on these lesions show pre-contrast, corticomedullary, nephrographic, and excretory phase HU of 13, 39, 144, and 50 for the chromophobe lesion and 29, 35, 42, and 25 for the papillary lesion, respectively.[6] (*From* Allgood E, Raman SS. Image Interpretation: Practical Triage of Benign from Malignant Renal Masses. Radiol Clin North Am. Sep 2020;58(5):875-884. https://doi.org/10.1016/j.rcl.2020.06.002.)

enhancement of background uninvolved cortex, which allows for control against variability of baseline renal perfusion from intrarenal causes such as kidney disease or extra-renal causes cardiac output or renal artery stenosis. Formula for relative enhancement is measured on the same phase: [(mass ROI − uninvolved cortex ROI)/uninvolved cortex ROI] x 100%.[16]

Corticomedullary phase relative enhancement >0% shows a 90% positive predictive value for ccRCC[16] (**Fig. 8**). Corticomedullary phase relative enhancement of <10% and >45 HU on the unenhanced phase shows a 97% negative predictive value for ccRCC.[16] The majority of all other renal lesions have < 10% relative enhancement compared with renal cortex.

Excretory phase relative enhancement also has been shown to be greater in type 2 pRCC compared with type 1 pRCC.[23]

In comparisons among different subtypes of indeterminate masses, greatest relative enhancement was observed in ccRCC compared with chromophobe and papillary RCC on CT,[21] on MRI[15] and CEUS,[11] although FP-AML and oncocytoma showed similar greater relative enhancement but with narrowing confidence intervals.[15]

Furthermore, corticomedullary phase relative enhancement has shown a correlation with aggressiveness of ccRCC with certain genes or chromosomes. For example, ccRCC shows higher enhancement in a subtype that lacks the expression of phosphatase and tension homolog (PTEN) compared with lower enhancement in ccRCC with retention of PTEN expression.[24] PTEN is a tumor suppressor gene, and lack of its expression is associated with decreased survival, worse response to anti-VEGF/EGF medications, higher Fuhrman grade, and a higher chance of metastasis to lymph nodes.[24] Nephrographic phase relative enhancement is lower in ccRCC with loss of Y chromosome versus lesion with retention of Y chromosome, with loss of Y

Clear cell RCC

Pre-contrast

Corticomedullary

Nephrographic

Delayed/
Excretory

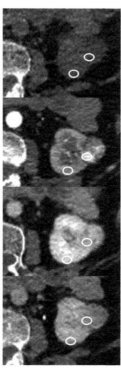

Fig. 8. Pre- and post-contrast CT showing relative enhancement of a clear cell RCC with ROIs placed over the area with peak corticomedullary enhancement and area of uninvolved cortex on all phases. The relative enhancement, as calculated with the formula described in the text, is 77% in the corticomedullary phase, −24% in the nephrographic phase, and −29% in the excretory phase.[6] (*From* Allgood E, Raman SS. Image Interpretation: Practical Triage of Benign from Malignant Renal Masses. Radiol Clin North Am. Sep 2020;58(5):875-884. https://doi.org/10.1016/j.rcl.2020.06.002.)

chromosome associated with higher T stage, Fuhrman grade, and risk of metastatic disease.[25] Nephrographic and excretory relative enhancement is lower in clear cell RCC with gain of chromosome 20 compared with lesion without gain of chromosome 20, where the gain is associated with an increased rate of tumor recurrence.[26]

Absolute De-enhancement

Absolute de-enhancement is defined as peak enhancement in the corticomedullary phase minus nephrographic peak enhancement, which is increased in ccRCC when compared with oncocytoma and shows <50 HU of absolute de-enhancement with 90% positive predictive value for ccRCC.[16]

Relative Washout

Relative washout as defined previously is a comparison of peak enhancement of the renal lesion against adjacent cortex with ccRCC most likely to have positive relative enhancement > 10%. Low levels of carbonic anhydrase-IX (CA-IX) in clear cell RCC has poor prognosis and high levels show good response to immunotherapy IL-2. When the level of CA-IX is high in ccRCC, there is higher nephrographic relative washout and trend toward high excretory relative washout compared with ccRCC with low CA-IX.[27]

Likelihood Scores to Aid Risk Stratification

To summarize these radiologic findings to help clinical decision-making, recent efforts in the radiology community have created several modality-specific algorithms that yield 5-point Likert scoring system that risk stratifies these indeterminate renal masses.

The MR clear cell likelihood score (ccLS) created by Pedrosa and colleagues[28] focus on qualitative data from MR that follows the algorithm in the following order: presence of enhancement, presence of macroscopic fat, amount of enhancing component, T2W signal intensity, corticomedullary phase mild, moderate or intense enhancement, microscopic fat, arterial-to-delayed enhancement ratio (ADER), and ancillary tiebreaker features of segmental enhancement inversion and restrict diffusion[28,29] (**Fig. 9**). Other relevant investigations from this group include assessment of performance in subset of small solid indeterminate renal masses <4 cm.[30–32] Examples of several ccLS with pathology correlation are shown in **Figs. 11–14**.

A more recently proposed and validated scoring algorithm, the UCLA MR score (UCLA MRS) is both qualitative and quantitative in this order: presence of macroscopic fat, presence of microscopic fat, T2w signal intensity (low, intermediate, high), absolute arterial enhancement index, relative arterial enhancement index, absolute delayed enhancement index, and arterial-to-delayed enhancement ratio[33] (**Fig. 10**). Ancillary MRI findings taken into consideration were angular interface sign, segmental enhancement inversion, tumor thrombus, distant metastasis, irregular contour, heterogeneous enhancement, neovascularity, calcification, marked diffusion restriction, and early peak enhancement. Examples of several UCLA MRS with pathology correlation are shown in **Figs. 11–14**.

Other MR algorithms also exist that follow algorithm order of T2w imaging (high, mid-low), microscopic fat, DWI/ADC (high, mid, low), dynamic contrast enhancement (fast and intense, mid and delayed, slow) and dynamic contrast wash out (yes, mid, no).[34]

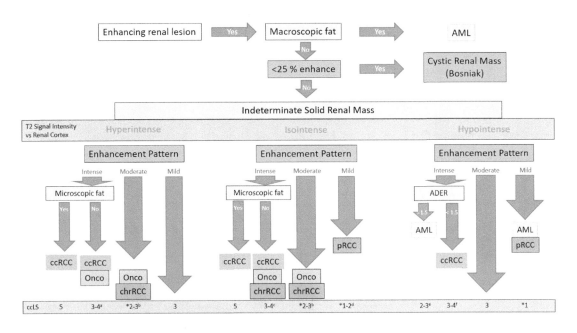

Tie-break rule if following are unequivocally present

[a]**ccLS3** if segmental enhancement inversion (SEI) present   [d]**ccLS1** if marked restricted diffusion on DWI
[b]**ccLS2** if segmental enhancement inversion (SEI) present   [e]**ccLS2** if homogeneous or marked restriction on DWI
[c]**ccLS3** if segmental enhancement inversion (SEI) present   [f]**ccLS3** if homogeneous or marked restriction on DWI. **ccLS3** if heterogeneous.
*Upgrade to **ccLS3** if unequivocal microscopic fat present

Corticomedullary Phase Enhancement

Intense: >75% vs cortex

Moderate: 40–75% vs cortex

Mild: <40% of cortex

Fig. 9. Clear cell likelihood score (ccLS) algorithm.[28] Absence of macroscopic fat and presence of enhancement in at least 25% of mass are eligibility criteria. T2 signal intensity, enhancement during corticomedullary phase, and presence of microscopic fat are major criteria. Other parameters such as DWI, segmental enhancement inversion (SEI), and arterial-to-delayed enhancement ratio (ADER) in the algorithm are assessed when indicated. AML, angiomyolipoma; ccRCC, clear cell renal cell carcinoma; chrRCC, chromophobe renal cell carcinoma; Onco, oncocytoma; pRCC, papillary renal cell carcinoma.

A more recent development is the qualitative and quantitative CT score (UCLA CTS) proposed by Tubtawee and colleagues,[34] which assigns points to quantitative and qualitative features. Quantitative features include absolute unenhanced attenuation, peak enhancement in the corticomedullary phase, absolute de-enhancement, and relative corticomedullary attenuation. Qualitative features include heterogeneity of enhancement or lesion, contour, neovascularity, dystrophic calcification, and angular interface. These parameters are assigned different points and are summarized in a clear cell RCC likelihood score (**Fig. 15**). Examples of several UCLA CTS with pathology correlation are shown in **Figs. 16–18**.

Novel Imaging Parameters and Artificial Intelligence

Besides conventional visual imaging characteristics, there are novel quantitative imaging parameters that are being investigated for further assistance with the identification of indeterminate renal masses. These include perfusion and single-photon emission tomography (SPECT). Other diagnostic approaches include radiomics features that rely on the heterogeneity of the grayscale images and artificial intelligence methodologies that rely on machine learning and deep learning to detect and characterize renal lesions.

Technetium 99m sestamibi single-photon emission tomography

Technetium 99m sestamibi (99mTc-sestamibi) SPECT imaging relies on the observation that benign renal lesions such as oncocytomas and less aggressive chrRCC have higher mitochondrial concentration compared with more aggressive ccRCC or pRCC, which have low mitochondrial concentration on histopathology.[36] When combining results from

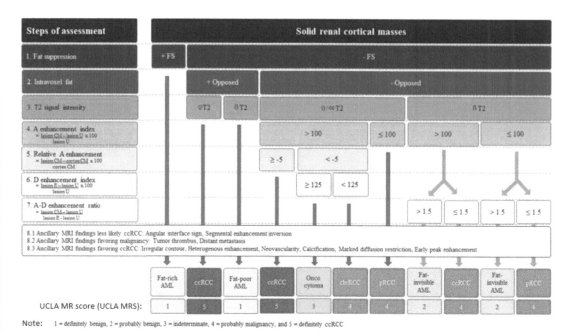

Steps of assessment	Solid renal cortical masses									
1. Fat suppression	+ FS	- FS								
2. Intravoxel fat		+ Opposed		- Opposed						
3. T2 signal intensity		↕T2	↓T2	↕/∞ T2			↓T2			
4. A enhancement index = $\frac{\text{lesion CM} - \text{lesion U}}{\text{lesion U}} \times 100$			> 100	≤ 100		> 100	≤ 100			
5. Relative A enhancement = $\frac{\text{lesion CM} - \text{cortex CM}}{\text{cortex CM}} \times 100$		≥ -5	< -5							
6. D enhancement index = $\frac{\text{lesion E} - \text{lesion U}}{\text{lesion U}} \times 100$		≥ 125	< 125							
7. A-D enhancement ratio = $\frac{\text{lesion CM} - \text{lesion U}}{\text{lesion E} - \text{lesion U}}$							> 1.5	≤ 1.5	> 1.5	≤ 1.5

8.1 Ancillary MRI findings less likely ccRCC: Angular interface sign, Segmental enhancement inversion
8.2 Ancillary MRI findings favoring malignancy: Tumor thrombus, Distant metastasis
8.3 Ancillary MRI findings favoring ccRCC: Irregular contour, Heterogenous enhancement, Neovascularity, Calcification, Marked diffusion restriction, Early peak enhancement

	Fat-rich AML	ccRCC	Fat-poor AML	ccRCC	Onco cytoma	chrRCC	pRCC	Fat-invisible AML	ccRCC	Fat-invisible AML	pRCC
UCLA MR score (UCLA MRS):	1	5	1	5	3	4	4	2	4	2	4

Note: 1 = definitely benign, 2 = probably benign, 3 = indeterminate, 4 = probably malignancy, and 5 = definitely ccRCC

Fig. 10. UCLA MR score (UCLA MRS) algorithm for assessing solid renal masses of any size and stage. Each step denotes characteristics that should be investigated in any part of the mass. The most likely diagnoses and likelihood scores are given at the bottom of each column. A, arterial; AML, angiomyolipoma; ccRCC, clear cell renal cell carcinoma; chrRCC, chromophobe RCC; CM, corticomedullary phase; D, delayed; E, excretory phase; +FS, presence of macroscopic fat; -FS, absence of macroscopic; fat, +Opposed, presence of intravoxel fat; -Opposed, absence of intravoxel fat; pRCC, papillary RCC; U, unenhanced phase.[33] (*Data from* Surawech C, Miao Q, Suvannarerg V. Differentiation Clear Cell Renal Cell Carcinoma from Other Common Renal Masses on Multiphasic MR.)

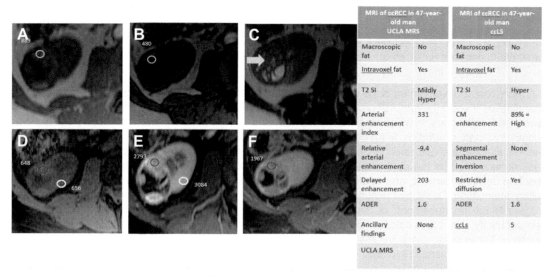

MRI of ccRCC in 47-year-old man UCLA MRS		MRI of ccRCC in 47-year-old man ccLS	
Macroscopic fat	No	Macroscopic fat	No
Intravoxel fat	Yes	Intravoxel fat	Yes
T2 SI	Mildly Hyper	T2 SI	Hyper
Arterial enhancement index	331	CM enhancement	89% = High
Relative arterial enhancement	-9.4	Segmental enhancement inversion	None
Delayed enhancement	203	Restricted diffusion	Yes
ADER	1.6	ADER	1.6
Ancillary findings	None	ccLS	5
UCLA MRS	5		

Fig. 11. UCLA MRS of 5 and clear cell likelihood score (ccLS) of 5 in a 47-year-old man with clear cell renal cell carcinoma (ccRCC). (*A, B*) On axial in phase and opposed-phase images, there is intravoxel fat within the 2 cm right upper pole renal mass (green circles). (*C*) On T2W HASTE, the lesion is mildly high signal relative to renal cortex (yellow arrow). On (*D*) unenhanced (U). (*E*) corticomedullary (CM). (*F*) excretory (*E*) phases, small ROIs were placed on the perceptibly most enhancing portion of the mass in CM phase and then in same location for U and E phases (*red circles*) and on the cortex in U and CM phases (*yellow circles*). The relevant parameters for each scoring system are shown.

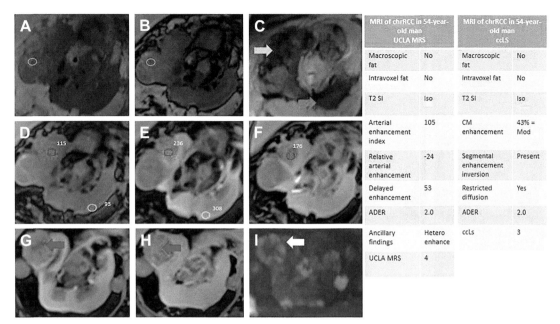

	MRI of chrRCC in 54-year-old man UCLA MRS		MRI of chrRCC in 54-year-old man ccLS	
Macroscopic fat	No		Macroscopic fat	No
Intravoxel fat	No		Intravoxel fat	No
T2 SI	Iso		T2 SI	Iso
Arterial enhancement index	105		CM enhancement	43% = Mod
Relative arterial enhancement	-24		Segmental enhancement inversion	Present
Delayed enhancement	53		Restricted diffusion	Yes
ADER	2.0		ADER	2.0
Ancillary findings	Hetero enhance		ccLS	3
UCLA MRS	4			

Fig. 12. UCLA MRS of 4 and clear cell likelihood score (ccLS) of 3 in a 54-year-old man with chromophobe renal cell carcinoma (chrRCC). (*A, B*) On axial in phase and opposed-phase images, there is no intravoxel fat within the right mid-pole renal mass (green circles). (*C*) On T2W HASTE, the lesion is isointense in signal (yellow arrow) relative to renal cortex (blue arrow). There is segmental enhancement inversion from CM phase on different part of lesion (*G*) and delayed phase (*H*) (red arrows) as well as restriction on diffusion-weighted imaging (white arrow) (*I*). The relevant parameters for each scoring system are shown.

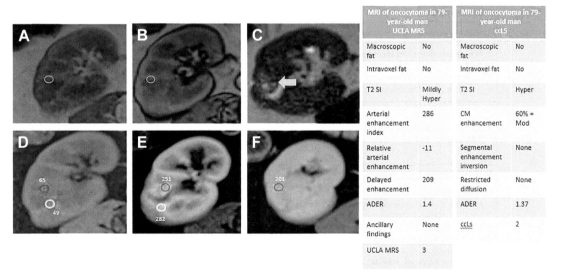

	MRI of oncocytoma in 79-year-old man UCLA MRS		MRI of oncocytoma in 79-year-old man ccLS	
Macroscopic fat	No		Macroscopic fat	No
Intravoxel fat	No		Intravoxel fat	No
T2 SI	Mildly Hyper		T2 SI	Hyper
Arterial enhancement index	286		CM enhancement	60% = Mod
Relative arterial enhancement	-11		Segmental enhancement inversion	None
Delayed enhancement	209		Restricted diffusion	None
ADER	1.4		ADER	1.37
Ancillary findings	None		ccLS	2
UCLA MRS	3			

Fig. 13. UCLA MRS of 3 and clear cell likelihood score (ccLS) of 2 in a 79-year-old man with oncocytoma. (*A, B*) On axial in phase and opposed-phase images, there is no intravoxel fat within the right mid-pole renal mass (green circles). (*C*) On T2W HASTE, the lesion is mildly high signal relative to renal cortex (yellow arrow). On (*D*) unenhanced (*U*). (*E*) corticomedullary (*CM*). (*F*) excretory (*E*) phases, small ROIs were placed on the perceptibly most enhancing portion of the mass in CM phase and then in same location for U and E phases (*red circles*) and on the cortex in U and CM phases (*yellow circles*). The relevant parameters for each scoring system are shown.

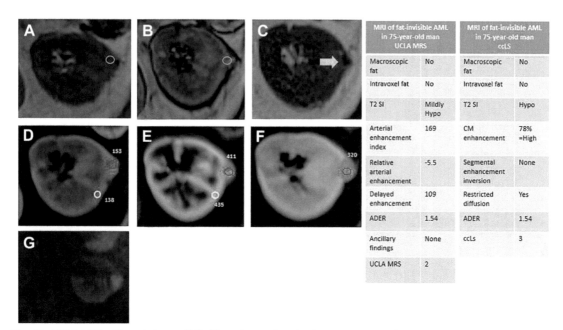

	MRI of fat-invisible AML in 75-year-old man UCLA MRS		MRI of fat-invisible AML in 75-year-old man ccLS	
Macroscopic fat	No	Macroscopic fat	No
Intravoxel fat	No	Intravoxel fat	No
T2 SI	Mildly Hypo	T2 SI	Hypo
Arterial enhancement index	169	CM enhancement	78% =High
Relative arterial enhancement	-5.5	Segmental enhancement inversion	None
Delayed enhancement	109	Restricted diffusion	Yes
ADER	1.54	ADER	1.54
Ancillary findings	None	ccLS	3
UCLA MRS	2		

Fig. 14. UCLA MRS of 2 and clear cell likelihood score (ccLS) of 3 in a 75-year-old man with fat-poor AML. (*A, B*) On axial in phase and opposed-phase images, there is no intravoxel fat within the left mid pole renal mass (green circles). (*C*) On T2W HASTE, the lesion is mildly hypointense in signal relative to renal cortex (yellow arrow). On (*D*) unenhanced (*U*). (*E*) corticomedullary (*CM*). (*F*) excretory (*E*) phases, small ROIs were placed on the perceptibly most enhancing portion of the mass in CM phase and then in same location for U and E phases (*red circles*) and on the cortex in U and CM phases (*yellow circles*). There is restriction on diffusion weight images (*G*). The relevant parameters for each scoring system are shown.

Quantitative features	UCLA CTS
1. Absolute unenhanced attenuation lesser than 45 HU	Yes = 1, No = 0
2. Peak enhancement in corticomedullary phase	
3. Absolute de-enhancement (= lesion ROI in corticomedullary phase - lesion ROI in nephrographic phase)	> 50 = 2 25-50 = 1 < 25 = 0
4. Relative corticomedullary attenuation (= [(lesion ROI-ipsilateral cortex ROI)/ipsilateral cortex ROI] x100)	< 0 = 0 1-10 = 1 10-20 = 2 >20 = 3
Qualitative features	
1. Heterogeneous enhancement: A mixture of solid enhancing areas and cystic/necrotic non-enhancing areas	Yes = 1, No = 0
2. Irregular contour	
3. Neovascularity: Presence of increased, irregular, and unnamed vessels in the Gerota fascia adjacent to the involved kidney	
4. Dystrophic calcification	
5. Angular interface sign	Yes = -1, No = 0

Fig. 15. UCLA CT score (UCLA CTS).[35] (*Data from* Tubtawee T. Multireader Diagnostic Accuracy of the Renal Mass CT Score (with Clear Cell RCC Likelihood Score) to Characterize Solid Renal Masses on Multiphasic MDCT.)

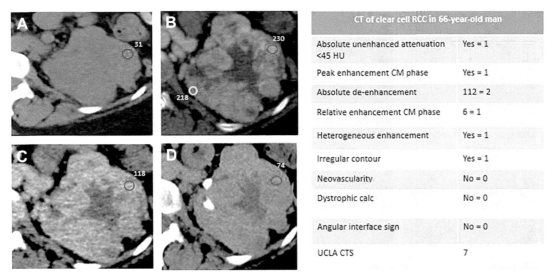

CT of clear cell RCC in 66-year-old man	
Absolute unenhanced attenuation <45 HU	Yes = 1
Peak enhancement CM phase	Yes = 1
Absolute de-enhancement	112 = 2
Relative enhancement CM phase	6 = 1
Heterogeneous enhancement	Yes = 1
Irregular contour	Yes = 1
Neovascularity	No = 0
Dystrophic calc	No = 0
Angular interface sign	No = 0
UCLA CTS	7

Fig. 16. UCLA CTS of 7 in a 66-year-old man with clear cell RCC. On (A) unenhanced (U), (B) corticomedullary (CM), (C) nephrographic (NG), and (D) excretory (E) phases. Small ROIs were placed on the perceptibly most enhancing portion of the mass in CM phase and then in same location for U, NG, and E phases (*red circles*) and on the cortex in CM phases (*yellow circle*). The relevant parameters for each scoring system are shown.

five recent studies, 94% of oncocytomas, 67% of AML, and 100% of hybrid oncocytic/chromophobe tumors were positive on SPECT and only 2% of non-chromophobe RCC were positive.[37] Also another retrospective review showed improvement of diagnostic performance in 30% of cases of indeterminate renal masses compared with conventional imaging alone.[38] SPECT imaging can potentially add value to the management of indeterminate renal masses for stratification of benign (oncocytoma) and less aggressive RCCs (chromophobe) versus more worrisome cell types of RCC.

Perfusion

Change of tissue attenuation on CT over time after administration of intravenous contrast can be measured in Hounsfield units (HU), and functional

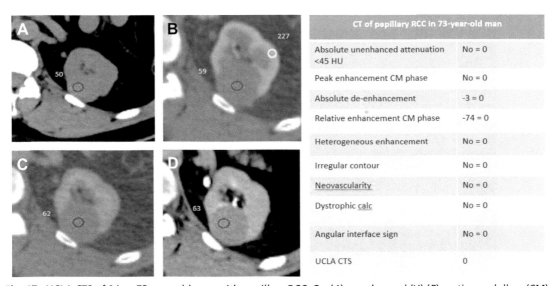

CT of papillary RCC in 73-year-old man	
Absolute unenhanced attenuation <45 HU	No = 0
Peak enhancement CM phase	No = 0
Absolute de-enhancement	-3 = 0
Relative enhancement CM phase	-74 = 0
Heterogeneous enhancement	No = 0
Irregular contour	No = 0
Neovascularity	No = 0
Dystrophic calc	No = 0
Angular interface sign	No = 0
UCLA CTS	0

Fig. 17. UCLA CTS of 0 in a 73-year-old man with papillary RCC. On (A) unenhanced (U) (B) corticomedullary (CM), (C) nephrographic (NG), and (D) excretory (E) phases. Small ROIs were placed on the perceptibly most enhancing portion of the mass in CM phase and then in the same location for U, NG, and E phases (*red circles*) and on the cortex in CM phases (*yellow circle*). The relevant parameters for each scoring system are shown.

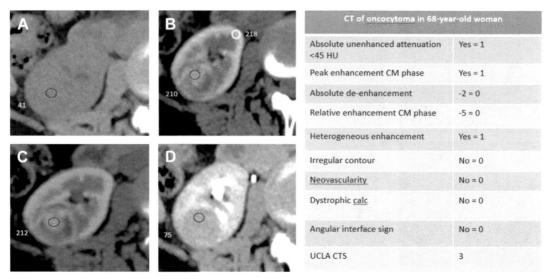

CT of oncocytoma in 68-year-old woman	
Absolute unenhanced attenuation <45 HU	Yes = 1
Peak enhancement CM phase	Yes = 1
Absolute de-enhancement	-2 = 0
Relative enhancement CM phase	-5 = 0
Heterogeneous enhancement	Yes = 1
Irregular contour	No = 0
Neovascularity	No = 0
Dystrophic calc	No = 0
Angular interface sign	No = 0
UCLA CTS	3

Fig. 18. UCLA CTS of 3 in a 68-year-old woman with oncocytoma. On (*A*) unenhanced (U) (*B*) corticomedullary (CM), (*C*) nephrographic (NG), and (*D*) excretory (*E*) phases; small ROIs were placed on the perceptibly most enhancing portion of the mass in CM phase and then in the same location for U, NG, and E phases (*red circles*) and on the cortex in CM phases (*yellow circle*). The relevant parameters for each scoring system are shown.

parameters can be generated based on enhancement curves depicting HU over time [39] (**Fig. 19**). As noted previously with four-phase scans, ccRCC tends to have rapid uptake and overall higher peak corticomedullary enhancement compared with normal renal cortex (**Fig. 20**), pRCC tends to have a slow uptake and delayed enhancement compared with the normal cortex (**Fig. 21**), and oncocytoma tends to show somewhat rapid uptake but enhancement lower than the normal renal cortex (**Fig. 22**). There have been efforts to characterize indeterminate renal masses as ccRCC, pRCC, chromophobe RCC, or oncocytoma using select relevant parameters derived from the enhancement curves such as blood volume (BV), blood flow (BF), flow extraction (FE), mean transit time (MTT), peak Hounsfield units (pHU), and time to peak (TTP) with promising results for specific parameters in lesion-to-lesion comparisons as well as lesion-to-cortex comparisons.[41]

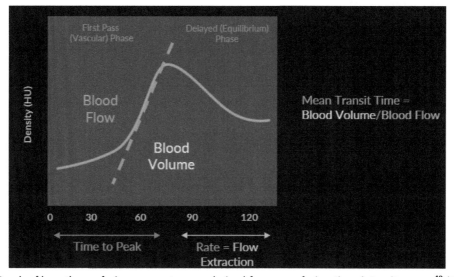

Fig. 19. Graph of how the perfusion parameters are derived from a perfusion time–intensity curve.[40] (*Data from* Chung A. Quantitative flow parameters differentiating oncocytoma and papillary renal cancer from clear cell renal cancer on perfusion MD CT.*)

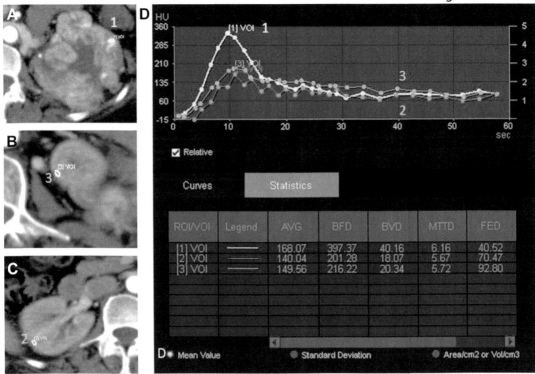

Fig. 20. Perfusion CT for a 68-year-old woman with clear cell RCC. The ROIs are placed on (*A*) lesion (1), (*B*) ipsilateral cortex (3), and (*C*) contralateral cortex (2) and the perfusion curve over time and parameters are attained (*D*).[40] (*Data from* Chung A. Quantitative flow Parameters Differentiating Oncocytoma and Papillary Renal Cancer from Clear Cell Renal Cancer on Perfusion MD CT.)

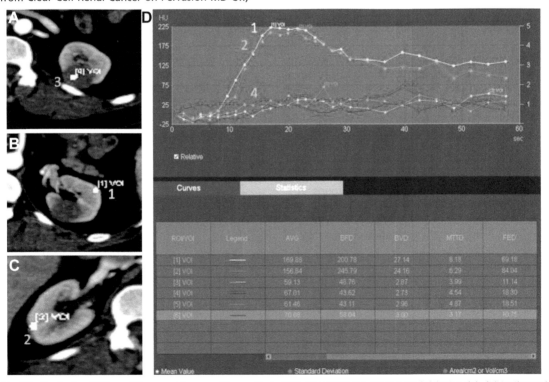

Fig. 21. Perfusion CT for a 59-year-old man with papillary RCC. The ROIs are placed on (*A*) lesion (3), (*B*) ipsilateral cortex (1), and (*C*) contralateral cortex (2) and the perfusion curve over time and parameters are attained (*D*).[40] (*Data from* Chung A. Quantitative flow Parameters Differentiating Oncocytoma and Papillary Renal Cancer from Clear Cell Renal Cancer on Perfusion MD CT.)

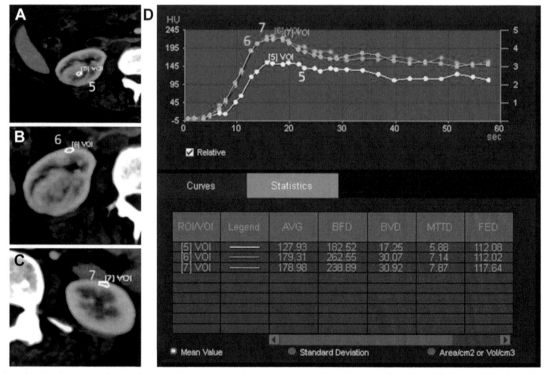

Fig. 22. Perfusion CT for a 60-year-old woman with oncocytoma. The ROIs are placed on (*A*) lesion (5), (*B*) ipsilateral cortex (6), and (*C*) contralateral cortex (7) and the perfusion curve over time and parameters are attained (*D*).[40] (*Data from* Chung A. Quantitative flow Parameters Differentiating Oncocytoma and Papillary Renal Cancer from Clear Cell Renal Cancer on Perfusion MD CT.)

An ongoing prospective study with a study cohort of 48 patients has corroborated several of these findings, with results showing significant differences between ccRCC and pRCC in a variety of parameters including BF, BV, TTP, and others. For example, between ccRCC and oncocytoma, significant differences exist in BV (*P* < .01) and TTP (*P* < .05) and between pRCC and oncocytoma significant differences exist in BF, BV, FE, and pHU (all *P* < .03) with similar MTT among all groups (37). Compared with ipsilateral cortex, ccRCC had less TTP, pRCC had lower BF, BV, FE, pHU, and higher TTP, and oncocytoma showed lower BV.[40]

Radiogenomics

The novel field of radiogenomics explores the idea that imaging is a biomarker of underlying genomic alterations with resulting phenotypic changes in the physiologic and molecular environment. Expanding on this idea in one study, a combination of imaging features predicted responders to a biological agent in advance of the actual result in a feasibility study with validation of a surrogate of molecular assay model[42] with ongoing research in the field. Several genes and groups of genes also have been targeted to evaluate for expression using radiomics, including survival-related genes[43] and specific genes like protein polybromo-1 gene (PBRM1).[44]

Artificial Intelligence

Artificial intelligence can be harnessed to help enhance the utilization of currently available parameters, and discover new types of nonconventional parameters and methods of analysis.

Select CT radionics parameters such as first-order, shape, and texture features have been investigated for utility in distinguishing benign lesions (such as AML) from types of RCC, differentiation among types of RCC, and distinguishing other non-RCC tumors such as oncocytoma and grading (Fuhrman and/or international society of urological pathology (ISUP)) and staging of RCC as well as treatment responses.[45] To distinguish between AML from RCC, Yan and colleagues[46] and Feng and colleagues[47] have shown high accuracy of texture analysis in differentiating AML from other RCC such as ccRCC and pRCC, and Cui and colleagues[48] have shown AML can be distinguished by automated computer-aided identification system for AML vs RCC differentiation. To characterize subtypes of RCC Yu and colleagues[49] used texture analysis to distinguish ccRCC vs oncocytoma AUC of 0.93 and pRCC vs oncocytoma with an AUC of 0.99. Meng and colleagues[50] showed radiomics analysis could differentiate sarcomatoid versus ccRCC.

Coy and colleagues[51] explored quantitative computer-aided diagnostic (CAD) methods on an available cohort with multiphasic CT imaging with known ccRCC, pRCC, oncocytomas, chrRCC, and fat-poor (FP)-AMLs, which showed similar performance of peak HU measurement between CAD and manual measurement. Furthermore, Coy and colleagues[52] used deep learning-based renal characterization to test if oncocytoma versus ccRCC could be distinguished at different layers with final layer positive predictive value of 82.5%.

Because of the importance of nuclear grade prediction of ccRCC in prognosis, many groups[53–59] have shown the ML algorithms analyzing texture features of CT can show predictive accuracy. Others have shown potential for radiomics in the staging of ccRCC with an AUC of 0.980 in low versus high TNM stages.[60]

Overall, there seems to be promising results for the discrimination of tumor types using radiomics although further assessment is needed to confirm the value added versus human assessment and in settings of treatment responses.[61]

Biopsy of Renal Masses

High-quality multiphasic renal mass imaging is inconclusive in 20% to 30% of cases and may require percutaneous CT and US tissue biopsy, which is now a well-established technique for providing a robust preoperative or preprocedural diagnosis, especially in non-clear cell lesions or lesions mimicking cancer such as infection or infiltration form IgG4.[62]

SUMMARY

There is a clear benefit of imaging-based differentiation of small indeterminate masses to its subtypes of clear cell RCC, chromophobe RCC, papillary RCC, fat poor AML, and oncocytoma because it helps determine the next step options for the patients. The work thus far in radiology has explored different parameters in CT, MRI, and CEUS with the discovery of many reliable imaging features that suggest certain tissue subtypes. Likert score-based risk stratification systems can help determine management, and new techniques such as perfusion, radiogenomics, SPECT, and artificial intelligence can add to imaging-based evaluation of indeterminate renal masses. With further improvement in accurate differentiation of indeterminate renal masses on imaging, it will allow for better triage of patients to active surveillance, biopsy, ablation or resection and ultimately improve patient care.

CLINICS CARE POINTS

- The combination of multiple imaging modalities can help diagnose and be used in active surveillance, especially in elderly patients or patients with multiple comorbidities precluding surgery or ablation.
- Several imaging modality-specific algorithms that yield 5-point Likert scoring system helps risk stratify indeterminate renal masses.
- Renal mass imaging is inconclusive in 20-30% of cases and may require tissue biopsy, which provide robust diagnosis.
- Additional imaging modalities beyond conventional imaging such as perfusion, single-photon emission tomography (SPECT) and other diagnostic approaches such as radiomics and artificial intelligence methods show early promising results.

DISCLOSURE

The authors have nothing to disclose.

Diagnostic criteria[6]

Clear Cell Renal Cell Carcinoma

- Heterogeneous, even at a small size
- Peak enhancement in the corticomedullary phase
- Relative enhancement in corticomedullary phase greater than 0
- Mild T2 hyperintensity
- Can have signal drop out on out-of-phase imaging, due to microscopic fat

Papillary Renal Cell Carcinoma

- More likely to be homogeneous than clear cell RCC
- Peak enhancement in the nephrographic phase
- Relative enhancement less than 0 in all phases
- Restricts diffusion
- T2 hypointense

Chromophobe Renal Cell Carcinoma

- Peak enhancement in the corticomedullary or nephrographic phase

- Relative enhancement less than 0 in all phases

Oncocytoma

- Mimic of clear cell RCC
- Peak enhancement in the corticomedullary phase
- Relative enhancement less than 0 in all phases

Fat-Poor Angiomyolipoma

- Peak enhancement in the corticomedullary phase
- Relative enhancement less than 0 in all phases
- Tends to be > 45 HU on unenhanced CT
- T2 hypointense

REFERENCES

1. Herts BR, Silverman SG, Hindman NM, et al. Management of the Incidental Renal Mass on CT: A White Paper of the ACR Incidental Findings Committee. J Am Coll Radiol 2018;15(2):264–73.
2. Frank I, Blute ML, Cheville JC, et al. Solid renal tumors: an analysis of pathological features related to tumor size. J Urol 2003;170(6 Pt 1):2217–20.
3. Gill IS, Aron M, Gervais DA, et al. Clinical practice. Small renal mass. N Engl J Med 2010;362(7):624–34.
4. Jewett MA, Mattar K, Basiuk J, et al. Active surveillance of small renal masses: progression patterns of early stage kidney cancer. Eur Urol 2011;60(1):39–44.
5. Motzer RJ, Jonasch E, Agarwal N, et al. Kidney Cancer, Version 3.2022, NCCN Clinical Practice Guidelines in Oncology. J Natl Compr Canc Netw 2022; 20(1):71–90.
6. Allgood E, Raman SS. Image Interpretation: Practical Triage of Benign from Malignant Renal Masses. Radiol Clin North 2020;58(5):875–84.
7. Wang ZJ, Davenport MS, Silverman SG, et al. (2018) CT renal mass protocols v1.0. Available at: https://c.ymcdn.com/sites/www.abdominalradiology.org/resource/resmgr/education_dfp/RCC/RCC.CTprotocolsfinal-7-15-17.pdf. Accessed February 12, 2023.
8. O'Connor SD, Silverman SG, Cochon LR, et al. Renal cancer at unenhanced CT: imaging features, detection rates, and outcomes. Abdom Radiol (NY) 2018;43(7):1756–63.
9. Costello JE, Cecava ND, Tucker JE, et al. CT radiation dose: current controversies and dose reduction strategies. AJR Am J Roentgenol Dec 2013;201(6):1283–90.
10. Wang ZJ, Davenport MS, Silverman SG, et al. (2018) MR renal mass protocols v1.0. Available at: https://c.ymcdn.com/sites/www.abdominalradiology.org/resource/resmgr/education_dfp/RCC/RCC.MRIprotocolfinal-7-15-17.pdf. Accessed February 12, 2023.
11. King KG, Gulati M, Malhi H, et al. Quantitative assessment of solid renal masses by contrast-enhanced ultrasound with time-intensity curves: how we do it. Abdom Imaging Oct 2015;40(7):2461–71.
12. Silverman SG, Pedrosa I, Ellis JH, et al. Bosniak Classification of Cystic Renal Masses, Version 2019: An Update Proposal and Needs Assessment. Radiology Aug 2019;292(2):475–88.
13. Young JR, Young JA, Margolis DJA, et al. Sarcomatoid Renal Cell Carcinoma and Collecting Duct Carcinoma: Discrimination From Common Renal Cell Carcinoma Subtypes and Benign RCC Mimics on Multiphasic MDCT. Acad Radiol 2017;24(10):1226–32.
14. Birnbaum BA, Jacobs JE, Ramchandani P. Multiphasic renal CT: comparison of renal mass enhancement during the corticomedullary and nephrographic phases. Radiology 1996;200(3):753–8.
15. Young JR, Coy H, Kim HJ, et al. Performance of Relative Enhancement on Multiphasic MRI for the Differentiation of Clear Cell Renal Cell Carcinoma (RCC) From Papillary and Chromophobe RCC Subtypes and Oncocytoma. AJR Am J Roentgenol 2017;208(4):812–9.
16. Lee-Felker SA, Felker ER, Tan N, et al. Qualitative and quantitative MDCT features for differentiating clear cell renal cell carcinoma from other solid renal cortical masses. AJR Am J Roentgenol 2014;203(5):W516–24.
17. Young JR, Margolis D, Sauk S, et al. Clear cell renal cell carcinoma: discrimination from other renal cell carcinoma subtypes and oncocytoma at multiphasic multidetector CT. Radiology 2013;267(2):444–53.
18. Bird VG, Kanagarajah P, Morillo G, et al. Differentiation of oncocytoma and renal cell carcinoma in small renal masses (<4 cm): the role of 4-phase computerized tomography. World J Urol Dec 2011;29(6):787–92.
19. Coy H, Young JR, Douek ML, et al. Association of qualitative and quantitative imaging features on multiphasic multidetector CT with tumor grade in clear cell renal cell carcinoma. Abdom Radiol (NY) 2019;44(1):180–9.
20. Coy H, Young JR, Pantuck AJ, et al. Association of tumor grade, enhancement on multiphasic CT and microvessel density in patients with clear cell renal cell carcinoma. Abdom Radiol (NY) 2020;45(10):3184–92.
21. Sun MR, Ngo L, Genega EM, et al. Renal cell carcinoma: dynamic contrast-enhanced MR imaging for differentiation of tumor subtypes–correlation with pathologic findings. Radiology 2009;250(3):793–802.
22. Young JR, Coy H, Douek M, et al. Clear cell renal cell carcinoma: identifying the gain of chromosome 12 on multiphasic MDCT. Abdom Radiol (NY) 2017;42(1):236–41.
23. Young JR, Coy H, Douek M, et al. Type 1 papillary renal cell carcinoma: differentiation from Type 2

papillary RCC on multiphasic MDCT. Abdom Radiol (NY) 2017;42(7):1911–8.

24. Young JR, Coy H, Kim HJ, et al. Clear cell renal cell carcinoma: identifying PTEN expression on multiphasic MDCT. Abdom Radiol (NY) 2018;43(12):3410–7.

25. Young JR, Coy H, Douek M, et al. Clear Cell Renal Cell Carcinoma: Identifying the Loss of the Y Chromosome on Multiphasic MDCT. AJR Am J Roentgenol 2017;209(2):333–8.

26. Young JR, Young JA, Margolis DJ, et al. Clear cell renal cell carcinoma: identifying the gain of chromosome 20 on multiphasic MDCT. Abdom Radiol (NY) 2016;41(11):2175–81.

27. Young JR, Coy H, Kim HJ, et al. Utility of multiphasic multidetector computed tomography in discriminating between clear cell renal cell carcinomas with high and low carbonic anhydrase-IX expression. Abdom Radiol (NY) 2018;43(10):2734–42.

28. Pedrosa I, Cadeddu JA. How We Do It: Managing the Indeterminate Renal Mass with the MRI Clear Cell Likelihood Score. Radiology 2022;302(2):256–69.

29. Steinberg RL, Rasmussen RG, Johnson BA, et al. Prospective performance of clear cell likelihood scores (ccLS) in renal masses evaluated with multiparametric magnetic resonance imaging. Eur Radiol 2021;31(1):314–24.

30. Schieda N, Davenport MS, Silverman SG, et al. Multicenter Evaluation of Multiparametric MRI Clear Cell Likelihood Scores in Solid Indeterminate Small Renal Masses. Radiology 2022;303(3):590–9.

31. Johnson BA, Kim S, Steinberg RL, et al. Diagnostic performance of prospectively assigned clear cell Likelihood scores (ccLS) in small renal masses at multiparametric magnetic resonance imaging. Urol Oncol 2019;37(12):941–6.

32. Rasmussen RG, Xi Y, Sibley RC, et al. Association of Clear Cell Likelihood Score on MRI and Growth Kinetics of Small Solid Renal Masses on Active Surveillance. AJR Am J Roentgenol 2022;218(1):101–10.

33. Surawech C, Miao Q, Suvannarerg V. Differentiation Clear Cell Renal Cell Carcinoma from Other Common Renal Masses on Multiphasic MRI: A Likert Based Multireader Analysis.

34. Cornelis F, Tricaud E, Lasserre AS, et al. Multiparametric magnetic resonance imaging for the differentiation of low and high grade clear cell renal carcinoma. Eur Radiol 2015;25(1):24–31.

35. Tubtawee T. Multireader Diagnostic Accuracy of the Renal Mass CT Score (with Clear Cell RCC Likelihood Score) to Characterize Solid Renal Masses on Multiphasic MDCT.

36. García-Figueiras R, Goh VJ, Padhani AR, et al. CT perfusion in oncologic imaging: a useful tool? AJR Am J Roentgenol 2013;200(1):8–19.

37. Mazzei FG, Mazzei MA, Cioffi Squitieri N, et al. CT perfusion in the characterisation of renal lesions: an added value to multiphasic CT. BioMed Res Int 2014;2014:135013.

38. Chung A. Quantitative flow Parameters Differentiating Oncocytoma and Papillary Renal Cancer from Clear Cell Renal Cancer on Perfusion MD CT.

39. Jamshidi N, Jonasch E, Zapala M, et al. The Radiogenomic Risk Score: Construction of a Prognostic Quantitative, Noninvasive Image-based Molecular Assay for Renal Cell Carcinoma. Radiology Oct 2015;277(1):114–23.

40. Johnson NB, Johnson MM, Selig MK, et al. Use of electron microscopy in core biopsy diagnosis of oncocytic renal tumors. Ultrastruct Pathol Aug 2010;34(4):189–94.

41. Wilson MP, Katlariwala P, Abele J, et al. A review of 99mTc-sestamibi SPECT/CT for renal oncocytomas: A modified diagnostic algorithm. Intractable Rare Dis Res 2022;11(2):46–51.

42. Sheikhbahaei S, Jones CS, Porter KK, et al. Defining the Added Value of 99mTc-MIBI SPECT/CT to Conventional Cross-Sectional Imaging in the Characterization of Enhancing Solid Renal Masses. Clin Nucl Med 2017;42(4):e188–93.

43. Coy H, Young JR, Douek ML, et al. Quantitative computer-aided diagnostic algorithm for automated detection of peak lesion attenuation in differentiating clear cell from papillary and chromophobe renal cell carcinoma, oncocytoma, and fat-poor angiomyolipoma on multiphasic multidetector computed tomography. Abdom Radiol (NY) 2017;42(7):1919–28.

44. Suarez-Ibarrola R, Basulto-Martinez M, Heinze A, et al. Radiomics Applications in Renal Tumor Assessment: A Comprehensive Review of the Literature. Cancers 2020;12(6). https://doi.org/10.3390/cancers12061387.

45. Yan L, Liu Z, Wang G, et al. Angiomyolipoma with minimal fat: differentiation from clear cell renal cell carcinoma and papillary renal cell carcinoma by texture analysis on CT images. Acad Radiol 2015;22(9):1115–21.

46. Feng Z, Rong P, Cao P, et al. Machine learning-based quantitative texture analysis of CT images of small renal masses: Differentiation of angiomyolipoma without visible fat from renal cell carcinoma. Eur Radiol 2018;28(4):1625–33.

47. Cui EM, Lin F, Li Q, et al. Differentiation of renal angiomyolipoma without visible fat from renal cell carcinoma by machine learning based on whole-tumor computed tomography texture features. Acta Radiol 2019;60(11):1543–52.

48. Yu H, Scalera J, Khalid M, et al. Texture analysis as a radiomic marker for differentiating renal tumors. Abdom Radiol (NY) 2017;42(10):2470–8.

49. Meng X, Shu J, Xia Y, et al. A CT-Based Radiomics Approach for the Differential Diagnosis of

Sarcomatoid and Clear Cell Renal Cell Carcinoma. BioMed Res Int 2020;2020:7103647.

50. Coy H, Hsieh K, Wu W, et al. Deep learning and radiomics: the utility of Google TensorFlow™ Inception in classifying clear cell renal cell carcinoma and oncocytoma on multiphasic CT. Abdom Radiol (NY) 2019;44(6):2009–20.

51. Bektas CT, Kocak B, Yardimci AH, et al. Clear Cell Renal Cell Carcinoma: Machine Learning-Based Quantitative Computed Tomography Texture Analysis for Prediction of Fuhrman Nuclear Grade. Eur Radiol 2019;29(3):1153–63.

52. Holdbrook DA, Singh M, Choudhury Y, et al. Automated Renal Cancer Grading Using Nuclear Pleomorphic Patterns. JCO Clin Cancer Inform 2018;2:1–12.

53. Ding J, Xing Z, Jiang Z, et al. CT-based radiomic model predicts high grade of clear cell renal cell carcinoma. Eur J Radiol 2018;103:51–6.

54. Kocak B, Yardimci AH, Bektas CT, et al. Textural differences between renal cell carcinoma subtypes: Machine learning-based quantitative computed tomography texture analysis with independent external validation. Eur J Radiol 2018;107:149–57.

55. Lin F, Cui EM, Lei Y, et al. CT-based machine learning model to predict the Fuhrman nuclear grade of clear cell renal cell carcinoma. Abdom Radiol (NY) 2019;44(7):2528–34.

56. Sun X, Liu L, Xu K, et al. Prediction of ISUP grading of clear cell renal cell carcinoma using support vector machine model based on CT images. Medicine (Baltim) 2019;98(14):e15022.

57. Shu J, Tang Y, Cui J, et al. Clear cell renal cell carcinoma: CT-based radiomics features for the prediction of Fuhrman grade. Eur J Radiol 2018;109:8–12.

58. Demirjian NL, Varghese BA, Cen SY, et al. CT-based radiomics stratification of tumor grade and TNM stage of clear cell renal cell carcinoma. Eur Radiol 2022;32(4):2552–63.

59. Li P, Ren H, Zhang Y, et al. Fifteen-gene expression based model predicts the survival of clear cell renal cell carcinoma. Medicine (Baltim) 2018;97(33):e11839.

60. Kocak B, Durmaz ES, Ates E, et al. Radiogenomics in Clear Cell Renal Cell Carcinoma: Machine Learning-Based High-Dimensional Quantitative CT Texture Analysis in Predicting PBRM1 Mutation Status. AJR Am J Roentgenol 2019;212(3):W55–63.

61. Mühlbauer J, Egen L, Kowalewski KF, et al. Radiomics in Renal Cell Carcinoma-A Systematic Review and Meta-Analysis. Cancers 2021;13(6). https://doi.org/10.3390/cancers13061348.

62. Marconi L, Dabestani S, Lam TB, Hofmann F, Stewart F, Norrie J, Bex A, Bensalah K, Canfield SE, Hora M, Kuczyk MA, Merseburger AS, Mulders PFA, Powles T, Staehler M, Ljungberg B, Volpe A. Systematic Review and Meta-analysis of Diagnostic Accuracy of Percutaneous Renal Tumour Biopsy. Eur Urol 2016 Apr;69(4):660–73. https://doi.org/10.1016/j.eururo.2015.07.072. Epub 2015 Aug 29. PMID: 26323946.

Evolution in the Pathologic Classification of Renal Neoplasia

Reza Alaghehbandan, MD[a], Steven C. Campbell, MD, PhD[b],
Jesse K. McKenney, MD[a],*

KEYWORDS

- Renal cell carcinoma • Pathology • WHO • Classification

KEY POINTS

- Pathologic classification of renal tumors is constantly evolving.
- Classification nomenclature is generally based on histologic features, anatomic location, underlying disease, familial syndromes, and/or specific genetic alterations.
- Despite advances in molecular characterization, most renal tumors can be diagnosed by morphology with or without using a limited set of immunohistochemical stains.
- In places with limited access to molecular resources and specific immunohistochemical markers, pathologists may face difficulties following an optimal algorithm to classify renal tumors.
- World Health Organization 2022 (fifth edition) represents the most up-to-date classification of renal tumors.

HISTORICAL PERSPECTIVES

The history of renal tumor classification is a unique example of evolution in medicine. The gradual recognition of kidney cancer as a heterogeneous disease has incrementally increased the complexity in classification. Tumor classification is a dynamic and complex process. In our opinion, historical background knowledge is critical to fully understanding current classification and future directions, ultimately leading to better patient care. In this article, our focus will be on the evolution in the pathologic classification of adult renal epithelial tumors.

1600 to 1900 Era

The first reference to renal tumors in recorded history dates to 1613, when German physician Daniel Sennert described a tumor arising in the kidney in *Practicae Medicinae*.[1] He stated, "moreover the hard swelling of the bad kidneys which has the capacity to throw a person into cachexia and dropsy, is of greater part incurable."[1]

The first well-documented case of renal cancer was reported by Miriel in 1810.[2] Fifteen years later, the first classification of renal tumors was proposed by Koenig,[2] based on gross (ie, macroscopic) findings and included the following categories: fungoid, medullary, scirrhous, and steatomatous types. A decade later, Rayer divided renal tumors into 3 categories based on morphologic and clinical features as follows: latent (no renal enlargement or hematuria), calyceal (renal pain and hematuria), and scirrhous cancers (hematuria).[2] Rayer's study led others to focus on histologic studies in the hope of identifying renal tumor origin.

For decades, the pathogenesis of renal tumors was debated. The first major "histogenesis" hypothesis was proposed by Paul Grawitz in 1883, when he published his adrenal rest theory (a popular misconception of renal tumor origin).[2,3]

[a] Department of Pathology, Robert J. Tomsich Pathology and Laboratory Medicine Institute, Cleveland Clinic, 2119 E. 96th Street, L25, Cleveland, OH 44106, USA; [b] Department of Urology, Glickman Urological and Kidney Institute, Cleveland Clinic, Q10-120, Glickman Tower, 9500 Euclid Avenue, Cleveland, OH 44195, USA
* Corresponding author.
E-mail address: mckennj@ccf.org

Urol Clin N Am 50 (2023) 181–189
https://doi.org/10.1016/j.ucl.2023.01.001

Grawitz concluded that "alveolar tumors" were of "intrarenal adrenal rest," whereas "papillary tumors" were originated from renal tissue. Grawitz initially called the small yellow cortical tumors "lipomas" and subsequently reclassified them as "adenomas," originating from adrenal rests.[2,3] Later, it was proposed that the so-called adenomas could undergo malignant transformation into carcinomas. Efforts were made to distinguish the two based on histologic features, although unsuccessfully.

1900 to 1980 Era

Scientific advancement in renal neoplasia was limited during the first half of the twentieth century (**Fig. 1**). In this timeframe, proposed classifications mainly included benign adenomas and malignant carcinomas, despite lack of specific defining features between the two. In general, small tumors (ie, <3 cm) were considered adenomas, irrespective of their architectural features.[2,3] Similarly, malignant tumors were grouped together regardless of histologic features (ie, no distinction was made between clear cell and papillary tumors in some classifications).

In 1976, Mancilla-Jimenez and colleagues[4] described clinical and histologic features of clear cell renal cell carcinoma (ccRCC) and papillary renal cell carcinoma (PRCC). This began the gradual description of other renal tumor entities and, ultimately, the first rather limited 1981 World Health Organization (WHO) classification of renal

tumors (**Box 1**).[5] In 1986, the Mainz classification led by Thoenes and colleagues[6] proposed 4 adenomas and 6 carcinomas based on cytologic and architectural features, providing a well-needed expansion to the 1981 WHO classification.

1980 to 2000 Era

The 1980s were important to the genetic understanding of renal cell carcinomas because classic cytogenetic techniques were used by researchers to further define classification (see **Fig. 1**). This included the discovery of mutations in chromosome 3p in ccRCC in 1987,[7] followed by trisomy of chromosomes 7 and 17 and loss of the Y chromosome in PRCCs in 1989,[8] and subsequently the frequent losses of multiple chromosomes in classic chromophobe RCC (ChRCC) in 1992.[9]

The importance of the 1997 Heidelberg-Rochester classification (**Box 2**) as the landmark event in modern renal tumor classification cannot be overstated, incorporating both morphologic and genetic features.[10,11] Importantly, it recognized that "granular RCC" included a heterogenous mixture of both benign and malignant tumors, and removed this historically ambiguous category. This single step allowed for the rapid identification of multiple novel tumor types in the following 2 decades. The second edition of the WHO classification was released in 1998 (see **Box 1**),[12] and while not adopting all proposals from the Heidelberg-Rochester classification, it

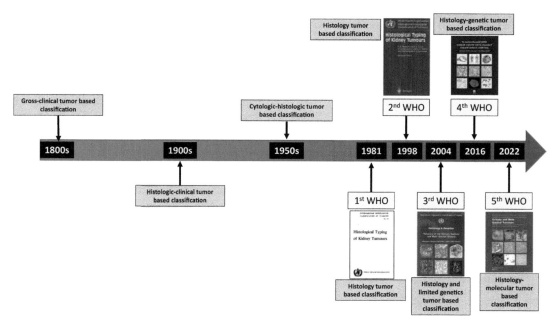

Fig. 1. Renal tumor classification timeline.

Box 1
World Health Organization epithelial renal tumor classification (1981 and 1998)

1981 WHO Classification (Histological typing of kidney tumors).

A. Adenoma

B. Carcinoma

   1. Renal cell carcinoma

   2. Others

1998 WHO Classification (Histological typing of kidney tumors).

1. Epithelial tumors of renal parenchyma

   1.1. Benign – adenoma

      1.1.1. Papillary/tubulopapillary adenoma

      1.1.2. Oncocytic adenoma (oncocytoma)

      1.1.3. Metanephric adenoma

   1.2. Malignant - carcinoma

      1.2.1. Renal cell carcinoma

         1.2.1.1. Clear cell carcinoma

         1.2.1.2. Granular cell carcinoma

         1.2.1.3. Chromophobe cell carcinoma

         1.2.1.4. Spindle cell carcinoma

         1.2.1.5. Cyst-associated renal cell carcinoma

            1.2.1.5.1 Renal cell carcinoma arising in a cyst

            1.2.1.5.2 Cystic renal cell carcinoma

            1.2.1.5.3 Papillary renal cell carcinoma

      1.2.2. Collecting duct carcinoma

Box 2
Heidelberg-Rochester classification of renal cell tumors 1997

Benign

1. Papillary adenoma

2. Renal oncocytoma

3. Metanephric adenoma/adenofibroma

Malignant

1. Conventional (clear cell) carcinoma

2. Papillary renal cell carcinoma

3. Chromophobe renal cell carcinoma

4. Collecting duct carcinoma

   a. Medullary carcinoma

5. Renal cell carcinoma, unclassified

shift in classification paradigm, using combined histology and genetics data (such as fluorescent in situ hybridization [FISH], a hallmark of molecular cytogenetics). This was underscored by the first inclusion of Xp11 translocation carcinoma (now *TFE3*-rearranged *RCC*) from specific molecular alterations.

The 2016 WHO classification of renal tumors shifted further toward "histomolecular" driven classification (**Box 4**).[14] It included 14 tumor subtypes and 4 emerging/provisional entities, including newly recognized entities such as hereditary leiomyomatosis and RCC syndrome-associated RCC (hereditary leiomyomatosis and

Box 3
2004 World Health Organization epithelial renal tumor classification

1. Clear cell renal cell carcinoma

2. Multi-locular clear cell renal cell carcinoma

3. Papillary renal cell carcinoma

4. Chromophobe renal cell carcinoma

5. Carcinoma of the collecting ducts of Bellini

6. Renal medullary carcinoma

7. Xp11 translocation carcinoma

8. Carcinoma associated with Neuroblastoma

9. Mucinous, tubular, and spindle cell carcinoma

10. Renal cell carcinoma, unclassified

11. Papillary adenoma

12. Oncocytoma

provided an initial step toward the 2004 WHO classification (**Box 3**).[13]

2000 to 2022 Era

Our understanding of renal neoplasia owes a large debt to the pioneers of morphological observations using conventional light microscopic techniques in the first half of the twentieth century, followed by ultrastructural studies and later basic genetic techniques (eg, classic cytogenetics) in the 1980 to 1990s (see **Fig. 1**). The 2004 WHO classification of renal tumors codified the major

---

Box 4
2016 World Health Organization epithelial renal tumor classification

1. Clear cell renal cell carcinoma
2. Multilocular cystic renal neoplasm of low malignant potential
3. Papillary renal cell carcinoma
4. Hereditary leiomyomatosis and renal cell carcinoma-associated renal cell carcinoma
5. Chromophobe renal cell carcinoma
6. Collecting duct carcinoma
7. Renal medullary carcinoma
8. MiT family translocation renal cell carcinoma
9. Succinate dehydrogenase-deficient renal carcinoma
10. Mucinous tubular and spindle cell carcinoma
11. Tubulocystic renal cell carcinoma
12. Acquired cystic disease-associated renal cell carcinoma
13. Clear cell papillary renal cell carcinoma
14. Renal cell carcinoma, unclassified
15. Papillary adenoma
16. Oncocytoma

---

renal cell cancer [HLRCC]), succinate dehydrogenase (SDH)-deficient RCC, tubulocystic RCC, acquired cystic disease-associated RCC, and clear cell papillary RCC.

In the last decade, the development of more advanced and efficient molecular techniques such as comparative genomic hybridization and next-generation sequencing (NGS) led to a tumor classification renaissance in identifying and reconsidering "old" and "new" entities.

WHAT IS NEW IN THE 2022 WORLD HEALTH ORGANIZATION CLASSIFICATION OF RENAL TUMORS?

Compared with previous editions, the recently published 2022 WHO classification of renal tumors incorporates even more molecular data with the introduction of additional tumors defined by genetic alterations.[15] The current edition includes changes and updates in established entities, novel distinct entities, a new category of molecularly defined tumors, and emerging provisional entities (**Box 5**).[15] A detailed list of pathologic updates in

the WHO classification of renal tumors was recently published.[16]

Updates in Established Entities

- The spectrum of PRCC continues to evolve, and some entities are now regarded as independent tumors with specific clinical and molecular features (ie, they are no longer classified as PRCC): fumarate hydratase (FH)-deficient RCC, tubulocystic RCC, and *TFE3/TFEB* alteration RCC. Thus, recent molecular and clinical outcome data no longer support subclassification of PRCC into type 1 and 2.[17] In our experience, a specific "microcystic" histologic pattern is associated with most adverse outcomes in PRCC, and we suspect its recognition may become more accepted in future classifications.[18]

- "Clear cell papillary renal cell carcinoma" was renamed "clear cell papillary renal cell *tumor* (CCPRCT)," given its consistently benign behavior. To date, no well-documented metastases are reported. These tumors are low-stage and low-grade with tubulopapillary and cystic architecture, and lack recurrent cytogenetic abnormalities or *VHL* gene alterations.

- ChRCC is recognized to have nonclassic (variant) morphologies such as trabecular, alveolar, papillary, microcystic or cystic architecture, none of which affect prognosis but are important for pathologists to recognize the correct diagnosis.

- "Oncocytic renal cell carcinoma occurring after neuroblastoma" was removed from the 2022 WHO classification. Recent studies show this is not a distinct tumor type but rather a heterogenous mixture of tumors including: sporadic tumors of any type, therapy-related *TFE3*-rearranged RCC, and eosinophilic solid and cystic (ESC) RCC. Any underlying genetic relationship between ESC RCC, originally called "oncocytoid RCC after neuroblastoma," and childhood neuroblastoma is unknown.[19–21]

- Historically, the spectrum of oncocytic renal tumors with a low risk for aggressive behavior has been classified as either renal oncocytoma or eosinophilic variant of ChRCC. It is now recognized that this may be more of a continuous spectrum of disease, and a subset of tumors may not precisely fit either specific type. Therefore, the term "oncocytic renal neoplasm of low malignant potential" is approved for histologically borderline cases.[22] This is a clinical management category

---

Box 5
2022 World Health Organization Epithelial Renal Tumor Classification

1. Clear cell renal cell tumors
   1.1. Clear cell renal cell carcinoma
   1.2. Multilocular cystic renal neoplasm of low malignant potential
2. Papillary renal tumors
   2.1. Renal papillary adenoma
   2.2. Papillary renal cell carcinoma
3. Oncocytic and chromophobe renal tumors
   3.1. Oncocytoma of the kidney
   3.2. Chromophobe renal cell carcinoma
   3.3. Other oncocytic tumors of the kidney
4. Collecting duct tumors
   4.1. Collecting duct carcinoma
5. Other renal tumors
   5.1. Clear cell papillary renal cell tumor
   5.2. Mucinous tubular and spindle cell carcinoma
   5.3. Tubulocystic renal cell carcinoma
   5.4. Acquired cystic disease-associated renal cell carcinoma
   5.5. Eosinophilic solid and cystic renal cell carcinoma
   5.6. Renal cell carcinoma NOS
6. Molecularly defined renal carcinomas
   6.1. *TFE3*-rearranged renal cell carcinomas
   6.2. *TFEB*-altered renal cell carcinomas
   6.3. *ELOC* (formerly *TCEB1*)-mutated renal cell carcinoma
   6.4. Fumarate hydratase-deficient renal cell carcinoma
   6.5. Succinate dehydrogenase-deficient renal cell carcinoma
   6.6. *ALK*-rearranged renal cell carcinomas
   6.7. SMARCB1-deficient renal medullary carcinoma
7. Emerging/provisional entities (still not part of the classification as definitive entities)
   7.1. Biphasic hyalinizing psammomatous renal cell carcinoma
   7.2. Papillary renal neoplasm with reverse polarity
   7.3. Thyroid-like follicular carcinoma
   7.4. Eosinophilic vacuolated tumor
   7.5. Low-grade oncocytic tumor

---

diagnosis that should be reserved for solitary and sporadic tumors. Of note, 2 "emerging" entities may fall within this spectrum: low-grade oncocytic tumor and eosinophilic vacuolated tumor. These have no documented risk of aggressive behavior; their recognition and place in current classification was recently reviewed.[23]

Molecularly Defined Renal Tumors

The following entities show significant tumor heterogeneity and overlapping morphologic features with other RCCs. Therefore, definitive diagnosis based on morphology alone may not be possible and molecular testing could be required (ie, FISH, NGS). Molecularly defined RCCs include the following:

- *TFE3*-rearranged *RCCs*: This tumor is heterogenous and shows a mixed histological pattern, often including papillary architecture and psammoma bodies; strong nuclear staining for *TFE3* by immunohistochemistry, or *TFE3* rearrangement identified by break-apart FISH, or *TFE3* gene fusion identified by RNA sequencing. These have the potential to behave aggressively. FISH testing (or sequencing) is needed for definitive diagnosis of these tumors.

- *ALK*-rearranged RCCs (novel entity): This tumor, which seems to be extremely rare, shows heterogenous morphologic spectrum with eosinophilic cytoplasm and mucinous features. Positive *ALK* IHC and/or FISH is essential for confirming the diagnosis. *ALK*-rearranged RCC may potentially be a clinically important diagnosis owing to the availability of *ALK* inhibitor–targeted therapies.[24] Although a minority of cases may have aggressive clinical course, the majority of *ALK*-rearranged RCCs have been indolent.

- *TFEB*-rearranged and *TFEB*-amplified RCC: *TFEB*-altered RCCs are less common than *TFE3*-rearranged RCC tumors. *TFEB*-translocated RCC is more indolent than *TFE3*-translocated RCC; however, *TFEB*-amplified RCCs are highly aggressive tumors. FISH testing is needed for definitive diagnosis of these tumors.

- *ELOC* (formerly *TCEB1*)-mutated RCC (novel entity): Most examples of these tumors have a distinct morphology reported as "RCC with fibromyomatous (or leiomyomatous) stroma." Based on limited data, the majority have an indolent behavior after resection. In our experience, morphologically identical tumors more frequently have underlying alterations in *TSC1*, *TSC2*, or *MTOR*.[25] Future classifications may combine these tumors into one group. Most importantly, it is our experience that these tumors are readily identified by combined morphology and immunohistochemistry without the need for molecular confirmation.

- SMARCB1 (INI1)-deficient Renal Medullary Carcinoma: This is a highly aggressive RCC, which is typically located within the renal medullary region. It frequently occurs in young patients with sickle cell trait (or other hemoglobinopathy). This diagnosis is readily made based on combined histologic, immunophenotypic, and clinical features.

- FH-deficient RCC (formerly HLRCC syndrome-associated RCC): FH-deficient RCCs typically demonstrate multiple admixed morphological patterns. Immunohistochemical loss of FH and overexpressed 2SC, and/or pathogenic FH mutation in the tumor is diagnostic. Most cases (over 85%) are associated with germline FH mutations, and patients may have personal and/or family history of skin and uterine leiomyomas with or without RCC. Appropriate genetic counseling and discussion of germline testing is important for patients with this tumor type. In familial cases, the term HLRCC syndrome-associated RCC is still acceptable. FH-deficient RCC has been targeted successfully in early-phase studies using erlotinib and bevacizumab.[26]

Novel Distinct Entities

ESC RCC was originally described in patients with tuberous sclerosis complex but more commonly occur sporadically due to somatic *TSC1* or *TSC2* mutations. ESC RCC is typically a solitary tumor, found in patients of broad age range, and mostly in women. Although the great majority of ESC RCCs have indolent behavior, rare tumors with metastatic disease have been reported.

Emerging/Provisional Entities

These tumors are not officially part of the classification because current data are limited. They include thyroid-like follicular carcinoma (with *EWSR1-PATZ1* fusion), biphasic hyalinizing psammomatous RCC (with *NF2* mutation), and papillary renal neoplasm with reverse polarity (with *KRAS* mutation but currently regarded as within spectrum of PRCC).

BEYOND 2022: FUTURE CLASSIFICATION AND THE ROLE OF MOLECULAR EVALUATION?

A major issue is (and will be) the overall availability of adjunctive molecular and immunohistochemical techniques for routine practice. We advocate for developing resource-stratified guidelines to provide a clinically relevant diagnostic approach for renal tumor subtyping with the use of ancillary tests that are feasible for pathologists and clinicians in low-resource settings.[27] Subclassification is only relevant if it has therapeutic significance in the setting it is diagnosed (which may be less often in underresourced countries). Fortunately, most RCCs (~75%) are relatively straightforward ccRCC, followed by PRCC and ChRCC. The majority of RCC subtypes may not be clinically relevant for treatment decisions. Some have prognostic significance but no therapeutic significance beyond grade and stage, and some are so rare that the average surgical pathologist may never see one in their career. However, as some subtypes become defined by unique molecular testing and distinct IHC findings that cannot be achieved in low-resource settings, a subset of cases may not be definitively subtyped.

Establishment of a pure molecular classification for renal tumors in the near future seems unlikely, in contrast to CNS and hematolymphoid tumor classifications, given that most renal tumors are easily diagnosable based on standard histologic examination. Morphology is a very sensitive test for identifying and classifying renal tumors without the need for expensive surrogate molecular or immunohistochemical confirmation in most cases. This is not surprising because almost all tumor subtypes were initially described by morphology and only later confirmed as distinct molecular groups when more sophisticated testing techniques became available. Moreover, the presence of different molecular pathways leading to the same tumor type makes molecular classification difficult and of questionable added benefit in many cases. More detailed molecular sequencing analyses are typically reserved for rare undifferentiated or difficult-to-classify tumors, where more specific subclassification or identification of targetable alterations might change treatment. At present, morphologic features are used to identify cases that might benefit from selective molecular testing (eg, *TFE3* and *TFEB* FISH). It is likely that even for rare and emerging entities in the future, the utility of standard routine gross and microscopic assessments will remain essential, but molecular studies will continue to provide insight into subtle differences, hereditary renal neoplasia, and rare esoteric tumor types.

STAGING AND GRADING SYSTEM

Flocks and Kadesky proposed a staging schema in 1958 as follows: Stage 1—limited to the renal capsule, Stage 2—invasion of the renal pedicle and/or renal fat, Stage 3—regional lymph node involvement, and Stage 4—distant metastasis.[28] Although staging renal cancers evolved during the next 6 decades, their initial recognition that invasion of perinephric tissue, metastasis to lymph nodes, and distant metastasis stratify patient outcomes, remains at the core of our staging system. Radical nephrectomy was initially proposed in 1963 as the treatment of RCC,[29] which led to modifications in staging. The modified staging system introduced confinement within Gerota's fascia as a criterion for stage II, and extension into the renal vein or vena cava as elements of stage III. Based largely on the detailed dissection studies of Dr Stephen Bonsib in the 2000s,[30–33] it is now well established that the primary route of extrarenal invasion

by renal cell carcinoma is through the blood vessels of the renal sinus. Therefore, microscopic confirmation of intravascular tumor within the small and/or large vessels of the renal sinus is the major determining factor of pT3 stage under current American Joint Committee on Cancer (AJCC) guidelines.[34]

Grading was initially applied in 1932, demonstrating that high-grade renal tumors were associated with poor survival.[35] Since then, other histologic grading systems have been introduced, based on architectural, cellular, and nuclear features.[35,36] However, it was the nuclear grading system by Fuhrman and colleagues[37] in 1985 that gained widespread recognition. In 2012, the International Society of Urological Pathology (ISUP) consensus conference proposed simplified/modified Fuhrman grading system by focusing only on nucleolar prominence. This was designated as the ISUP grade, which was subsequently recognized by the 2016 WHO classification to become the WHO/ISUP grade.[38] WHO/ISUP grading is only recommended for ccRCC and PRCC. For other RCC subtypes, there is currently no grading system recommended. Specifically, multiple studies show histologic grading of ChRCC does not correlate with prognosis, short of sarcomatoid differentiation.[39–43]

2022 WORLD HEALTH ORGANIZATION CLASSIFICATION APPLICATION IN RENAL MASS BIOPSY

Small renal masses (less than 4 cm) usually have low metastatic risk. The incidence of such tumors has increased due to increased utilization of cross-sectional imaging for a variety of unrelated concerns.[44,45] Percutaneous renal tumor biopsy continues to be a useful tool for oncologic risk stratification for a subset of patients who are candidates for active surveillance, tumor ablation, or surgical management.[44,46–48]

However, there are several challenges to classifying renal tumors on core biopsy. First, core biopsy material may be limited/inadequate or not representative of the lesion. The nondiagnostic rate of renal mass biopsy has been approximately 10% to 15% in recent studies.[47] Second, certain types of renal tumors can only be definitively diagnosed after review of the entire resection (eg, low-risk oncocytic neoplasms and predominantly cystic clear cell tumors). Third, other renal neoplasms, including ccRCC may be morphologically heterogenous across the entire tumor, which can potentially create diagnostic difficulties due to sampling bias. Although classification of tumor histology seems to be relatively accurate (>95%)

with renal mass biopsy, discordance of tumor grade between the biopsy and final pathology is seen in 30%-40% of cases.[47]

Many prototypical examples of renal neoplasia can be definitively diagnosed on biopsy, including common types such as urothelial carcinoma, ccRCC, ChRCC, and PRCC. Under the 2022 WHO classification, definitive diagnosis of multilocular cystic neoplasm of low malignant potential (MCNLMP), CCPRCT, and oncocytoma is, for most practical purposes, not possible on biopsy because each requires evaluation of the entire tumor. MCNLMP has a significant overlap with predominantly cystic ccRCC and even solid ccRCC with a focal cystic/degenerative component. Additionally, CCPRCT can manifest as a nearly entirely cystic tumor and mimic MCNLMP or ccRCC. In scenarios where there is strong/diffuse expression of CK7 in tumors suspicious for ccRCC, we tend to err on side of caution and avoid rendering an unequivocal diagnosis of ccRCC based on core biopsies alone. Similarly, in our opinion, a definitive diagnosis of oncocytoma cannot be made on a core biopsy because ChRCC may show intratumoural heterogeneity, including areas essentially identical to oncocytoma. Furthermore, "other oncocytic tumors of the kidney" in the 2022 WHO classification are a heterogeneous group with overlapping or borderline features between oncocytoma and ChRCC. These tumors are typically small, well-circumscribed and indolent, so it is often sufficient at biopsy to recognize a tumor in the family of low-risk oncocytic tumors and simply exclude the possibility of higher-risk types. Clinical decisions about suitability of active surveillance or less aggressive management strategies, such as thermal ablation rather than surgical excision, do not necessarily require a definitive subclassification.

SUMMARY

The 2022 WHO classification of renal tumors provides the most current approach, incorporating recent genomic discoveries. Global efforts in comprehensive sequencing with more advanced technologies will result in better understanding of renal tumors and their proper place in upcoming classifications. However, morphology will continue to play a primary role in standard daily renal tumor diagnosis. Ultimately, tumor classification, as a dynamic and complex process, will continue to evolve in the pursuit of optimizing clinical care for our patients.

DISCLOSURE

The authors declare no conflict of interest.

REFERENCES

1. Hansel DE, Kane CJ, Paner GP, et al. The kidney: a comprehensive guide to pathologic diagnosis and management. New York, NY: Springer; 2016.
2. Delahunt B, Eble JN. History of the development of the classification of renal cell neoplasia. Clin Lab Med 2005;25(2):231–46.
3. Young RH, Eble JN. The history of urologic pathology: an overview. Histopathology 2019;74(1):184–212.
4. Mancilla-Jimenez R, Stanley RJ, Blath RA. Papillary renal cell carcinoma: a clinical, radiologic, and pathologic study of 34 cases. Cancer 1976;38(6):2469–80.
5. Mostofi FK, Sesterhenn IA, and Sobin LH. Histological typing of kidney tumours, 1981, World Health Organization; Geneva, Switzerland.
6. Thoenes W, Storkel S, Rumpelt HJ. Histopathology and classification of renal cell tumors (adenomas, oncocytomas and carcinomas). The basic cytological and histopathological elements and their use for diagnostics. Pathol Res Pract 1986;181(2):125–43.
7. Szucs S, Muller-Brechlin R, DeRiese W, et al. Deletion 3p: the only chromosome loss in a primary renal cell carcinoma. Cancer Genet Cytogenet 1987;26(2):369–73.
8. Kovacs G, Wilkens L, Papp T, et al. Differentiation between papillary and nonpapillary renal cell carcinomas by DNA analysis. J Natl Cancer Inst 1989;81(7):527–30.
9. Kovacs A, Kovacs G. Low chromosome number in chromophobe renal cell carcinomas. Genes Chromosomes Cancer 1992;4(3):267–8.
10. Storkel S, Eble JN, Adlakha K, et al. Classification of renal cell carcinoma: Workgroup No. 1. Union Internationale Contre le Cancer (UICC) and the American Joint Committee on Cancer (AJCC). Cancer 1997;80(5):987–9.
11. Kovacs G, Akhtar M, Beckwith BJ, et al. The Heidelberg classification of renal cell tumours. J Pathol 1997;183(2):131–3.
12. Mostofi FK, Davis CJ, Sobin LH. Histological typing of kidney tumors. 2nd edition. Springer; Geneva, Switzerland; 1998.
13. Eble JN, Sauter G, Epstein JI, et al. World Health Organization classification of tumours. Pathology and genetics of tumours of the urinary system and male genital organs. IARC; Lyon, France; 2004.
14. Moch H, Humphrey PA, Ulbright TM, et al. 4th edition. WHO classification of tumours of the urinary system and male genital organs, 8. Lyon, France: IARC; 2016.
15. Board WcoTE. Urinary and male genital tumours (WHO classification of tumours). Lyon, France: IARC; 2022.
16. Moch H, Amin MB, Berney DM, et al. The 2022 World Health Organization Classification of tumours of the urinary system and male genital organs-part a: renal, penile, and testicular tumours. Eur Urol 2022;82(5):458–68.
17. Ricketts CJ, Linehan WM, Spellman PT, et al, Cancer Genome Atlas Research Network. Comprehensive molecular characterization of papillary renal-cell carcinoma. N Engl J Med 2016;374(2):135–45.

18. Chan E, Stohr BA, Butler RS, et al. Papillary renal cell carcinoma with microcystic architecture is strongly associated with extrarenal invasion and metastatic disease. Am J Surg Pathol 2022;46(3):392–403.

19. Palsgrove DN, Li Y, Pratilas CA, et al. Eosinophilic Solid and Cystic (ESC) renal cell carcinomas harbor tsc mutations: molecular analysis supports an expanding clinicopathologic spectrum. Am J Surg Pathol 2018;42(9):1166–81.

20. Falzarano SM, McKenney JK, Montironi R, et al. Renal cell carcinoma occurring in patients with prior neuroblastoma: a heterogenous group of neoplasms. Am J Surg Pathol 2016;40(7):989–97.

21. Medeiros LJ, Palmedo G, Krigman HR, et al. Oncocytoid renal cell carcinoma after neuroblastoma: a report of four cases of a distinct clinicopathologic entity. Am J Surg Pathol 1999;23(7):772–80.

22. Trpkov K, Williamson SR, Gill AJ, et al. Novel, emerging and provisional renal entities: The Genitourinary Pathology Society (GUPS) update on renal neoplasia. Mod Pathol 2021;34(6):1167–84.

23. Amin MB, McKenney JK, Martignoni G, et al. Low grade oncocytic tumors of the kidney: a clinically relevant approach for the workup and accurate diagnosis. Mod Pathol 2022;35:1306–16.

24. Tao JJ, Wei G, Patel R, et al. ALK fusions in renal cell carcinoma: response to entrectinib. JCO Precis Oncol 2018;2:1–8.

25. Shah RB, Stohr BA, Tu ZJ, et al. "Renal cell carcinoma with leiomyomatous stroma" harbor somatic mutations of TSC1, TSC2, MTOR, and/or ELOC (TCEB1): clinicopathologic and molecular characterization of 18 sporadic tumors supports a distinct entity. Am J Surg Pathol 2020;44(5):571–81.

26. Srinivasan R, Su D, Stamatakis L, et al. 5 Mechanism based targeted therapy for hereditary leiomyomatosis and renal cell cancer (HLRCC) and sporadic papillary renal cell carcinoma: interim results from a phase 2 study of bevacizumab and erlotinib. Eur J Cancer 2014;50(6):8.

27. Anglade F, Milner DA Jr, Brock JE. Can pathology diagnostic services for cancer be stratified and serve global health? Cancer 2020;126(Suppl 10):2431–8.

28. Flocks RH, Kadesky MC. Malignant neoplasms of the kidney; an analysis of 353 patients followed five years or more. J Urol 1958;79(2):196–201.

29. Robson CJ, Churchill BM, Anderson W. The results of radical nephrectomy for renal cell carcinoma. J Urol 1969;101(3):297–301.

30. Bonsib SM, Gibson D, Mhoon M, et al. Renal sinus involvement in renal cell carcinomas. Am J Surg Pathol 2000;24(3):451–8.

31. Bonsib SM. The renal sinus is the principal invasive pathway: a prospective study of 100 renal cell carcinomas. Am J Surg Pathol 2004;28(12):1594–600.

32. Bonsib SM. T2 clear cell renal cell carcinoma is a rare entity: a study of 120 clear cell renal cell carcinomas. J Urol 2005;174(4 Pt 1):1199–202.

33. Bonsib SM. Renal veins and venous extension in clear cell renal cell carcinoma. Mod Pathol 2007;20(1):44–53.

34. Amin MB, Edge S, Greene F, et al. AJCC cancer staging manual. 8th edition. Springer International Publishing: American Joint Committee on Cancer; Chicago, IL; 2017.

35. Paner GP, Chumbalkar V, Montironi R, et al. Updates in grading of renal cell carcinomas beyond clear cell renal cell carcinoma and papillary renal cell carcinoma. Adv Anat Pathol 2022;29(3):117–30.

36. Delahunt B, Eble JN, Egevad L, et al. Grading of renal cell carcinoma. Histopathology 2019;74(1):4–17.

37. Fuhrman SA, Lasky LC, Limas C. Prognostic significance of morphologic parameters in renal cell carcinoma. Am J Surg Pathol 1982;6(7):655–63.

38. Moch HHP, Ulbright TM, Reuter VE. *WHO classification of tumours of the urinary system and male genital organs*, . WHO Classification of Tumours. 4th edition8. Lyon, France: IARC; 2016.

39. Ohashi R, Martignoni G, Hartmann A, et al. Multi-institutional re-evaluation of prognostic factors in chromophobe renal cell carcinoma: proposal of a novel two-tiered grading scheme. Virchows Arch 2020;476(3): 409–18.

40. Volpe A, Novara G, Antonelli A, et al. Chromophobe renal cell carcinoma (RCC): oncological outcomes and prognostic factors in a large multicentre series. BJU Int 2012;110(1):76–83.

41. Lopez-Beltran A, Montironi R, Cimadamore A, et al. Grading of chromophobe renal cell carcinoma: do we need it? Eur Urol 2021;79(2):232–3.

42. Avulova S, Cheville JC, Lohse CM, et al. Grading chromophobe renal cell carcinoma: evidence for a four-tiered classification incorporating coagulative tumor necrosis. Eur Urol 2021;79(2):225–31.

43. Cheville JC, Lohse CM, Sukov WR, et al. Chromophobe renal cell carcinoma: the impact of tumor grade on outcome. Am J Surg Pathol 2012;36(6):851–6.

44. Wilcox Vanden Berg RN, Basourakos SP, LaRussa S, et al. Management of the small renal mass: a 2020 update. Curr Oncol Rep 2020;22(7):69.

45. Shen SS, Ro JY. Histologic diagnosis of renal mass biopsy. Arch Pathol Lab Med 2019;143(6):705–10.

46. Campbell RA, Scovell J, Rathi N, et al. Partial versus radical nephrectomy: complexity of decision-making and utility of AUA guidelines. Clin Genitourin Cancer 2022;20(6):501–9.

47. Campbell SC, Clark PE, Chang SS, et al. Renal mass and localized renal cancer: evaluation, management, and follow-up: AUA guideline: part I. J Urol 2021;206(2):199–208.

48. Campbell SC, Uzzo RG, Karam JA, et al. Renal mass and localized renal cancer: evaluation, management, and follow-up: AUA guideline: part II. J Urol 2021;206(2):209–18.

Biomarkers for the Detection and Surveillance of Renal Cancer

José Ignacio Nolazco, MD[a,b],*, Simon John Christoph Soerensen, MD[c,d], Benjamin I. Chung, MD, MS[c]

KEYWORDS

- Renal cell carcinoma • Biomarkers • Diagnosis • Screening

KEY POINTS

- Currently, no validated biomarkers are incorporated in clinical guidelines for screening and follow-up of patients with RCC.
- Renal cancer is a heterogeneous disease, and finding a single biomarker capable of detecting these tumors with high sensitivity and specificity is challenging.
- Characterizing the nature of small renal masses through renal cell carcinoma biomarkers may enable more effective treatment selection between surgery and active surveillance.
- Such markers could also provide valuable insights into new cancer therapies, aiding the development of personalized treatments tailored to individual patients' genetic signatures.
- Further prospective clinical trials are warranted to validate biomarkers and assess their utility in clinical practice.

INTRODUCTION

Renal cell carcinoma (RCC) is one of the most commonly diagnosed cancers in the United States. It accounts for approximately 4.0% of new cancers and 2.3% of cancer-specific deaths in the United States alone.[1] Advances in imaging technologies and the widespread use of computed tomography (CT) and MRI have led to an increase in the detection of the disease and an increased percentage of cases diagnosed with early-stage RCC.[2,3] Stage migration toward early-stage kidney cancer has enabled the utilization of active surveillance to a greater extent than previously, especially in elderly or frail patients.[4] However, due to genetic, clinical, and pathological heterogeneity of RCC, it is difficult to assess whether a suspicious mass is benign or malignant by using imaging alone.[5] Usually, diagnosis and treatment indications do not represent a clinical challenge for large tumors. However, for small renal masses (often defined as < 4 cm) that are usually asymptomatic, it might not be evident to clinicians what the best diagnostic and treatment approaches are, for example, follow-up or treatment. Moreover, approximately 20% of small renal masses are benign[6] and those that are malignant might have an indolent evolution and a low risk of progression or metastasis.[7]

Radical or partial nephrectomy is the gold standard for patients diagnosed with RCC. After surgery, the standard of care is observation and follow-up to eventually identify recurrence or progression to metastatic disease.[8] Leibovich and

[a] Division of Urological Surgery, Brigham and Women's Hospital, Harvard Medical School, 45 Francis Street, Boston, MA 02115, USA; [b] Servicio de Urología, Hospital Universitario Austral, Universidad Austral, Av Juan Domingo Perón 1500, B1629AHJ Pilar, Argentina; [c] Department of Urology, Stanford University School of Medicine, Stanford, CA, USA; [d] Department of Epidemiology and Population Health, Stanford University School of Medicine, Stanford, USA
* Corresponding author.
E-mail address: JNolazco@bwh.harvard.edu

Urol Clin N Am 50 (2023) 191–204
https://doi.org/10.1016/j.ucl.2023.01.009

colleagues[9] found a relapse rate of 29% in a cohort of patients diagnosed with localized RCC. Therefore, although there is no consensus about follow-up,[10] it is critically important to observe these patients with imaging after surgery. However, imaging has an associated risk of cumulative radiation exposure.[11]

Incorporating biological markers into clinical practice could address issues related to diagnosing, prognoses, and surveillance of patients with RCC.

1. They can be collected noninvasively in the serum or urine.
2. They are less expensive than biopsies or other more invasive interventions that might require hospitalization.
3. Biomarkers can be objectively measured and do not rely on professional expertise.
4. They could significantly influence patient care, because RCC is curable when detected early, similar to many solid cancers.
5. Biomarkers may help identify patients who are candidates for targeted therapies, which may have improved efficacy and fewer side effects than traditional chemotherapy.
6. They can be helpful in monitoring response to treatment and detecting the recurrence or progression of RCC.

However, further investigation is warranted to improve patient selection and validate the cost-effectiveness of these tools. Because RCC encompasses a highly heterogeneous group of tumors, identifying a single biomarker that can diagnose all or most of the different tumors is challenging.

Currently, there are no validated biomarkers for patients with RCC. In this review, we aim to understand better some potential biomarkers for the detection and surveillance of RCC.

Serum Biomarkers

The use of serum biomarkers as tools for detecting and in the surveillance of RCC has recently been gaining traction. Ideally, such markers are noninvasive, easily obtained, and provide objective measurements, which make them attractive alternatives or augments to imaging techniques. Furthermore, they have the potential to identify patients who could benefit from targeted therapies with increased efficacy compared with traditional chemotherapy but with fewer side effects. Numerous serum biomarkers such as circulating tumor DNA (ctDNA), heat shock protein 27 (HSP27), serum amyloid A (SAA), matrix metalloproteinase-7 (MMP-7), and osteopontin (OPN), among many others, have been studied in patients with both early-stage and metastatic RCC (mRCC); however, none have yet been established as a reliable tool for clinical practice. This review will examine the current evidence promising serum markers that might aid in diagnosing RCC and detecting its recurrence or progression after treatment.

ctDNA a promising biomarker for diagnosing RCC does not require invasive sample collection, thus posing nearly no risk associated with it. Additionally, ctDNA enables serial testing to monitor disease status, which allows tracking clonal evolution over time while identifying resistance mechanisms and detecting residual or recurring disease. Compared with tissue biopsies obtained through invasive interventions, excellent safety profile of ctDNA, coupled with its lower cost, make it a cost-effective alternative tool in localized RCC cases where it has proven helpful as a surveillance biomarker for disease recurrence.[12] Similarly, in mRCC cases where most patients have detectable ctDNA levels, using next-generation sequencing of such molecules possesses considerable potential in predicting tumor responses to immunotherapy by acting as surrogates for measuring tumor mutational burden.[13]

HSP27 is a protein associated with tumor growth and has antioxidant and antiapoptotic functions. Because it is implicated in multiple cellular processes, HSP27 responds to stress conditions of oxidative and chemical stress. Studies have found that it could lower the concentration of reactive oxygen species by raising intracellular glutathione levels and lowering intracellular iron concentration.[14] In general, overexpression of HSPs, especially HSP27, is associated with poor prognosis in multiple cancers because it protects malignant cells from undergoing apoptosis.[15] White and colleagues found significant differences in blood concentrations of HSP27 in patients with RCC compared with control individuals. Moreover, the authors found a correlation between the level of HSP27 expression and RCC tumor grade. Additionally, this biomarker can also be acquired through urine samples.[16]

SAA is an acute-phase protein with the potential for detecting RCC, particularly in advanced stages. Studies have indicated that serum levels of SAA correlate with tumor stage, suggesting it may not be suitable for identifying early-stage RCC. However, a study found SAA to be more sensitive than interleukin 6 and C-reactive protein when used to detect the later stages of RCC.[17]

Ramankulov and colleagues[18] found SAA to be an independent factor of survival in patients with RCC and concluded that it could be useful as a predictor for survival. An additional study also found SAA to be a robust and independent prognosticator for progression-free survival and overall survival in patients with mRCC.[19] However, further research is needed to understand how well SAA can diagnose and monitor the disease before its utility as a biomarker can be established definitively. Additionally, elevated SAA levels are associated with other conditions, such as infections or inflammatory diseases,[20] which could reduce its specificity as a marker for RCC diagnosis. Nevertheless, preliminary evidence suggests that measuring and interpreting SAA levels could prove valuable in conjunction with other diagnostic tests when managing patients suffering from the disease, although further studies will be required for confirmation.

MMP-7 is a zinc-containing enzyme involved in degrading extracellular matrix components. It is found to be overexpressed in RCC, and its levels are correlated with higher tumor grade, cancer invasion, and metastasis, as well as worse cancer-specific survival.[21] In addition, Lu and colleagues[22] found a positive correlation between serum levels of MMP-7 and RCC pathological grade and clinical stage. Ramankulov and colleagues[23] reported that higher levels of MMP-7 correlated with metastatic disease and poor prognosis in patients with RCC.

OPN is a chemokine-like protein involved in many cell functions, including bone remodeling, inflammatory response, and cell adhesion. OPN regulates hypoxia-inducible factor-1α-dependent VEGF expression and plays critical roles in cell pathways involved in tumor growth, angiogenesis, and metastasis.[24]

OPN plasma concentrations were an independent predictor for decreased cancer-specific survival in patients with renal cancer.[25,26] In addition, high levels of OPN have been found to be associated with a more aggressive and advanced stage of RCC.[27] OPN expression has also been shown to be correlated with the degree of tumor angiogenesis, invasiveness, and metastasis in RCC.[28] These findings suggest that OPN may be a potential therapeutic target for the treatment of RCC, as inhibiting OPN activity or blocking its signaling pathways may slow or prevent the progression of the disease.[24,29]

Urinary Biomarkers

Urinary biomarkers are a promising tool for detecting and monitoring RCC. Through their minimally invasive nature, urinary tests provide a reliable, cost-effective alternative to more expensive imaging modalities such as CT scans and MRIs. Urinary biomarkers present in the urine can be used to diagnose or monitor RCC at its earliest stages before any symptoms manifest. These markers may include proteins, hormones, enzymes, or other substances that either originate from the body or are byproducts caused by certain conditions associated with RCC. In this review article, we will focus on aquaporin-1 (AQP1), perilipin 2 (PER2; PLIN2), carbonic anhydrase IX (CA-IX), kidney injury molecule-1 (KIM-1), and neutrophil gelatinase-associated lipocalin (NGAL), which have been identified as potential urinary biomarkers for detecting and monitoring renal cancer.

AQP1 is a transmembrane protein expressed in many different cells that facilitates water movement and is associated with angiogenesis and tumor progression.[30] Although it is not specific to renal cells and can be upregulated in other organs, it is expressed in the proximal tubule cells, and its secretion is associated with a pathological process, making it a candidate for RCC detection.[31] In addition, common underlying kidney pathologic conditions such as diabetic nephropathy, glomerulonephritis, and urinary tract infections did not confound the ability of AQP-1 to screen for renal cancer.[32] Morrissey and colleagues[33] showed that urinary AQP-1 could distinguish between RCC and healthy surgical controls with an area under the receiver operating characteristic (AUROC) of 1.0 and also reported a correlation between the urinary AQP-1 concentrations and the tumor prognosis.[34] However, some reports have shown a decrease in AQP-1 concentrations in patients with RCC compared with healthy controls.[35,36] Therefore, more studies are needed to validate AQP-1 usefulness as a biomarker for detecting RCC.

PER2 (PLIN2) is also known as adipophilin. Overexpression of PLIN2 is seen in Von Hippel-Lindau/hypoxia-inducible factor pathway alterations.[37] PLIN2 is elevated in patients with RCC compared with healthy controls. A study found that urinary PLIN2 differentiated RCC from a healthy control with a specificity and a sensitivity of 100% (AUROC: 1.0).[32] Urinary PLIN2 concentrations were also correlated with prognosis.[34] When combined, PLIN2 and AQP-1 significantly increase the test's specificity compared with each one alone.[38]

CA-IX is a cell membrane protein expressed in various human tumors, including RCC, but it has low specificity for RCC. However, it has been proposed as a biomarker for early cancer detection. Under normal conditions, it is only expressed in the mucosa of the digestive tube and mainly in the stomach.[39] An upregulation of the expression of this protein has been observed in highly hypoxic tumors, and it is associated with poor prognosis.[40]

Immunohistochemical studies have shown that CA-IX is expressed in 94% to 100% of RCC tumors.[41] It has been hypothesized that CA-IX plays an essential role in maintaining the extracellular acidic pH in tumors—a fundamental property in malignant phenotypes—creating an optimal microenvironment for tumor growth under hypoxic conditions.[42]

KIM-1 is a sensitive urine marker for proximal renal tubule injury. Clear cell and papillary RCCs and their metastatic lesions, which originate from proximal renal tubules, stain positively for KIM-1. In contrast, chromophobe RCC and oncocytoma originate in the distal nephron and stain negatively for this biomarker.[43] KIM-1 is absent in healthy kidneys, and therefore it might have a role in the post-nephrectomy setting where KIM-1 should be undetectable. Its finding may indicate either remaining RCC in the operated or contralateral kidney or other renal disease involving proximal tubules.[44]

NGAL is another sensitive biomarker for tubular injury and indicates a highly elevated histological grade of ccRCC and papillary RCC.[45] A prospective cohort study evaluated its use for clear cell and papillary kidney cancer subtypes in 67 patients who underwent kidney cancer surgery and 55 controls who did not undergo kidney cancer surgery. In patients with kidney cancer, the excretion rate of NGAL was 0.52 ng/mg (IQR: 0.28–0.82) urinary creatinine before nephrectomy compared with 0.15 (IQR: 0.04–0.031) ng/mg urinary creatinine in controls. There was also a 30% decrease in excretion after the nephrectomy. However, the authors did not find it to correlate with tumor size or stage and the NGAL concentration range for patients with kidney cancer and controls overlapped. Therefore, the authors concluded that it is not a sensitive or specific urinary biomarker for kidney cancer.[46] Nonetheless, some evidence suggests that NGAL could be a biomarker for follow-up in patients diagnosed with mRCC to predict progression-free survival. It is hypothesized that it has an accurate prediction value even higher than the Motzer criteria, which may warrant their inclusion in future scoring systems/prognostic nomograms.[47]

Nuclear matrix protein 22 (NMP-22) is currently used to detect transitional cell carcinoma of the bladder.[48] NMP-22 plays a role in DNA replication, gene organization, and expression. Huang and colleagues evaluated a cohort of patients with renal cancer and reported an elevation of NMP-22 in 40% of those patients. They concluded that since this biomarker is typically assessed in patients with bladder cancer, it is important to also keep in mind the association between renal cancer and NMP-22 when this biomarker is present without the evidence of transitional cell carcinoma.[49]

Imaging Biomarkers

Imaging biomarkers can be critical in detecting and monitoring RCC. Cross-sectional and molecular imaging techniques provide a noninvasive means of obtaining biomarkers that can assist in the accurate diagnosis and staging of RCC. These techniques can help differentiate potentially aggressive from indolent local tumors and predict disease progression and response to systemic therapy.[50]

The combination of radiomics and radiogenomics, 2 closely related fields, has explored computational machine learning to improve the accuracy and reproducibility of imaging biomarkers in RCC.[51] Radiomics involves the extraction of quantitative imaging features from medical images. In contrast, radiogenomics consists in integrating genomic data with imaging data to better understand the underlying biological processes that drive the disease. Radiomics and radiogenomics can predict the likelihood of a positive response to systemic therapy and identify potential predictors of disease progression in RCC.[52–54]

These efforts have the potential to significantly improve patient outcomes by helping to guide treatment decisions and optimize therapy selection. In addition to their role in diagnosis and staging, imaging biomarkers can also be used to monitor the response to treatment and detect early signs of disease recurrence in RCC.[55,56]

MAGNETIC RESONANCE IMAGING

MRI is a valuable imaging modality that has gained increasing attention in assessing renal cancer. Unlike CT, MRI does not rely on ionizing radiation and can provide detailed anatomic and functional information about the kidneys and surrounding structures. Additionally, MRI can differentiate between different types of tissue, including fat, muscle, and tumor, which can help distinguish aggressive RCC from benign growths such as fat-poor angiomyolipomas (AMLs) and oncocytomas. This is especially relevant given the limitations of CT in accurately differentiating between these types of masses and a rate of benign pathologic condition after surgery of approximately 10% to 20% for small renal masses.[6,57]

Multiparametric MRI (mpMRI) allows for evaluating multiple MRI sequences and techniques in a single imaging session, providing a more comprehensive assessment of kidney masses. One of the critical advantages of mpMRI is the ability to assess the functional characteristics of a renal mass, such as perfusion and diffusion, which can provide valuable information about the nature and behavior of the mass. In particular, diffusion-weighted imaging (DWI) and dynamic contrast-enhanced (DCE) MRI techniques have been explored as imaging biomarkers to differentiate between different types of renal tumors and assess response to treatment.[58]

DWI MRI allows for the assessment of the movement of water molecules within the tissue, which can be used to differentiate between benign and malignant tumors based on their cellular density and organization.[59] A systematic review found that DWI had a sensitivity of 86% and a specificity of 78% for differentiating between malignant and nonmalignant renal lesions. DWI also had a moderate accuracy in differentiating between high-grade and low-grade RCC.[60] In addition, diffusion MRI techniques such as parenchymal wash index and apparent diffusion coefficient ratio were found to be correlated with Furhman grade in clear cell RCC (ccRCC).[61]

DCE MRI involves the injection of a contrast agent and can be used to assess tumor perfusion, providing information about tumor aggressiveness and response to treatment.[62] Additionally, the presence or absence of contrast enhancement on DCE MRI was found to be correlated with tumor grade in ccRCC.[63]

Overall, mpMRI is an effective imaging modality for assessing renal tumors and can provide valuable information about their functional characteristics. DWI and DCE MRI techniques have been demonstrated to reliably differentiate between benign and malignant lesions and high-grade from low-grade tumors.[64] As such, mpMRI should be considered in both the initial assessment and follow-up evaluation of suspected renal cancer.

Molecular Imaging Biomarkers

Positron emission tomography

[18]F-2-fluoro-2-deoxy glucose/positron emission tomography-CT (FDG PET/CT) is a noninvasive imaging modality that allows for the evaluation of glucose metabolism in the body and is a useful prognostic biomarker in various cancer types. This technique enables in vivo visualization of biological processes at cellular and molecular levels by using radiopharmaceutical compounds that bind to specific molecules.[50]

In a study, FDG PET/CT was prospectively evaluated as a prognostic indicator in patients with advanced RCC. A total of 101 patients, including those with recurrent and stage IV disease, were enrolled in the study between 2008 and 2014

and underwent pretreatment FDG PET/CT. The maximum standardized uptake value (SUVmax) was recorded and compared with various clinical risk factors as prognostic indicators. The median observation period was 18 months, and during this time, patients received various systematic therapies, including targeted therapies and interferon-α. The study's results showed that patients with high SUVmax had a poor prognosis, with multivariate analysis revealing that SUVmax was an independent predictor of survival. In addition, a cutoff value of 8.8 for SUVmax was highly significant in predicting the overall survival.[65]

In a phase II trial, FDG-PET was explored as a predictive biomarker for response to everolimus (mTOR inhibition) in mRCC, baseline average SUVmax was correlated with the overall survival.[66]

FDG-PET/CT activity was associated with tumor aggressiveness characteristics; higher Furhman grade, tumor, nodes, and metastases. (TNM) staging, and sarcomatoid features aiding clinical decision-making.[67,68]

According to a meta-analysis, the use of FDG-PET/CT can improve the sensitivity and specificity of detecting extrarenal metastasis in patients with RCC. The study analyzed 14 relevant studies published since 2001 and found that the use of FDG-PET alone had a sensitivity of 79% and a specificity of 90% in detecting extrarenal lesions, whereas the use of FDG-PET/CT increased the sensitivity to 91% and the specificity to 88%. FDG-PET was found to have a lower sensitivity and specificity in detecting primary renal lesions, with a pooled sensitivity of 62% and a pooled specificity of 88%. The authors conclude that the use of FDG-PET/CT may be more useful for detecting extrarenal metastasis in RCC compared with FDG-PET alone.[69]

Another review, which included 158 relevant articles, found that most studies used ^{18}F-fluorodeoxyglucose as the radiotracer, with a sensitivity range of 31.5% to 77% for diagnosing RCCs. However, higher success rates were observed for the diagnosis of clear cell carcinomas, which can be detected using a radiolabeled antibody to CA-IX called 124I-girentuximab, with a sensitivity of 86.2% and a specificity of 85.9%. PET/CT was also found to be more accurate than CT alone for the diagnosis of metastases, with a sensitivity of 94%. In predicting response to targeted therapy, PET/CT can be used to assess changes in ^{18}F-fluorodeoxyglucose uptakes before and after treatment, with low uptake before treatment and decreased uptake after 2 cycles associated with better survival. The review concluded that PET/CT with ^{18}F-fluorodeoxyglucose has lower sensitivity than enhanced

CT for diagnosing primary renal masses but higher sensitivity for diagnosing metastases.[70]

These findings suggest that FDG PET/CT may be useful prognostically in advanced RCC and may provide helpful information for clinical decision-making in the era of molecular-targeting therapies.

Iodine-124-cG250 (girentuximab) to carbonic anhydrase IX

Iodine-124-cG250, also known as girentuximab, is a radioimmunoconjugate used for molecular imaging of RCC. It consists of a monoclonal antibody cG250 that is specific for the CA-IX antigen, which is overexpressed in RCC, conjugated to the radionuclide iodine-124 (I-124).[71] CA-IX is a transmembrane enzyme involved in regulating pH and bicarbonate metabolism in normal cells but is highly expressed in RCC and other types of cancer.[72] The overexpression of CA-IX in RCC makes it an attractive target for cancer imaging and therapy.

Divgi and colleagues studied 195 patients with renal masses who were scheduled for resection and received an intravenous injection of I-124-girentuximab, a PET tracer, followed by PET/CT and contrast-enhanced CT (CECT) imaging. Three blinded readers interpreted the images and a blinded central pathologist determined the tumor histology. The results showed that PET/CT had higher average sensitivity and specificity for detecting ccRCC than CECT. Interreader and intrareader agreement for PET/CT was also higher than for CECT. These findings suggest that PET/CT with I-124-girentuximab is an accurate and noninvasive method for identifying ccRCC in patients with renal masses, with potential utility for designing the best management approaches for these patients.[73]

Hekman evaluated the feasibility and safety of the CAIX-targeting antibody ^{111}In-DOTA-girentuximab-IRDye800CW for intraoperative imaging in patients with ccRCC. The study included 15 patients, 12 of whom had ccRCC and 3 with CAIX-negative tumors. The antibody was administered intravenously and imaging was performed after 4 days. Seven days later, surgery was performed using a gamma probe and near-infrared fluorescence camera. The results showed that all ccRCC tumors were visualized by single-photon emission computed tomography-computed tomography (SPECT/CT) and localized by intraoperative gamma probe detection, whereas CAIX-negative tumors were not. ccRCC tumors were also hyperfluorescent and could be detected by fluorescence imaging, which was helpful for intraoperative tumor delineation and assessment of the

surgical cavity and margins. The study concluded that dual-modality imaging using ^{111}In-DOTA-girentuximab-IRDye800CW is safe and effective for intraoperative guidance of ccRCC resection.

Girentuximab has shown promising results as a molecular imaging biomarker for RCC. It has high sensitivity and specificity for the detection of RCC, and it has the potential to be used for guiding treatment decisions and surgery. However, further studies are needed to fully establish the role of girentuximab in managing RCC.

Technetium-99m-sestamibi single-photon emission computed tomography-computed tomography

[99]Tc-sestamibi is a nuclear imaging agent that can differentiate between oncocytomas and chromophobe RCC through their mitochondrial content.[74] ^{99}Tc-sestamibi accumulates in cells with high levels of mitochondria and low MDR pump expression, which are characteristic of oncocytomas. In contrast, clear cell and chromophobe RCC have higher MDR pump expression and lower mitochondrial activity, although chromophobe RCC tends to have higher activity than ccRCC.[75]

In a prospective study, ^{99}Tc-sestamibi SPECT/CT had a sensitivity of 87.5% and a specificity of 95.2% in differentiating oncocytomas and hybrid oncocytic/chromophobe tumors.[76]

Another study evaluated the utility of ^{99m}Tc-sestamibi (MIBI) SPECT-CT in the assessment and risk stratification of renal masses. The study included 29 patients with 31 renal masses, and the imaging results were compared with histopathology. The results showed that all oncocytic lesions, including oncocytomas and hybrid oncocytic chromophobe tumors, were positive for MIBI. One chromophobe RCC showed low-grade MIBI uptake, whereas the remaining RCC subtypes were MIBI-negative. The quantitative relative tumor uptake was statistically significantly higher in low-risk/oncocytic lesions compared with RCCs. The combination of MIBI uptake on SPECT and lesion density on noncontrast CT was useful for risk stratification of renal masses.[77]

In conclusion, Tc-MIBI SPECT/CT has been demonstrated to be a valuable tool in detecting and monitoring renal cancer. Its ability to differentiate oncocytomas from chromophobe RCC, as well as other RCC subtypes, through their mitochondrial content, has proven effective with high sensitivity and specificity. Its combination with noncontrast CT allows for risk stratification of renal masses, potentially reducing the need for further imaging or biopsy and allowing for more patients to be followed with active surveillance. These findings suggest that Tc-MIBI SPECT/CT can play a significant role in managing renal cancer.

Prostate-specific membrane antigen-targeted positron emission tomography/computed tomography

Prostate-specific membrane antigen (PSMA) is a protein found on the surface of cells that is mainly expressed in prostate tissue and the neovasculature of some types of solid tumors, such as RCC.[78] Researchers have explored PSMA-targeted imaging in metastatic and localized tumor settings. PSMA may be a promising theragnostic target in RCC, with data suggesting a potential role for PSMA-targeting radiopharmaceuticals in improving the staging of patients with ccRCC at risk of nodal involvement and oligometastatic disease through complementary use with conventional imaging.[79]

Morgantetti and colleagues found that PSMA had a consistently higher expression in the vena cava renal tumor thrombus than in the intrarenal tumor mass. This suggests that PSMA may be involved in the neoangiogenesis and local progression of ccRCC and could be used as a biomarker for diagnostic and therapeutic purposes.[80]

Rhee and colleagues found that gallium-68 PSMA-binding ligand and PET had a role in detecting metastatic lesions in patients with renal tumors, leading to changes in surgical strategies in some patients. This imaging technique detected multiple histologically proven metastatic lesions missed by CT scanning.[81]

Therapy response monitoring with PSMA PET/CT in RCC has also been explored in a few studies. In one study, Mittlmeier and colleagues used ^{18}F-PSMA-1007 PET to assess treatment response in patients with mRCC receiving either tyrosine kinase inhibitors or immune checkpoint inhibitors. The PET tracer and CT scanning were performed before the initiation of systemic treatment and again 8 weeks after treatment initiation. The PSMA PET and CT results were concordant in only 2 of the 11 patients, with the majority of cases showing that the PSMA PET indicated a partial or complete response, whereas the CT showed stable disease. The authors suggested that ^{18}F-PSMA-1007 PET may be able to assess treatment response at a molecular level earlier than morphological changes appear on CT imaging. However, the study was limited by a small and heterogeneous patient population.[82]

Siva and colleagues also used 68Ga-PSMA PET to evaluate treatment response after stereotactic radiotherapy in 8 RCC patients. They found that the uptake of the PSMA ligand was typically more intense than the uptake of FDG PET, and both imaging modalities showed metabolic changes and an earlier response than morphological appearances on CT or MRI imaging, with FDG the fastest.[83]

Although limited evidence exists, several studies have demonstrated that PSMA PET consistently outperforms conventional imaging modalities in staging and restaging ccRCC and may assist in selecting patients for metastasis-directed therapy. PSMA imaging has shown potential for use in RCC clinical management. However, its utility in this context is not yet fully understood.

Radiomics and Radiogenomics Biomarkers

Radiomics

Radiomics is a medical research field involving the extraction of quantitative data from medical images using mathematical algorithms. It can improve the diagnostic accuracy of medical imaging, particularly in oncology, by providing more detailed and specific information about the tumor and its characteristics. This technique has been applied to various medical conditions, including cancer, to improve diagnosis, prognosis, and treatment planning.[84]

The diagnosis and management of RCC can be challenging due to the high prevalence of benign renal masses, the complex assessment of treatment response to ST in mRCC, and the limited accuracy of traditional radiological imaging in predicting the histology or natural history of small renal tumors.[85]

Radiomics can improve the diagnostic accuracy of medical imaging in kidney cancer by providing more detailed and specific information about the tumor and its characteristics.[55] This can be particularly useful in the diagnosis and staging of RCC, as well as in the assessment of treatment response. In addition, radiomics may be able to identify biomarkers that can be used to predict patient outcomes, such as disease-free survival or overall survival.[86]

Given the limitations of traditional radiological imaging in the diagnosis and management of RCC, there is a need for alternative approaches to improve diagnostic accuracy and treatment response assessment. Radiomics may be able to address these challenges by providing additional information on the spatial distribution of signal intensities and pixel relationships within the affected tissue. A systematic review and meta-analysis of studies on the use of radiomics in RCC found that it may be a promising tool for the discrimination of AML, oncocytoma, and unspecified benign tumors from RCC, with an odds ratio (OR) of 2.89,

Table 1
A summary of biomarkers for the diagnosis and monitoring of renal cell carcinoma

SERUM

Circulating tumor DNA	ctDNA	It enables serial testing to monitor disease status, track clonal evolution over time, identify resistance mechanisms, and detect residual or recurrent disease. Additionally, it has the potential to predict tumor responses to immunotherapy by acting as a surrogate for measuring tumor mutational burden
Heat shock protein 27	HSP27	Associated with tumor growth, antioxidant, and antiapoptotic functions. Overexpression of HSPs is associated with a poor prognosis in multiple cancers, including RCC, because it protects malignant cells from undergoing apoptosis. Additionally, this biomarker can be acquired through urine samples
Serum amyloid A	SAA	An acute-phase protein with the potential for detecting RCC, particularly in advanced stages. SAA levels correlate with advanced tumor stage and can be used as an independent survival factor in patients with RCC. However, SAA levels are also associated with other conditions, such as infections and inflammatory diseases, which could reduce its specificity as a marker for RCC diagnosis
Matrix metalloproteinase-7	MMP-7	Overexpressed in RCC. Its levels are correlated with high tumor grade, cancer invasion, metastasis, and worse cancer-specific survival. Not yet established as a reliable tool for clinical practice
Osteopontin	OPN	Associated with aggressive and advanced stage RCC. OPN expression correlates with the degree of tumor angiogenesis, invasiveness, and metastasis. Not yet established as a reliable tool for clinical practice

URINARY

Aquaporin-1	AQP1	Transmembrane protein that facilitates water movement and is associated with angiogenesis and tumor progression. It was found to distinguish between RCC and healthy surgical controls with high accuracy
Perilipin 2 (Adipophilin)	PER2	Protein overexpressed in RCC, differentiating RCC from healthy controls. It is also associated with a worse prognosis in patients with RCC. When combined with another biomarker, AQP1, the test specificity increases significantly compared with using each one alone

Carbonic anhydrase IX	*CA-IX*	Cell membrane protein expressed in RCC and upregulation of the expression of this protein has been observed in highly hypoxic tumors, which is associated with a poor prognosis. It has low specificity but is proposed as a biomarker for early cancer detection
Kidney injury molecule-1	*KIM-1*	A sensitive urine marker for proximal renal tubule injury. Expressed in clear cell and papillary RCCs, which originate from proximal renal tubules, it is not present in healthy kidneys
Neutrophil gelatinase-associated lipocalin	*NGAL*	Indicates a highly elevated histological grade of ccRCC and papillary RCC. However, it has very low sensitivity and specificity
Nuclear matrix protein 22	*NMP-22*	Potential use as a biomarker for detecting renal cancer in addition to its established use for detecting transitional cell carcinoma of the bladder
IMAGING		
Magnetic resonance imaging	*MRI*	An imaging modality, that does not use ionizing radiation, that provides detailed anatomic and functional information about the kidneys and surrounding structures and differentiates between different types of tissue, such as fat, muscle, and tumor, to help distinguish aggressive RCC from benign growths
[18]F-2-fluoro-2-deoxy glucose/Positron emission tomography-CT	*FDG PET/CT*	A noninvasive imaging modality that allows for the evaluation of glucose metabolism in the body, using radiopharmaceutical compounds that bind to specific molecules. It is a useful prognostic biomarker in RCC, where it can be used for the detection of extrarenal metastasis to predict response to targeted therapy and as a prognostic indicator for overall survival
Girentuximab	*I-124-cG250*	Is a radioimmunoconjugate that specifically targets the CA-IX antigen, which is overexpressed in RCC and is conjugated to the radionuclide I-124 making it a useful molecular imaging biomarker for RCC with high sensitivity and specificity for the detection of RCC and the potential to be used for guiding treatment decisions and surgery

| Technetium-99m-sestamibi single-photon emission computed tomography-computed tomography | Tc-MIBI SPECT/CT | Imaging modality that uses 99Tc-sestamibi, a nuclear imaging agent, to differentiate between oncocytomas and chromophobe RCC by assessing the levels of mitochondria and MDR pump expression in cells, which are characteristic of oncocytomas. It has been demonstrated to be a valuable tool in detecting and monitoring renal cancer with high sensitivity and specificity. In combination with noncontrast CT allows for risk stratification of renal masses, potentially reducing the need for further imaging or biopsy and allowing for more patients to be followed with active surveillance |
| PSMA-targeted | PET/CT | It is a noninvasive imaging modality that evaluates PSMA expression in the body, a protein found mainly in prostate tissue and the neovasculature of some types of solid tumors, such as RCC. PSMA may also be involved in the neoangiogenesis and local progression of RCC and could be used as a biomarker for diagnostic and therapeutic purposes. However, its utility in this context has yet to be fully understood |

3.08, and 3.57, respectively (all $P < .001$). The meta-analysis also found that radiomics may be useful for the general discrimination of benign tumors from RCC, with a log OR of 3.17 (95% CI 2.73–3.62, $P < .001$). However, the authors caution that these results should be interpreted with care due to the poor quality of many of the included studies and the inconsistency in using radiomics in clinical practice.[87]

Future research should focus on developing standardized protocols and algorithms for radiomics analysis and conducting large, well-designed clinical trials to validate the use of radiomics in the diagnosis, staging, and treatment of kidney cancer. In addition, further research is needed to determine the long-term effectiveness of radiomics in detecting and monitoring kidney cancer progression.[86]

Radiogenomics

Radiogenomics has experienced significant growth in recent years, particularly concerning its application to the diagnosis and surveillance of ccRCC. This type of kidney cancer is well suited for radiogenomic analysis due to its relatively low number of mutated genes. As a result, associations between gene expression patterns and imaging features can be more easily identified.[88]

A few studies have thus far examined the link between image characteristics and single gene mutations in ccRCC cases, such as those involving VHL, KDM5C, and BAP1 genes.[89,90] Intriguingly, certain image features—including intratumoral vascularity—were significantly associated with specific gene mutations.[91] Although this progress is promising, several limitations must still be addressed before radiogenomics becomes a reliable biomarker for detecting and monitoring renal cancer; these include the need for larger validation sets and standardization across various methods used for feature extraction from images.[92]

Given that radiogenomics offers additional information regarding diagnosis, prognostic stratification, and treatment response assessment in patients with ccRCC, further research into this field may prove beneficial in improving patient management strategies moving forward. To this end, it will be essential to continue pursuing advances that address existing challenges related to external validation sets or standardizing image-processing techniques so that the potential clinical implications of this approach may eventually become realized on a broader scale (**Table 1**).

SUMMARY

Using biomarkers to detect and monitor renal cancer (RCC) can significantly improve patient outcomes by providing noninvasive, accurate, reproducible information about the presence and progression of the disease. To date, no validated serum or urinary biomarker for RCC diagnosis has been incorporated into clinical practice; however, cross-sectional and molecular imaging techniques have improved our ability to differentiate between different types of tissue. Molecular (serum or urinary) biomarkers could enable earlier detection before the onset of symptoms in order to improve clinical outcomes. In addition, advanced imaging techniques such as radiomics and radiogenomics can be used to predict a positive response to systemic therapy while also identifying potential predictors of disease progression. Moreover, molecular imaging biomarkers such as PSMA-targeted PET/CT may provide further insight into RCC detection and monitoring.

Biomarkers might have a promising role to play in the future of "personalized medicine," revealing specific tumor characteristics and providing a better understanding of the disease in a particular patient. As the research field continues to advance, biomarkers will continue to emerge, and ultimately, it is likely that they will find their place in the precision medicine landscape. Different kidney tumors could be treated differently depending on their genomic signature, proteomics, and transcriptomics, which will help to "update" the old paradigm of "one size fits all" toward individualized treatments according to a patient's unique profile.

DECLARATION OF INTERESTS

There are no disclosures. The authors declare no competing interests.

REFERENCES

1. Sun M, Thuret R, Abdollah F, et al. Age-adjusted incidence, mortality, and survival rates of stage-specific renal cell carcinoma in North America: a trend analysis. Eur Urol 2011;59(1):135–41.
2. Israel GM, Bosniak MA. Renal imaging for diagnosis and staging of renal cell carcinoma. Urol Clin North Am 2003;30(3):499–514.
3. Kane CJ, Mallin K, Ritchey J, et al. Renal cell cancer stage migration: analysis of the National Cancer Data Base. Cancer 2008;113(1):78–83.
4. Mir MC, Capitanio U, Bertolo R, et al. Role of active surveillance for localized small renal masses. Eur Urol Oncol 2018;1(3):177–87.
5. Bechtold RE, Zagoria RJ. Imaging approach to staging of renal cell carcinoma. Urol Clin North Am 1997; 24(3):507–22.
6. Johnson DC, Vukina J, Smith AB, et al. Preoperatively misclassified, surgically removed benign renal masses: a systematic review of surgical series and United States population level burden estimate. J Urol 2015;193(1):30–5.
7. Lee H, Lee JK, Kim K, et al. Risk of metastasis for T1a renal cell carcinoma. World J Urol 2016;34(4): 553–9.
8. Ljungberg B, Bensalah K, Canfield S, et al. EAU guidelines on renal cell carcinoma: 2014 update. Eur Urol 2015;67(5):913–24.
9. Leibovich BC, Blute ML, Cheville JC, et al. Prediction of progression after radical nephrectomy for patients with clear cell renal cell carcinoma: a stratification tool for prospective clinical trials. Cancer 2003; 97(7):1663–71.
10. Dabestani S, Beisland C, Stewart GD, et al. Increased use of cross-sectional imaging for follow-up does not improve post-recurrence survival of surgically treated initially localized R.C.C.: results from a European multicenter database (R.E.C.U.R. Scand J Urol 2019;53(1):14–20.
11. Lipsky MJ, Shapiro EY, Hruby GW, et al. Diagnostic radiation exposure during surveillance in patients with pT1a renal cell carcinoma. Urology 2013; 81(6):1190–5.
12. Cimadamore A, Gasparrini S, Massari F, et al. Emerging Molecular Technologies in Renal Cell Carcinoma: Liquid Biopsy. Cancers 2019;11(2). https://doi.org/10.3390/cancers11020196.
13. Bergerot PG, Hahn AW, Bergerot CD, et al. The Role of Circulating Tumor DNA in Renal Cell Carcinoma. Curr Treat Options Oncol 2018;19(2):10.
14. Lianos GD, Alexiou GA, Mangano A, et al. The role of heat shock proteins in cancer. Cancer Lett 2015; 360(2):114–8.
15. Vidyasagar A, Wilson NA, Djamali A. Heat shock protein 27 (HSP27): biomarker of disease and therapeutic target. Fibrogenesis Tissue Repair 2012;5(1): 7.
16. White NMA, Masui O, Desouza LV, et al. Quantitative proteomic analysis reveals potential diagnostic markers and pathways involved in pathogenesis of renal cell carcinoma. Oncotarget 2014;5(2):506–18.
17. Fischer K, Theil G, Hoda R, et al. Serum amyloid A: a biomarker for renal cancer. Anticancer Res 2012; 32(5):1801–4.
18. Ramankulov A, Lein M, Johannsen M, et al. Serum amyloid A as indicator of distant metastases but not as early tumor marker in patients with renal cell carcinoma. Cancer Lett 2008;269(1):85–92.
19. Vermaat JS, Gerritse FL, van der Veldt AA, et al. Validation of serum amyloid α as an independent biomarker for progression-free and overall survival in metastatic renal cell cancer patients. Eur Urol 2012;62(4):685–95.
20. Lannergård A, Larsson A, Kragsbjerg P, et al. Correlations between serum amyloid A protein and C-reactive protein in infectious diseases. Scand J Clin Lab Invest 2003;63(4):267–72.

21. Miyata Y, Iwata T, Ohba K, et al. Expression of matrix metalloproteinase-7 on cancer cells and tissue endothelial cells in renal cell carcinoma: prognostic implications and clinical significance for invasion and metastasis. Clin Cancer Res 2006;12(23): 6998–7003.

22. Lu H, Yang Z, Zhang H, et al. The expression and clinical significance of matrix metalloproteinase 7 and tissue inhibitor of matrix metalloproteinases 2 in clear cell renal cell carcinoma. Exp Ther Med 2013;5(3):890–6.

23. Ramankulov A, Lein M, Johannsen M, et al. Plasma matrix metalloproteinase-7 as a metastatic marker and survival predictor in patients with renal cell carcinomas. Cancer Sci 2008;99(6):1188–94.

24. Bandopadhyay M, Bulbule A, Butti R, et al. Osteopontin as a therapeutic target for cancer. Expert Opin Ther Targets 2014;18(8):883–95.

25. Sim SH, Messenger MP, Gregory WM, et al. Prognostic utility of pre-operative circulating osteopontin, carbonic anhydrase IX and CRP in renal cell carcinoma. Br J Cancer 2012;107(7):1131–7.

26. Papworth K, Bergh A, Grankvist K, et al. Osteopontin but not parathyroid hormone-related protein predicts prognosis in human renal cell carcinoma. Acta Oncol 2013;52(1):159–65.

27. Ramankulov A, Lein M, Kristiansen G, et al. Elevated plasma osteopontin as marker for distant metastases and poor survival in patients with renal cell carcinoma. J Cancer Res Clin Oncol 2007;133(9):643–52.

28. Ramchandani D, Weber GF. Interactions between osteopontin and vascular endothelial growth factor: Implications for cancer. Biochim Biophys Acta 2015;1855(2):202–22.

29. Ahmed M, Behera R, Chakraborty G, et al. Osteopontin: a potentially important therapeutic target in cancer. Expert Opin Ther Targets 2011;15(9): 1113–26.

30. Verkman AS. More than just water channels: unexpected cellular roles of aquaporins. J Cell Sci 2005;118(Pt 15):3225–32.

31. Grebe SK, Erickson LA. Screening for kidney cancer: is there a role for aquaporin-1 and adipophilin? Mayo Clin Proc 2010;85(5):410–2.

32. Morrissey JJ, Kharasch ED. The specificity of urinary aquaporin 1 and perilipin 2 to screen for renal cell carcinoma. J Urol 2013;189(5):1913–20.

33. Morrissey JJ, London AN, Luo J, et al. Urinary biomarkers for the early diagnosis of kidney cancer. Mayo Clin Proc 2010;85(5):413–21.

34. Morrissey JJ, Mobley J, Song J, et al. Urinary concentrations of aquaporin-1 and perilipin-2 in patients with renal cell carcinoma correlate with tumor size and stage but not grade. Urology 2014;83(1). 256.e9–14.

35. Raimondo F, Morosi L, Corbetta S, et al. Differential protein profiling of renal cell carcinoma urinary exosomes. Mol Biosyst 2013;9(6):1220–33.

36. Mijugković M, Stanojević I, Milović N, et al. Urinary KIM-1 and AQP-1 in patients with clear renal cell carcinoma: Potential noninvasive biomarkers. Vojnosanit Pregl 2016;73(3):266–72.

37. Cao Q, Ruan H, Wang K, et al. Overexpression of PLIN2 is a prognostic marker and attenuates tumor progression in clear cell renal cell carcinoma. Int J Oncol 2018;53(1):137–47.

38. Song JB, Morrissey JJ, Mobley JM, et al. Urinary aquaporin 1 and perilipin 2: Can these novel markers accurately characterize small renal masses and help guide patient management? Int J Urol 2019;26(2):260–5.

39. Závada J, Závadová Z, Zaťovicová M, et al. Soluble form of carbonic anhydrase IX (CA IX) in the serum and urine of renal carcinoma patients. Br J Cancer 2003;89(6):1067–71.

40. Giatromanolaki A, Koukourakis MI, Sivridis E, et al. Expression of hypoxia-inducible carbonic anhydrase-9 relates to angiogenic pathways and independently to poor outcome in non-small cell lung cancer. Cancer Res 2001;61(21):7992–8.

41. Bui MHT, Seligson D, Han K-R, et al. Carbonic anhydrase IX is an independent predictor of survival in advanced renal clear cell carcinoma: implications for prognosis and therapy. Clin Cancer Res 2003; 9(2):802–11.

42. Ivanov S, Liao SY, Ivanova A, et al. Expression of hypoxia-inducible cell-surface transmembrane carbonic anhydrases in human cancer. Am J Pathol 2001;158(3):905–19.

43. Lin F, Zhang PL, Yang XJ, et al. Human kidney injury molecule-1 (hKIM-1): a useful immunohistochemical marker for diagnosing renal cell carcinoma and ovarian clear cell carcinoma. Am J Surg Pathol 2007;31(3):371–81.

44. Han WK, Alinani A, Wu C-L, et al. Human kidney injury molecule-1 is a tissue and urinary tumor marker of renal cell carcinoma. J Am Soc Nephrol 2005;16(4):1126–34.

45. Carlo DI. A. Evaluation of neutrophil gelatinase-associated lipocalin (NGAL), matrix metalloproteinase-9 (MMP-9) and their complex MMP-9/NGAL in sera and urine of patients with kidney tumors. Oncol Lett 2013;5(5):1677–81.

46. Morrissey JJ, London AN, Lambert MC, et al. Sensitivity and specificity of urinary neutrophil gelatinase-associated lipocalin and kidney injury molecule-1 for the diagnosis of renal cell carcinoma. Am J Nephrol 2011;34(5):391–8.

47. Porta C, Paglino C, De Amici M, et al. Predictive value of baseline serum vascular endothelial growth factor and neutrophil gelatinase-associated lipocalin in advanced kidney cancer patients receiving sunitinib. Kidney Int 2010;77(9):809–15.

48. Wang Z, Que H, Suo C, et al. Evaluation of the NMP22 BladderChek test for detecting bladder

cancer: a systematic review and meta-analysis. Oncotarget 2017;8(59):100648–56.

49. Huang S, Rhee E, Patel H, et al. Urinary NMP22 and renal cell carcinoma. Urology 2000;55(2):227–30.

50. Roussel E, Capitanio U, Kutikov A, et al. Novel Imaging Methods for Renal Mass Characterization: A Collaborative Review. Eur Urol 2022;81(5):476–88.

51. Bodalal Z, Trebeschi S, Nguyen-Kim TDL, et al. Radiogenomics: bridging imaging and genomics. Abdom Radiol (NY) 2019;44(6):1960–84.

52. de Leon AD, Kapur P, Pedrosa I. Radiomics in Kidney Cancer: MR Imaging. Magn Reson Imaging Clin N Am 2019;27(1):1–13.

53. Khaleel S, Katims A, Cumarasamy S, et al. Radiogenomics in clear cell renal cell carcinoma: a review of the current status and future directions. Cancers 2022;14(9). https://doi.org/10.3390/cancers14092085.

54. Negreros-Osuna AA, Ramírez-Mendoza DA, Casas-Murillo C, et al. Clinical-radiomic model in advanced kidney cancer predicts response to tyrosine kinase inhibitors. Oncol Lett 2022;24(6):446.

55. Suarez-Ibarrola R, Basulto-Martinez M, Heinze A, et al. Radiomics Applications in Renal Tumor Assessment: A Comprehensive Review of the Literature. Cancers 2020;12(6). https://doi.org/10.3390/cancers12061387.

56. Kang B, Sun C, Gu H, et al. T1 stage clear cell renal cell carcinoma: A CT-based radiomics nomogram to estimate the risk of recurrence and metastasis. Front Oncol 2020;10:579619.

57. Sasaguri K, Takahashi N. CT and MR imaging for solid renal mass characterization. Eur J Radiol 2018;99:40–54.

58. Farber NJ, Kim CJ, Modi PK, et al. Renal cell carcinoma: the search for a reliable biomarker. Transl Cancer Res 2017;6(3):620–32.

59. Gilet AG, Kang SK, Kim D, et al. Advanced renal mass imaging: diffusion and perfusion MRI. Curr Urol Rep 2012;13(1):93–8.

60. Kang SK, Zhang A, Pandharipande PV, et al. DWI for renal mass characterization: systematic review and meta-analysis of diagnostic test performance. AJR Am J Roentgenol 2015;205(2):317–24.

61. Cornelis F, Tricaud E, Lasserre AS, et al. Multiparametric magnetic resonance imaging for the differentiation of low and high grade clear cell renal carcinoma. Eur Radiol 2015;25(1):24–31.

62. Choyke PL, Dwyer AJ, Knopp MV. Functional tumor imaging with dynamic contrast-enhanced magnetic resonance imaging. J Magn Reson Imaging 2003; 17(5):509–20.

63. Padhani AR. Dynamic contrast-enhanced MRI in clinical oncology: current status and future directions. J Magn Reson Imaging 2002;16(4):407–22.

64. Serter A, Onur MR, Coban G, et al. The role of diffusion-weighted MRI and contrast-enhanced MRI for differentiation between solid renal masses and renal cell carcinoma subtypes. Abdom Radiol (NY) 2021;46(3):1041–52.

65. Nakaigawa N, Kondo K, Tateishi U, et al. FDG PET/CT as a prognostic biomarker in the era of molecular-targeting therapies: max SUVmax predicts survival of patients with advanced renal cell carcinoma. BMC Cancer 2016;16:67.

66. Chen JL, Appelbaum DE, Kocherginsky M, et al. FDG-PET as a predictive biomarker for therapy with everolimus in metastatic renal cell cancer. Cancer Med 2013;2(4):545–52.

67. Takahashi M, Kume H, Koyama K, et al. Preoperative evaluation of renal cell carcinoma by using 18F-FDG PET/CT. Clin Nucl Med 2015;40(12):936–40.

68. Ferda J, Ferdova E, Hora M, et al. 18F-FDG-PET/CT in potentially advanced renal cell carcinoma: a role in treatment decisions and prognosis estimation. Anticancer Res 2013;33(6):2665–72.

69. Wang H-Y, Ding H-J, Chen J-H, et al. Meta-analysis of the diagnostic performance of [18F]FDG-PET and PET/CT in renal cell carcinoma. Cancer Imag 2012; 12(3):464–74.

70. Gofrit ON, Orevi M. Diagnostic challenges of kidney cancer: a systematic review of the role of positron emission tomography-computerized tomography. J Urol 2016;196(3):648–57.

71. Lam JS, Pantuck AJ, Belldegrun AS, et al. G250: a carbonic anhydrase IX monoclonal antibody. Curr Oncol Rep 2005;7(2):109–15.

72. Benej M, Pastorekova S, Pastorek J. Carbonic anhydrase IX: regulation and role in cancer. Subcell Biochem 2014;75:199–219.

73. Divgi CR, Uzzo RG, Gatsonis C, et al. Positron emission tomography/computed tomography identification of clear cell renal cell carcinoma: results from the REDECT trial. J Clin Oncol 2013;31(2):187–94.

74. Campbell SP, Tzortzakakis A, Javadi MS, et al. Tc-sestamibi SPECT/CT for the characterization of renal masses: a pictorial guide. Br J Radiol 2018; 91(1084):20170526.

75. Rowe SP, Gorin MA, Solnes LB, et al. Correlation of Tc-sestamibi uptake in renal masses with mitochondrial content and multi-drug resistance pump expression. EJNMMI Res 2017;7(1):80.

76. Gorin MA, Rowe SP, Baras AS, et al. Prospective Evaluation of (99m)Tc-sestamibi SPECT/CT for the Diagnosis of Renal Oncocytomas and Hybrid Oncocytic/Chromophobe Tumors. Eur Urol 2016;69(3): 413–6.

77. Sistani G, Bjazevic J, Kassam Z, et al. The value of Tc-sestamibi single-photon emission computed tomography-computed tomography in the evaluation and risk stratification of renal masses. Can Urol Assoc J 2021;15(6):197–201.

78. Rowe SP, Gorin MA, Allaf ME, et al. PET imaging of prostate-specific membrane antigen in prostate cancer: current state of the art and future

challenges. Prostate Cancer Prostatic Dis 2016; 19(3):223–30.

79. Pozzessere C, Bassanelli M, Ceribelli A, et al. Renal cell carcinoma: the oncologist asks, can PSMA PET/CT answer? Curr Urol Rep 2019;20(11):68.

80. Morgantetti G, Ng KL, Samaratunga H, et al. Prostate specific membrane antigen (PSMA) expression in vena cava tumour thrombi of clear cell renal cell carcinoma suggests a role for PSMA-driven tumour neoangiogenesis. Transl Androl Urol 2019;8(Suppl 2):S147–55.

81. Rhee H, Blazak J, Tham CM, et al. Pilot study: use of gallium-68 PSMA PET for detection of metastatic lesions in patients with renal tumour. EJNMMI Res 2016;6(1):76.

82. Mittlmeier LM, Unterrainer M, Rodler S, et al. F-PSMA-1007 PET/CT for response assessment in patients with metastatic renal cell carcinoma undergoing tyrosine kinase or checkpoint inhibitor therapy: preliminary results. Eur J Nucl Med Mol Imaging 2021;48(6):2031–7.

83. Siva S, Callahan J, Pryor D, et al. Utility of Ga prostate specific membrane antigen - positron emission tomography in diagnosis and response assessment of recurrent renal cell carcinoma. J Med Imaging Radiat Oncol 2017;61(3):372–8.

84. Lambin P, Leijenaar RTH, Deist TM, et al. Radiomics: the bridge between medical imaging and personalized medicine. Nat Rev Clin Oncol 2017;14(12):749–62.

85. Diaz de Leon A, Pirasteh A, Costa DN, et al. Current challenges in diagnosis and assessment of the response of locally advanced and metastatic renal cell carcinoma. Radiographics 2019;39(4):998–1016.

86. Rallis KS, Kleeman SO, Grant M, et al. Radiomics for renal cell carcinoma: predicting outcomes from immunotherapy and targeted therapies-a narrative review. Eur Urol Focus 2021;7(4):717–21.

87. Mühlbauer J, Egen L, Kowalewski K-F, et al. Radiomics in renal cell carcinoma-a systematic review and meta-analysis. Cancers 2021;13(6). https://doi.org/10.3390/cancers13061348.

88. Alessandrino F, Shinagare AB, Bossé D, et al. Radiogenomics in renal cell carcinoma. Abdom Radiol (NY) 2019;44(6):1990–8.

89. Karlo CA, Di Paolo PL, Chaim J, et al. Radiogenomics of clear cell renal cell carcinoma: associations between CT imaging features and mutations. Radiology 2014;270(2):464–71.

90. Shinagare AB, Vikram R, Jaffe C, et al. Radiogenomics of clear cell renal cell carcinoma: preliminary findings of The Cancer Genome Atlas-Renal Cell Carcinoma (TCGA-RCC) Imaging Research Group. Abdom Imaging 2015;40(6):1684–92.

91. Choudhary S, Sudarshan S, Choyke PL, et al. Renal cell carcinoma: recent advances in genetics and imaging. Semin Ultrasound CT MR 2009;30(4):315–25.

92. Gopal N, Yazdian Anari P, Turkbey E, et al. The next paradigm shift in the management of clear cell renal cancer: radiogenomics-definition, current advances, and future directions. Cancers 2022;14(3). https://doi.org/10.3390/cancers14030793.

Diseases of Hereditary Renal Cell Cancers

Othon Iliopoulos, MD[a,b,c,d],*

KEYWORDS

- Hereditary kidney cancers • Von Hippel–Lindau (VHL) • Birt–Hogg–Dubé (BHD) • Folliculin
- Hereditary leiomyomatosis and renal cell carcinoma (HLRCC) • Fumarate hydratase (FH)
- Succinate dehydrogenase (SDH) • Germline mutations

KEY POINTS

- A significant number of patients with renal cell cancers (RCCs) harbor a germline mutation.
- Identification of germline mutation carriers and their relatives at risk allows for surveillance and early detection of developing RCCs.
- Insights into the molecular mechanism of hereditary renal cell carcinomas allows for effective targeted therapy of advanced disease.

VON HIPPEL–LINDAU DISEASE (OMIM 193300)

The disease takes its name after the German ophthalmologist Eugen von Hippel who described the presence of angiomas in the retina in 1904, and Dr Arnold Lindau, a Swedish pathologist who conducted postmortem studies of patients with cerebellar hemangioblastomas and cysts in the pancreas, liver, and kidneys. The incidence of the disease is estimated at 1:34,000 births. Approximately 95% of patients with a clinical diagnosis of Von Hippel–Lindau (VHL) disease harbor a germline mutation in the *VHL* gene,[1,2] which was cloned in 1992.[3] The rest of the patients who have a compelling clinical diagnosis for VHL disease (two VHL-related lesions or one lesion and a family history of VHL disease) may be mosaic for a VHL pathogenic variant.[4] Recently, a de novo germline pathogenic variant in Elongin C (*ELOC*) gene was identified in a proband with clinical features of VHL disease but no mutation in the *VHL* gene, suggesting that such patients should also undergo ELOC germline sequencing.[5]

Clinical Manifestations

Patients with VHL are at a lifetime high risk for developing any of the following lesions: (1) hemangioblastomas (HB) of the central nervous system (CNS) and the retina, (2) multiple and bilateral renal cysts and renal cell carcinoma (RCC), (3) pheochromocytomas and/or paragangliomas, (4) pancreatic cysts and neuroendocrine tumors of the pancreas, and (5) serous cystadenomas of the endolymphatic sac of the ear, the pancreas, the epididymis, and the adnexal organs.[6] The clinical diagnosis of VHL disease was based on the presence of two VHL-associated lesions or one lesion in a patient with a known family dx of VHL disease.

Central Nervous System Hemangioblastomas

These most frequent VHL disease-associated neoplasms are the CNS and retinal HB. They are nonmetastatic, hyper-vascular, benign lesions of the CNS developing in approximately 80% of the patients with VHL.[7] The cell of origin for HBs is currently unknown. HB may present in four different forms: (a) as solid very vascular tumors,

[a] VHL Comprehensive Clinical Care Center and Hemangioblastoma Center; [b] Division of Hematology-Oncology, Department of Medicine, Massachusetts General Hospital; [c] Center for Cancer Research, Massachusetts General Hospital Cancer Center, 149 13th Street, Charlestown, MA 02129, USA; [d] Harvard Medical School, Boston, MA, USA
* Corresponding author. Center for Cancer Research, Massachusetts General Hospital Cancer Center, 149 13th Street, Charlestown, MA 02139.
E-mail address: oiliopoulos@mgh.harvard.edu

Urol Clin N Am 50 (2023) 205–215
https://doi.org/10.1016/j.ucl.2023.01.010

(b) as a cyst with a solid nodule, (c) as a mixture of solid and cystic components, or (d) as a simple cyst, in which the solid nodule is not visible. They develop more often in the cerebellum (75%), spine (20%) and they present as single or multiple, synchronous or metachronous lesions.[8] HBs are nonmetastatic, noninfiltrating tumors but they have been responsible for a major morbidity or even mortality of patients with VHL, because of their space-occupying nature. Symptoms depend on the total size of the lesion(s) (both cystic and solid component), anatomic location in the CNS, and velocity of growth. They typically cause headaches, hiccups, nausea, vomiting, ataxia, peripheral motor, and sensory symptoms.[8] Retinal HBs (formerly reported as retinal angiomas) may cause retinal detachment heralded by changes in vision. HBs of the optic nerve may lead to a decrease in visual acuity and eventually loss of vision.[9,10] Rare HB locations in the skin, liver, or sacral bone have been reported. The *VHL* gene is inactivated in both VHL disease-associated and sporadic HBs.[11,12]

Renal Cell Cancers

Patients with VHL are at a lifetime risk (40% to 60%) of developing synchronous and/or metachronous RCC, exclusively of clear cell type (ccRCC), arising at multiple and bilateral renal cysts or from the noncystic parenchyma.[13] Renal cysts may present radiographically as simple cysts without enhancing components or complex cysts with varying degrees of solid components ranging from enhancing septa to majorly solid lesions. Nevertheless, the cyst is not an obligatory premalignant stage, as most of the RCCs in the patients with VHL develop as solid tumors from a noncystic parenchyma. The number and size of the cysts in VHL are not associated with a malignant potential.[14]

Pheochromocytomas and Paragangliomas

Patients with VHL with clinical type 2 disease (see below genotype–phenotype correlations) may develop pheochromocytoma and very rarely paragangliomas. Pheochromocytomas may be present in early childhood, warranting biochemical screening of children at risk. Pheochromocytomas may release catecholamines and therefore cause symptoms such as sweating, tremor, palpitations, and high blood pressure.

Pancreatic Lesions

Patients with VHL are not at high risk for classic adenocarcinoma of the pancreas, nor the premalignant mucinous cystadenoma.[7] They may develop multiple pancreatic cysts, pancreatic neuroendocrine tumors (pNETs), or serous cystadenomas.[15] Pancreatic cysts and serous cystadenomas may seem radiographically dramatic; nevertheless, they are most of the time asymptomatic. Symptoms of epigastric discomfort are very rare. Imaging of the pancreatic lesions is usually sufficiently characteristic to lead to the diagnosis; biopsy of pNETs or other pancreatic lesions can usually be avoided.

Serous Cystadenomas

These characteristic lesions may develop in the middle ear (called endolymphatic sac tumors [ELST]), the epididymis, or the female adnexal organs. As ELST they may cause tinnitus, decreased hearing, or acute bleeding resulting in hearing loss.[16,17] Epididymal and adnexal lesions may lead to discomfort or pain during intercourse or at rest.[18]

Genetic considerations
The VHL disease is characterized by almost complete penetrance by the sixth decade of life. Typically, VHL disease-associated lesions are detected during the second decade of life, with the exception of pheochromocytomas and retinal HBs that may develop in early childhood. The expressivity of the disease may vary significantly among individuals with the same germline mutation, even among members of the same family. This is most likely influenced by each individual's genetic makeup which places the VHL mutation in the context of coexisting modifier genes and polymorphisms.

There is a phenotype-genotype correlation for VHL disease. Patients with Type 1 VHL develop HB and RCC but not pheochromocytoma. In contrast, patients with Type 2 VHL may develop pheochromocytoma and are subdivided into three subtypes. Type 2 A is at low risk for RCC and type 2B is at high risk for RCC. Type 2 C patients present as cases of familial pheochromocytoma only, without the development of RCC or HB. Germline mutations in the VHL gene consist of large or small deletions, nonsense mutations, missense mutations, or silencing of the gene by methylation.[19,20] Mutations that result in total protein deletion or its unfolding lead to Type 1 disease, whereas missense mutations that are predicted to preserve the partial function of the protein lead to Type 2 disease.[19,20]

Two homozygous VHL mutations (R200 W, known as Chuvash mutation, and H191D, known as Croatian mutation) lead to increased erythropoietin and primary erythrocytosis,[21,22] without predisposing to typical VHL-related tumors in the reported populations. Nevertheless, there is anecdotal evidence that heterozygous pathogenic germline VHL$^{R200W/WT}$ mutations in VHL families segregate with the development of ccRCC and pheochromocytoma; therefore, the surveillance protocol for Chuvash VHL patients should be individualized.

Mechanisms of Disease

The quest for the function of the *VHL* gene is an example of a departure from the established notion of the function of tumor suppressor genes and it has been based on clinical observations. Iliopoulos and colleagues[23] showed that reintroduction of the VHL gene in VHL-deficient human RCC cells did not change their growth in vitro but dramatically suppressed their growth as tumors xenografted in mice, putting forward the hypothesis that the function of VHL gene is not limited to a cell autonomous role but regulates angiogenesis and the tumor microenvironment. They went into showing that the VHL gene regulates the expression of hypoxia and angiogenesis genes, such as VEGF.[24] MaxwelL and colleagues[25] discovered that VHL degrades a master regulation of angiogenesis, the transcription factors Hypoxia Inducible genes 1α and 2α (HIF1α and HIF2α). The pVHL protein acts as the substrate receptor for an E3 ubiquitin ligase multi-protein complex consisting of RBX1, ELonginC, ElonginB, and Cullin2.[26] HIF1α and HIF2α are the main substrates degraded by VHL, and the regulation of their expression is now regarded as the canonical function of the pVHL protein. The pVHL-HIF interaction depends on the prolyl-hydroxylation of HIF1/2α subunits by the cellular oxygen-responding oxoglutarate-dependent oxygenases EGLNs.[27,28] The alpha subunits of HIF1 and HIF2 are required to heterodimerize with the beta subunits (HIF1β and HIF2β) for the dimer to bind DNA and activate growth factor and metabolism genes. A small molecule that specifically disrupts the HIF2α-HIF2β interaction inhibits activity and it has been approved for the treatment of VHL disease (see below). Although the HIF1α and HIF2α paralogs both respond to hypoxia, compelling evidence suggest that, at least for RCC, HIF2α acts as an oncogene and HIF1α acts as a tumor suppressor gene.[29,30] In vivo xenograft experiments and in vivo genetically engineered mice were used to prove that inactivation of HIF2α by pVHL is necessary and sufficient for the tumor suppression function of *VHL*.[31–33] HIF2α reprograms RCC metabolism by promoting anaerobic glycolysis and glutamine reductive carboxylation,[34] and inhibition of glutaminase 1 (GLS1) alone or in combination with PARP inhibitors dramatically suppresses RCC growth in preclinical models.[35,36]

Treatment of Von Hippel–Lindau Disease: Belzutifan and the Need to Optimize Its Use

The goals of treating VHL-disease-related tumors are to prevent metastasis and/or symptom development while preserving the functional parenchyma of the target organ. Treatment is based on close annual surveillance to detect early-onset tumors. Surveillance for each tumor type is based on the reported earliest age of onset for the specific tumor. For retinal HBs and pheochromocytomas, it starts in infancy, for CNS HBs at the age of 9 to 10 years old, and for pNETs and ccRCCs at age of 16 to 17 years old.

The treatment of VHL disease entered a new era in August of 2021, when FDA approved the first class, oral inhibitor of HIF2a, belzutifan (Welireg, Merck and Co.) for VHL-related RCC, pNET, and CNS HB (https://www.fda.gov/drugs/resources-information-approved-drugs/fda-approves-belzutifan-cancers-associated-von-hippel-lindau-disease). Before belzutifan approval treatment of VHL disease was based on timely surgical interventions. RCCs were observed without intervention until they reached 3-cm maximum cross-sectional diameter, to preserve renal parenchyma; no risk for metastasis exists in tumors less than 3 cm.[37,38] Tumors larger than 3 cm were treated with partial nephrectomy or, alternatively, with radiofrequency ablation or cryoablation. A consensus statement about evaluation, diagnosis, and surveillance of renal masses in the setting of VHL disease summarizes the practice of VHL experts before belzutifan approval.[39] To avoid metastasis of pNET tumors, surgical intervention was recommended for tumors greater than 3 cm (or >2 cm for lesions in the head of the pancreas), and/or a doubling time is less than 500 days or there is a mutation in exon 3.[40,41] There has been no size cut-off for Hbs of the CNS, as the symptoms depend on size, location and growth rate. Approval of belzutifan for VHL-related ccRCC, HB, and pNETs changed the treatment paradigm. The drug was approved based on a Phase 2 trial in which, after a follow-up time of 21.8 months, it was shown that patients with VHL had an objective response in RCCs (49%), pancreatic NETs (77%) and CNS Hbs (30%).[42] The optimal time to start therapy with this medication, the duration of treatment, and the subset of patients that derive the most benefit from treatment with belzutifan are questions that will need to be answered with well-designed future clinical trials.

SUCCINATE DEHYDROGENASES AND THE HEREDITARY PHEOCHROMOCYTOMA/ PARAGANGLIOMA DISEASES
Clinical Manifestations

Germline mutations in the succinate dehydrogenase (*SDHx*) genes (*SDHA, SDHB, SDHC, SDHD, and SDHAF2*), which encode the subunits of the mitochondrial enzyme succinate dehydrogenase (SDH), predispose carriers to hereditary phaeochromocytoma and/or paragangliomas (HPPG), adenoma of the hypophysis, gastrointestinal stromal tumors (GIST), differentiated thyroid cancers, and RCC.[43] There is a genotype-phenotype correlation in SDH-deficient tumors with regard to malignant potential and the target organ. SDHB-deficient tumors have the highest malignant potential with SDHC, SDHD, and SDHA following in order of decreasing malignant potential. SDHB-deficient tumors develop as intra-abdominal paragangliomas (PGL), RCCs, or head and neck PGL (HNPGL) with a penetrance of 50%, 20%, and 30% accordingly by the age of 80. SDHC-deficient tumors tend to present as solitary HNPGL. *SDHD* or *SDHAF2*-deficient tumors present as multiple HNPGL. The SDHD P81 L pathogenic variant has a high malignant potential.[43–45]

Comprehensive review of the clinical heterogeneity and stage-dependent treatment of HPPGs is beyond the scope of this review and here we will focus on the manifestations of RCC in HPPG diseases. SDH-deficient RCCs have characteristic histologic features, marked by eosinophilic cells with cytoplasmic inclusions and/or vacuoles, with tumors often presenting papillary, solid, and tubular architecture. Typically, they stain negative for the expression of SDHB protein. In addition, SDH-deficient RCCs are negative for CD117, cytokeratin 7, carbonic anhydrases 9/12, and S100.[46–49] RCCs develop in younger patients and the lifetime risk was estimated at 15% to 20%. In a genotype-phenotype correlation study by Evenepoel at al. 83% of RCCs were linked to SDHB, 10% to SDHC, and 7% to SDHD germline pathogenic variants.[43]

An international consensus statement on initial testing and follow-up surveillance of asymptomatic individuals with SDHx germline mutations was issued in 2021.[50] Panelist recommended germline screening for SDHx family mutations in all patients with the diagnosis of pheochromocytoma/paraganglioma, followed by surveillance imaging (MRI of the head, neck, abdomen and pelvis and chest mediastinal imaging by CT) of all individuals at risk, starting at the age of 6 year old (for asymptomatic *SDHB* carriers) or 10 year old for the rest of individuals with other SDHx gene pathogenic variants.

Mechanisms of Disease

Loss of SDH mitochondrial complex function results in cellular accumulation of succinate. Succinate competes with a-ketoglutarate and inhibits the enzymatic activity of the oxoglutarate-dependent oxygenases. TETs and JMJDs proteins are such O-dependent oxygenases demethylating DNA and histone residues correspondingly. Loss of SDHx function promotes DNA and histone hypermethylation and establishes a migratory phenotype, which was shown to be reversed by the pyrimidine nucleoside analog decitabine.[51] Succinate has also a paracrine function; it is released in the tumor environment and may affect immune cell function through uptake by the cognate receptor.[52]

RENAL CELL CARCINOMA AND MELANOMA DISEASES: *MITF* (OMIM 614456) AND *BAP1* (OMIM 614327) GENES

Patients with a personal or family history of RCC and melanoma (skin or uveal) may have a germline mutation in the MITF or the BAP1 gene and they need germline mutation testing.

MITF Germline Mutations

Patients with a SUMOylation (secondary modification of a protein) whereby a SUMO molecule is covalently attached to the target protein, in this case the transcription factor MITF, MITF (Mi-E318 K) are predisposed to skin melanoma and RCC.[53] Carriers had a higher than fivefold increased risk of developing melanoma, RCC or both cancers. MITF codon 318 is located with a consensus site for SUMO attachment and mutant MITF was shown to have increased binding to the HIF1A promoter and increased HIF1A transcription. There seems to be no increased risk for other cancer than melanoma and RCC.[54]

BAP1 Germline Mutations

Individuals with germline inactivating mutations in the BAP1 tumor suppressor gene are at high risk of developing uveal and skin melanoma (Spitz tumors), basal cell carcinoma, ccRCC, thoracic and peritoneal mesothelioma, and high-grade rhabdoid meningiomas.[55–59] It seems that BAP1-deficient tumors are sensitive to EZH2 inhibitors.[60]

PBRM1

Germline inactivating mutations in the *PBRM1* tumor suppressor gene predispose to the development of ccRCC, without extrarenal manifestations.[61] The gene should be included in the panel of genes predisposing to HRCC diseases.

HEREDITARY PAPILLARY RENAL CELL CARCINOMA TYPE 1 (OMIM 1447000)
Clinical Manifestations

HPRCC 1 patients develop multiple and bilateral papillary Type 1 RCC at a much younger age than those with sporadic papillary type 1 RCC. The disease is autosomal dominant. The frequency of HPRCC type 1 is estimated 1 in one million.[62] Approximately 80% of the families presenting with the phenotype of the disease harbor an activating germline mutation in *c-MET* oncogene.[63] Sporadic papillary RCC tumors are characterized by trisomy of ch.7 and mutation of the duplicate c-MET proto-oncogene.[64] No extrarenal clinical manifestations have been described in the HPRCC Type 1 patients so far. It seems that HPRCC1 results in a "field defect" of the kidney parenchyma. The presence of "microadenomatosis" in the renal parenchyma around papillary type 1 RCC points to a high probability of HPRCC1.[65]

Mechanism of Disease and Therapeutic Advances

The *c-MET* oncogene-encoded protein is a heterodimeric transmembrane receptor tyrosine kinase, stimulated by the ligand hepatocyte growth factor/scatter factor (HGF/SF).[66,67] Mutations induce ligand-independent activation of the *c-MET* receptor, leading to aberrant activation of Ras and PI3K pathways, which are responsible for the invasive and metastatic phenotype[63] (3).[68] Clinical trials with c-Met inhibitors for the treatment of metastatic disease are underway.[69]

HEREDITARY LEIOMYOMATOSIS WITH RENAL CELL CARCINOMA (OMIM 150800)
Clinical Manifestations

HLRCC is caused by inactivating germline mutations in one copy of the fumarate Hydratase (*FH*) gene.[70] HLRCC patients are at high risk of developing skin leiomyomas, uterine fibroids, pheochromocytomas/paragangliomas, and RCC. The typical FH-deficient RCCs are papillary type 2 tumors,[70–72] although cases of FH-deficient clear cell and collecting duct RCC were reported.[73] HLRCC-associated RCCs are very aggressive tumors, with high metastatic potential. They usually present as single unilateral tumors and they require immediate surgical intervention independently of their size[72].[74] Patients with FH germline mutations should be screened, at least annually,

with MRI of the abdomen. We recommend that patients with personal and/or family history of a single skin leiomyoma, multiple uterine fibroids (especially FH-negative in routine immunohistochemistry), pheochromocytoma/paraganglioma, or papillary type 2 RCC be tested, among other genes, for germline *FH* mutations.[75]

Mechanisms of Disease

FH is a mitochondrial enzyme catalyzing the hydration of fumarate to malate. Germline inactivation and second-hit somatic loss of the wild-type allele lead to tumor formation. Loss of FH metabolic activity results in increased levels of fumarate in the cell. Fumarate is an oncometabolite, which inactivates several enzyme members of the family of a-ketoglutarate-dependent oxygenases, including HIF prolyl-hydroxylases (EGLNs), histone demethylases (KDMs), and the TET family of DNA demethylases. In addition, fumarate binds covalently to cellular proteins containing cysteine-disulfide bonds, forming S-(2-succino)-cysteines.[76] This modification, called protein succination, modifies the function of targeted cellular proteins, contributing to cellular transformation.[77] The formation of S-(2-succino)-cysteines can be detected by IHC of tumors by an antibody recognizing the covalent bond.[78]

Treatment of Localized and Advanced Disease

HLRCC RCCs require aggressive surgical intervention and resection immediately after detection. Locally advanced and metastatic tumors have a very unfavorable prognosis, usually not responding to TKI therapies indicated for clear cell RCC. Recently, combination treatment with the EGFR inhibitor erlotinib with the anti-VEGF antibody bevacizumab leads to impressive response rates and PFS and presents as an appealing first-line therapy.[79]

Research Directions

In the era of targeted therapy, the profound metabolic changes induced by FH deficiency approaches provide attractive opportunities for proposed synthetic lethality treatments. High throughput screens suggested that inactivation genes of the heme pathway (heme oxygenase HOMX1), adenylate cyclase (*ADCY*), ferroptosis (*GPX4*), and phosphogluconate dehydrogenase (PGD) provide synthetic lethality with FH-deficient tumors.[80–82]

BIRT–HOGG–DUBE DISEASE (OMIM 135150)
Clinical Manifestations

Birt, Hogg, and Dube initially described an inherited dermatologic condition characterized by multiple fibrofolliculomas, trichodiscomas, and acrochordons.[83] These lesions are benign hamartomatous tumors of the base of the hair follicle.[84] They present as multiple skin-colored papules of the face (including oral mucosa), neck, scalp, and upper trunk. Angiofibromas, lipomas, and collagenomas are less characteristic but they have been described in patients with BHD. Patients with BHD have a lifetime high risk of developing (a) these skin lesions, (b) renal tumors, and (c) spontaneous pneumothoraxes. In contrast to other inherited kidney cancers, where a certain histologic type is characteristic of the disease, RCC tumors in patients with BHD display a mixture of histologic types that coexist in the same individual and even in the same tumor. The predominant histology is chromophobe RCC, followed by chromophobe/oncocytic hybrids, and less frequently, clear and/or papillary-type mixtures.[85] Often pathologists report "RCC" but cannot subclassify histologically the kidney tumor of a patient with BHD. Patients with BHD have lung cysts and suffer from spontaneous pneumothorax.[86,87] Patients with BHD may present with any combination of skin lesions, RCCs, and spontaneous pneumothoraxes, or with a single one of these manifestations. Patients presenting with a primary spontaneous pneumothorax without other manifestations of BHD disease may harbor a germline FLCN mutation, and therefore warrant genetic testing.[88] The earliest onset of RCC disease in a patient with BHD was reported at the age of 15 years old and therefore we recommend clinical surveillance to begin in early adolescence.[89] Colonic polyps and a higher risk of colon cancer, although initially suspected as part of the disease, they are not currently considered part of it.[90]

Mechanisms of Disease

Approximately 85% of the patients with BHD harbor a germline mutation in the Folliculin (*FLCN*) tumor suppressor gene, located on ch.17[91,92].[93] Germline mutations are mainly nonsense mutations leading to frameshift and early protein truncation as well as intragenic or larger deletions. Point mutations exist.[85] List of FLCN mutations as well as clinical and research updates can be found on the BHD Foundation webpage: https://bhdsyndrome.org/for-families/skin/rare-skin-symptoms-of-bhd/

Folliculin is 57-kDa phosphoprotein that localizes to the nucleus and the cytoplasm. It forms complexes with Folliculin Interacting Proteins 1 and 2 (FNIP1, FNIP2),[94] through its C-terminal domain. The heterodimeric complex acts as a GTPase activating protein (GAP, in case of FLCN) and GTP exchange factor (GEF, in the case of FNIP1/2).[95] The GAP/GEF dimer enhances the function of targeted cellular GTPases and suppresses tumor growth. FLCN/FNIP targets several cellular Rab GTPases,[96] including Rab7A: the latter promotes the degradation of EGFR and other RTK receptors through the lysosomal pathway.[96] FLCN pathogenic mutations inactivate its GAP function and enhance signaling through EGFR, c-MET, and other RTKs, leading to growth-factor-dependent activation of MAPK/ERK, mTOR, and other signaling pathways.[96] FLCN also acts as GAP for the RagC/d GTPases that recruit to the surface of the lysosome the transcription factors TFE3/TFEB/TFEC for phosphorylation by mTORC1. Phosphorylated TFE3 is retained in the cytoplasm. FLCN mutations result in RagC/d inactivation, hypo-phosphorylated TFE3, and translocation to the nucleus where it acts as a growth-promoting factor. Elegant structural studies explain how FLCN-RagD/C interactions may provide substrate specificity for mTORC1 toward TFE3.[97]

PTEN Hamartoma Tumor Syndrome

Individuals with phosphatase and tensin homolog (PTEN) hamartoma tumor syndrome (PHTS), including Cowden syndrome (CS), are at high risk for multiple benign hamartomas and an increased risk of breast, endometrial, and thyroid cancers. Kim and colleagues[98] reported an increased risk for RCC, starting at the third decade of life, an observation that calls for RCC surveillance programs in patients with PTEN inactivating mutations.

Tuberous Sclerosis Complex 1/2

A detailed description of the clinical manifestations of people with TSC1/2 disease is beyond the scope of this restricted space review. The reader is referred to updated diagnostic criteria and guidelines for the treatment of TSC disease.[99] Patients with TSC21/2 disease may develop multiple and bilateral angiomyolipoma (AML, 80%), renal cysts (30%–40%), impaired kidney function, and, more rarely, RCC (3%), papillary type. In contrast to VHL disease, TSC-associated renal cysts may lead to kidney failure and hypertension.[100] In the case of TSC2 and PKD1 contiguous gene-deletion syndrome, where both TSC2 and PKD genes are co-deleted, the kidney function is further compromised. AML complication rates (bleeding, pain, hypertension, and renal insufficiency) depend on the size of AML; tumors larger than 3 cm may be surgically excised or treated with TORC1 inhibitors.[101]

RHABDOID TUMOR PREDISPOSING SYNDROMES RHABDOID TUMOR PREDISPOSING SYNDROME-1 AND RHABDOID TUMOR PREDISPOSING SYNDROME-2 (OMIM 609322 AND OMIM 613325)

Rhabdoid malignant tumors of the CNS, kidney, and ovaries in infants, children, and young adults, are caused by inactivating germline mutations in the *SMARCB1* (Rhabdoid tumor predisposing syndrome RTPS1) and *SMARCA4* (Rhabdoid tumor predisposing syndrome RTPS2) genes. SMARCB1-deficient tumors seem sensitive to the proteasome and possibly PARP inhibitors.

CHALLENGES IN GENETIC DIAGNOSIS OF HEREDITARY RENAL CELL CARCINOMA

Box 1 list the criteria we use in MGH to refer RCC patients for genetic testing. Similar criteria are included in a consensus statement issued before.[75]

Calo and colleagues[102] examined the prevalence of germline mutations in 254 patients that presented with metastatic RCC. They discovered germline mutations in 16% of these patients. Patients with nonclear cell RCC were significantly more likely to have an RCC-associated gene germline mutation than ccRCC patients. Interestingly, there was a significant association with CHEK2 mutations; this gene has not been previously described in HRCC cases, it is possible though that CHEK2 carriers do have an increased risk for RCC. These findings suggest that, like metastatic prostate cancer, patients presenting with metastatic RCC may warrant germline testing independently of other criteria. Further studies are needed to confirm these observations.

Lastly, patients with a typical clinical presentation of an HRCC but a negative germline testing present a diagnostic challenge. It is possible that these patients are mosaics for the suspected germline mutation; in this case testing of the offspring may reveal the presence of the mutation and confirm mosaicism. Alternatively, the cause of HRCC may be a mutation in a yet unknown gene linked to HRCC (eg, ELOC in patients with VHL).

CLINICS CARE POINTS

The following patients should be referred for risk assessment of hereditary renal cell carcinoma (HRCC):

- All members at risk of an HRCC family
- Patients with more than one synchronous or metachronous RCCs
- RCC patients with a family history of RCC
- Patients with RCC and a personal or family history of at least *one extra-renal manifestation associated with HRCC*[a]
- Early onset RCC (younger than 45 years old)
- Any patient with even a single hemangioblastoma of the central nervous system or the retinal, rhabdoid malignant tumor, choroidal melanoma, pheochromocytoma or paraganglioma.

Patients presenting with metastatic RCC (mRCC) may have an increased possibility of harboring a germline mutation.

The absence of a germline mutations in patients with a strong clinical HRCC phenotype may be explained by mosaicism of a de novo mutation. Genomic analysis of the tumor or other tissue of the patient (ie, skin biopsy) may help diagnose mosaicism in HRCC patients.

Established guidelines for clinical surveillance of HRCC patient exist, and they depend on the type of HRCC.

^a*Extra-renal manifestations of HRCC include*: CNS or retinal hemangioblastoma, extra lymphatic sac tumor of the middle ear (ELST), pancreatic neuro-endocrine tumor, serous cystadenoma (of the pancreas, adnexal organs of the uterus or epididymis), pheochromocytoma or paraganglioma, uterine fibroid negative for expression of FH by immunohistochemistry, spontaneous pneumothorax, choroidal or cutaneous melanoma, cutaneous fibrofolliculomas or leiomyomas.

DISCLOSURE

Merck (Advisory Board), Pfizer (consultant), C4 (consultant), and CALITHERA, USA (research support).

REFERENCES

1. Gossage L, Eisen T, Maher ER. VHL, the story of a tumour suppressor gene. Nat Rev Cancer 2015; 15(1):55–64.
2. Melmon KL, Rosen SW. Lindau's Disease. Review of the Literature and Study of a Large Kindred. Am J Med 1964;36:595–617.
3. Latif F, et al. Identification of the von Hippel-Lindau disease tumor suppressor gene. Science 1993; 260(5112):1317–20.
4. Coppin L, et al. VHL mosaicism can be detected by clinical next-generation sequencing and is not restricted to patients with a mild phenotype. Eur J Hum Genet 2014;22(9):1149–52.
5. Andreou A, et al. Elongin C (ELOC/TCEB1)-associated von Hippel-Lindau disease. Hum Mol Genet 2022;31(16):2728–37.
6. Iliopoulos O. von Hippel-Lindau disease: genetic and clinical observations. Front Horm Res 2001; 28:131–66.
7. Lonser RR, et al. von Hippel-Lindau disease. Lancet 2003;361(9374):2059–67.
8. Wanebo JE, et al. The natural history of hemangioblastomas of the central nervous system in patients with von Hippel-Lindau disease. J Neurosurg 2003; 98(1):82–94.
9. Wong WT, et al. Genotype-phenotype correlation in von Hippel-Lindau disease with retinal angiomatosis. Arch Ophthalmol 2007;125(2):239–45.
10. Wong WT, Chew EY. Ocular von Hippel-Lindau disease: clinical update and emerging treatments. Curr Opin Ophthalmol 2008;19(3):213–7.
11. Lee JY, et al. Loss of heterozygosity and somatic mutations of the VHL tumor suppressor gene in sporadic cerebellar hemangioblastomas. Cancer Res 1998;58(3):504–8.
12. Shankar GM, et al. Sporadic hemangioblastomas are characterized by cryptic VHL inactivation. Acta Neuropathol Commun 2014;2:167.
13. Lubensky IA, et al. Allelic deletions of the VHL gene detected in multiple microscopic clear cell renal lesions in von Hippel-Lindau disease patients. Am J Pathol 1996;149:2089–94.
14. Poston CD, et al. Characterization of the renal pathology of a familial form of renal cell carcinoma associated with von Hippel-Lindau disease: clinical and molecular genetic implications. J Urol 1995; 153(1):22–6.
15. Choyke PL, et al. von Hippel-Lindau disease: genetic, clinical and imaging features. Radiology 1995;194:629–42.
16. Manski TJ, et al. Endolymphatic sac tumors. A source of morbid hearing loss in von Hippel-Lindau disease. JAMA 1997;277(18):1461–6.
17. Kim HJ, et al. Tumors of the endolymphatic sac in patients with von Hippel-Lindau disease: implications for their natural history, diagnosis, and treatment. J Neurosurg 2005;102(3):503–12.
18. Choyke PL, et al. Epididymal cystadenomas in von Hippel-Lindau disease. Urology 1997;49(6):926–31.
19. Crossey PA, et al. Identification of intragenic mutations in the von Hippel-Lindau disease tumour suppressor gene and correlation with disease phenotype. Hum Mol Genet 1994;3(8):1303–8.
20. Chen F, et al. Germline mutations in the von hippel-lindau disease tumor suppressor gene:correlations with phenotype. Hum Mutat 1995;5:66–75.
21. Ang SO, et al. Disruption of oxygen homeostasis underlies congenital Chuvash polycythemia. Nat Genet 2002;32(4):614–21.
22. Pastore Y, et al. Mutations of von Hippel-Lindau tumor-suppressor gene and congenital polycythemia. Am J Hum Genet 2003;73(2):412–9.
23. Iliopoulos O, et al. Tumour suppression by the human von Hippel-Lindau gene product. Nat Med 1995;1(8):822–6.
24. Iliopoulos O, et al. Negative regulation of hypoxia-inducible genes by the von Hippel-Lindau protein. Proc Natl Acad Sci U S A 1996;93(20):10595–9.
25. Maxwell PH, et al. The tumour suppressor protein VHL targets hypoxia-inducible factors for oxygen-dependent proteolysis. Nature 1999;399(6733):271–5.
26. Kibel A, et al. Binding of the von Hippel-Lindau tumor suppressor protein to Elongin B and C. Science 1995;269(5229):1444–6.
27. Jaakkola P, et al. Targeting of HIF-alpha to the von Hippel-Lindau ubiquitylation complex by O2-regulated prolyl hydroxylation. Science 2001; 292(5516):468–72.
28. Ivan M, et al. HIFalpha targeted for VHL-mediated destruction by proline hydroxylation:

implications for O2 sensing. Science 2001; 292(5516):464–8.

29. Shen C, et al. Genetic and functional studies implicate HIF1alpha as a 14q kidney cancer suppressor gene. Cancer Discov 2011;1(3):222–35.

30. Hoefflin R, et al. HIF-1alpha and HIF-2alpha differently regulate tumour development and inflammation of clear cell renal cell carcinoma in mice. Nat Commun 2020;11(1):4111.

31. Zimmer M, et al. Inhibition of hypoxia-inducible factor is sufficient for growth suppression of VHL-/- tumors. Mol Cancer Res 2004;2(2):89–95.

32. Kondo K, et al. Inhibition of HIF is necessary for tumor suppression by the von Hippel-Lindau protein. Cancer Cell 2002;1(3):237–46.

33. Rankin EB, Tomaszewski JE, Haase VH. Renal cyst development in mice with conditional inactivation of the von Hippel-Lindau tumor suppressor. Cancer Res 2006;66(5):2576–83.

34. Metallo CM, et al. Reductive glutamine metabolism by IDH1 mediates lipogenesis under hypoxia. Nature 2012;481(7381):380–4.

35. Gameiro PA, et al. In vivo HIF-mediated reductive carboxylation is regulated by citrate levels and sensitizes VHL-deficient cells to glutamine deprivation. Cell Metab 2013;17(3):372–85.

36. Okazaki A, et al. Glutaminase and poly(ADP-ribose) polymerase inhibitors suppress pyrimidine synthesis and VHL-deficient renal cancers. J Clin Invest 2017;127(5):1631–45.

37. Walther MM, et al. Renal cancer in families with hereditary renal cancer: prospective analysis of a tumor size threshold for renal parenchymal sparing surgery. J Urol 1999;161(5):1475–9.

38. Duffey BG, et al. The relationship between renal tumor size and metastases in patients with von Hippel-Lindau disease. J Urol 2004;172(1):63–5.

39. Chahoud J, et al. Evaluation, diagnosis and surveillance of renal masses in the setting of VHL disease. World J Urol 2021;39(7):2409–15.

40. Keutgen XM, et al. Evaluation and management of pancreatic lesions in patients with von Hippel-Lindau disease. Nat Rev Clin Oncol 2016;13(9):537–49.

41. Tirosh A, et al. Association of VHL Genotype With Pancreatic Neuroendocrine Tumor Phenotype in Patients With von Hippel-Lindau Disease. JAMA Oncol 2018;4(1):124–6.

42. Jonasch E, et al. Belzutifan for Renal Cell Carcinoma in von Hippel-Lindau Disease. N Engl J Med 2021;385(22):2036–46.

43. Evenepoel L, et al. Toward an improved definition of the genetic and tumor spectrum associated with SDH germ-line mutations. Genet Med 2015; 17(8):610–20.

44. Andrews KA, et al. Tumour risks and genotype-phenotype correlations associated with germline variants in succinate dehydrogenase subunit genes SDHB, SDHC and SDHD. J Med Genet 2018;55(6):384–94.

45. Ricketts C, et al. Germline SDHB mutations and familial renal cell carcinoma. J Natl Cancer Inst 2008; 100(17):1260–2.

46. Gill AJ, et al. Succinate dehydrogenase (SDH)-deficient renal carcinoma: a morphologically distinct entity: a clinicopathologic series of 36 tumors from 27 patients. Am J Surg Pathol 2014; 38(12):1588–602.

47. Fuchs TL, et al. Expanding the clinicopathological spectrum of succinate dehydrogenase-deficient renal cell carcinoma with a focus on variant morphologies: a study of 62 new tumors in 59 patients. Mod Pathol 2022;35(6):836–49.

48. Tsai TH, Lee WY. Succinate Dehydrogenase-Deficient Renal Cell Carcinoma. Arch Pathol Lab Med 2019;143(5):643–7.

49. Williamson SR, et al. Succinate dehydrogenase-deficient renal cell carcinoma: detailed characterization of 11 tumors defining a unique subtype of renal cell carcinoma. Mod Pathol 2015;28(1):80–94.

50. Amar L, et al. International consensus on initial screening and follow-up of asymptomatic SDHx mutation carriers. Nat Rev Endocrinol 2021;17(7):435–44.

51. Letouze E, et al. SDH mutations establish a hypermethylator phenotype in paraganglioma. Cancer Cell 2013;23(6):739–52.

52. Wu JY, et al. Cancer-Derived Succinate Promotes Macrophage Polarization and Cancer Metastasis via Succinate Receptor. Mol Cell 2020;77(2): 213–227 e5.

53. Bertolotto C, et al. A SUMOylation-defective MITF germline mutation predisposes to melanoma and renal carcinoma. Nature 2011;480(7375):94–8.

54. Guhan SM, et al. Cancer risks associated with the germline MITF(E318K) variant. Sci Rep 2020; 10(1):17051.

55. Popova T, et al. Germline BAP1 mutations predispose to renal cell carcinomas. Am J Hum Genet 2013;92(6):974–80.

56. Testa JR, et al. Germline BAP1 mutations predispose to malignant mesothelioma. Nat Genet 2011;43(10):1022–5.

57. Mochel MC, et al. Loss of BAP1 Expression in Basal Cell Carcinomas in Patients With Germline BAP1 Mutations. Am J Clin Pathol 2015;143(6): 901–4.

58. de la Fouchardiere A, et al. Germline BAP1 mutations predispose also to multiple basal cell carcinomas. Clin Genet 2015;88(3):273–7.

59. Carbone M, et al. Biological Mechanisms and Clinical Significance of BAP1 Mutations in Human Cancer. Cancer Discov 2020;10(8):1103–20.

60. LaFave LM, et al. Loss of BAP1 function leads to EZH2-dependent transformation. Nat Med 2015; 21(11):1344–9.

61. Benusiglio PR, et al. A germline mutation in PBRM1 predisposes to renal cell carcinoma. J Med Genet 2015;52(6):426–30.

62. Zbar B. Inherited epithelial tumors of the kidney: old and new diseases. Semin Cancer Biol 2000; 10(4):313–8.

63. Schmidt L, et al. Germline and somatic mutations in the tyrosine kinase domain of the MET proto-oncogene in papillary renal carcinomas. Nat Genet 1997;16:68–73.

64. Zhuang Z, et al. Trisomy 7-harbouring non-random duplication of the mutant MET allele in hereditary papillary renal carcinomas. Nat Genet 1998;20(1): 66–9.

65. Lubensky IA, et al. Hereditary and sporadic papillary renal carcinomas with c-met mutations share a distinct morphological phenotype. Am J Pathol 1999;155(2):517–26.

66. Bottaro DP, et al. Identification of the hepatocyte growth factor receptor as the c-met proto-oncogene product. Science 1991;251(4995): 802–4.

67. Ponzetto C, et al. A multifunctional docking site mediates signaling and transformation by the hepatocyte growth factor/scatter factor receptor family. Cell 1994;77(2):261–71.

68. Giordano S, et al. Transfer of mitogenic and invasive response to scatter factor/hepatocyte growth factor by transfection of human MET protoonco-gene. Proc Natl Acad Sci 1993;90(2):649–53.

69. Comoglio PM, Giordano S, Trusolino L. Drug development of MET inhibitors: targeting oncogene addiction and expedience. Nat Rev Drug Discov 2008;7(6):504–16.

70. Consortium TML. Germline mutations in FH predispose to dominantly inherited uterine fibroids, skin leiomyomata and papillary renal cell cancer. Nat Genet 2002;30(4):306–10.

71. Launonen V, et al. Inherited susceptibility to uterine leiomyomas and renal cell cancer. Proc Natl Acad Sci 2001;98(6):3387–92.

72. Toro JR, et al. Mutations in the fumarate hydratase gene cause hereditary leiomyomatosis and renal cell cancer in families in North America. Am J Hum Genet 2003;73(1):95–106.

73. Shyu I, et al. Clues to recognition of fumarate hydratase-deficient renal cell carcinoma: Findings from cytologic and limited biopsy samples. Cancer Cytopathol 2018;126(12):992–1002.

74. Sudarshan S, et al. Mechanisms of disease: hereditary leiomyomatosis and renal cell cancer–a distinct form of hereditary kidney cancer. Nat Clin Pract Urol 2007;4(2):104–10.

75. Bratslavsky G, et al. Genetic risk assessment for hereditary renal cell carcinoma: Clinical consensus statement. Cancer 2021;127(21):3957–66.

76. Schmidt C, Sciacovelli M, Frezza C. Fumarate hydratase in cancer: A multifaceted tumour suppressor. Semin Cell Dev Biol 2020;98:15–25.

77. Yang M, et al. The Succinated Proteome of FH-Mutant Tumours. Metabolites 2014;4(3):640–54.

78. Reyes C, et al. Uterine smooth muscle tumors with features suggesting fumarate hydratase aberration: detailed morphologic analysis and correlation with S-(2-succino)-cysteine immunohistochemistry. Mod Pathol 2014;27(7):1020–7.

79. Choi Y, et al. Bevacizumab Plus Erlotinib Combination Therapy for Advanced Hereditary Leiomyomatosis and Renal Cell Carcinoma-Associated Renal Cell Carcinoma: A Multicenter Retrospective Analysis in Korean Patients. Cancer Res Treat 2019; 51(4):1549–56.

80. Frezza C, et al. Haem oxygenase is synthetically lethal with the tumour suppressor fumarate hydratase. Nature 2011;477(7363):225–8.

81. Boettcher M, et al. High throughput synthetic lethality screen reveals a tumorigenic role of adenylate cyclase in fumarate hydratase-deficient cancer cells. BMC Genom 2014;15:158.

82. Sun Y, et al. Functional Genomics Reveals Synthetic Lethality between Phosphogluconate Dehydrogenase and Oxidative Phosphorylation. Cell Rep 2019;26(2):469–482 e5.

83. Birt AR, Hogg GR, Dube WJ. Hereditary multiple fibrofolliculomas with trichodiscomas and acrochordons. Arch. Derm. 1977;113:1674–7.

84. Scalvenzi M, et al. Hereditary multiple fibrofolliculomas, trichodiscomas and acrochordons: syndrome of Birt-Hogg-Dube. J Eur Acad Dermatol Venereol 1998;11(1):45–7.

85. Toro JR, et al. BHD mutations, clinical and molecular genetic investigations of Birt-Hogg-Dube syndrome: a new series of 50 families and a review of published reports. J Med Genet 2008;45(6):321–31.

86. Ayo DS, et al. Cystic lung disease in Birt-Hogg-Dube syndrome. Chest 2007;132(2):679–84.

87. Toro JR, et al. Lung cysts, spontaneous pneumothorax, and genetic associations in 89 families with Birt-Hogg-Dube syndrome. Am J Respir Crit Care Med 2007;175(10):1044–53.

88. Sriram JD, et al. Birt-Hogg-Dube syndrome in apparent primary spontaneous pneumothorax patients; results and recommendations for clinical practice. BMC Pulm Med 2022;22(1):325.

89. Schneider M, et al. Early onset renal cell carcinoma in an adolescent girl with germline FLCN exon 5 deletion. Fam Cancer 2018;17(1):135–9.

90. Zbar B, et al. Risk of renal and colonic neoplasms and spontaneous pneumothorax in the Birt-Hogg-Dube syndrome. Cancer Epidemiol Biomarkers Prev 2002;11(4):393–400.

91. Khoo SK, et al. Birt-Hogg-Dube syndrome: mapping of a novel hereditary neoplasia gene to chromosome 17p12-q11.2. Oncogene 2001;20(37):5239–42.

92. Schmidt LS, et al. Birt-Hogg-Dube syndrome, a genodermatosis associated with spontaneous pneumothorax and kidney neoplasia, maps to chromosome 17p11.2. Am J Hum Genet 2001; 69(4):876–82.

93. Nickerson ML, et al. Mutations in a novel gene lead to kidney tumors, lung wall defects, and benign tumors of the hair follicle in patients with the Birt-Hogg-Dube syndrome. Cancer Cell 2002;2(2):157–64.

94. Baba M, et al. Folliculin encoded by the BHD gene interacts with a binding protein, FNIP1, and AMPK, and is involved in AMPK and mTOR signaling. Proc Natl Acad Sci U S A 2006;103(42):15552–7.

95. Tsun ZY, et al. The folliculin tumor suppressor is a GAP for the RagC/D GTPases that signal amino acid levels to mTORC1. Mol Cell 2013;52(4):495–505.

96. Laviolette LA, et al. Negative regulation of EGFR signalling by the human folliculin tumour suppressor protein. Nat Commun 2017;8:15866.

97. Jansen RM, et al. Structural basis for FLCN RagC GAP activation in MiT-TFE substrate-selective mTORC1 regulation. Sci Adv 2022;8(37):eadd2926.

98. Kim RH, et al. Early-onset renal cell carcinoma in PTEN harmatoma tumour syndrome. NPJ Genom Med 2020;5:40.

99. Northrup H, et al. Updated International Tuberous Sclerosis Complex Diagnostic Criteria and Surveillance and Management Recommendations. Pediatr Neurol 2021;123:50–66.

100. Kingswood JC, et al. Renal Manifestations of Tuberous Sclerosis Complex: Key Findings From the Final Analysis of the TOSCA Study Focussing Mainly on Renal Angiomyolipomas. Front Neurol 2020;11:972.

101. Kingswood JC, et al. Renal angiomyolipoma in patients with tuberous sclerosis complex: findings from the TuberOus SClerosis registry to increase disease Awareness. Nephrol Dial Transplant 2019;34(3):502–8.

102. Carlo MI, et al. Prevalence of Germline Mutations in Cancer Susceptibility Genes in Patients With Advanced Renal Cell Carcinoma. JAMA Oncol 2018;4(9):1228–35.

The Changing Role of Renal Mass Biopsy

Sohrab Naushad Ali, MD, MSc, FRCSC[1], Zachary Tano, MD[1], Jaime Landman, MD*

KEYWORDS

- Renal mass • Biopsy • Kidney cancer

KEY POINTS

- Renal mass biopsy (RMB) is a safe and effective diagnostic procedure with the rate of complications including hematoma, macroscopic hematuria, and clinically significant pain at only 4.9%, 1.0%, and 1.2%, respectively.
- RMB has a sensitivity of 96.7%, specificity of 94.4%, and a positive predictive value (PPV) of 98.8% making it a reliable diagnostic test.
- RMB has a nondiagnostic rate of approximately 14%, which can be improved with repeat biopsy or a multidisciplinary approach including urologist-, interventional radiologist-, and gastroenterologist-directed biopsy techniques.
- Histologic grade concordance for RMB is approximately 62% and remains a limitation of RMB.
- RMB is an effective risk stratification tool and can increase the number of patients undergoing active surveillance and reduce the risk of benign pathology after surgical extirpation.

INTRODUCTION

The management of an incidentally detected small (<4 cm) renal mass (SRM) is a common clinical scenario for urologists, with the incidence increasing over the past two decades mostly due to the widespread use of cross-sectional imaging.[1,2] The management of SRMs is an area of great controversy with significant variation in practice patterns worldwide.[3,4] This is of concern for several reasons. First, most SRMs are asymptomatic and incidentally detected.[5] Second, all surgically fit patients with an enhancing renal mass were historically presumed to harbor malignancy and recommended surgical management, usually with radical nephrectomy (RN). However, we now acknowledge the heterogeneity in tumor biology of these lesions with data suggesting that approximately 26% of SRMs are benign and would likely never require therapy.[5–8] A retrospective analysis of 2770 patients who underwent surgery for an incidentally detected renal mass showed that approximately 20% of masses between 1 and 4 cm were benign, and that approximately 46% of masses ≤1 cm were nonmalignant.[9] Lastly, most malignant SRMs tend to be of lower histologic grade and some are less aggressive renal cell carcinoma subtypes; both factors with a favorable prognosis and could be considered for less invasive thermal ablative therapies or active surveillance (AS) in what is often an older population with comorbidities.[10] The increasing grade with size relationship is supported by a retrospective analysis using the Surveillance, Epidemiology, and End Results (SEER) database that identified 19,932 patients with localized renal masses having an overall distribution of 80% low grade and 20% high grade with an odds ratio (OR) of high-grade disease increasing by 13% for each 1 cm of growth (OR 1.13, $p < 0.001$).[11] Despite the above, there has been a concomitant increase in surgical procedures performed for SRMs with negligible improvement in overall survival.[2,12] This is mostly in part due to loss of functional nephrons and

Department of Urology, University of California, Irvine, CA, USA
[1] Present address: 3800 West Chapman Avenue Suite 7200, Orange, CA 92868.
* Corresponding author. 3800 West Chapman Avenue Suite 7200, Orange, CA 92868.
E-mail address: landmanj@hs.uci.edu

Urol Clin N Am 50 (2023) 217–225
https://doi.org/10.1016/j.ucl.2023.01.002
0094-0143/23/© 2023 Elsevier Inc. All rights reserved.

sequalae such as chronic kidney disease (CKD), the need for dialysis, increased cardiovascular risk, and thus, an overall reduction in lifespan.[13] The initial survival advantage independent of tumor size seen in the 1990s has been lost in more contemporary studies.[14] As such, there has been an increased effort for risk stratification of SRMs and this has been reflected in most recent versions of clinical practice guidelines.[13,15,16]

Classically, imaging has been the mainstay for the diagnosis of SRMs and is used for the decision to intervene and/or surveil. Renal mass biopsy (RMB) is a clinical tool that serves as an important adjunct for patients with a renal mass suspicious of malignancy and allows for risk stratification. RMB can provide important information regarding cell type, histologic grade, degree of differentiation, plus molecular and genomic markers that can ultimately be used to inform diagnosis, prognosis, and guide medical/surgical decision-making. Multiple management options are now available for the treatment of renal masses including RN, partial nephrectomy (PN), thermal ablation (TA), and AS.[13,17,18] To fully appreciate the role of RMB in the management of SRMs, this review examines the historical context, controversies, current landscape, improvements in technique and outcomes, and future directions with regard to RMB in the management of SRMs.

History of Renal Mass Biopsy

The first percutaneous RMB was performed by Iverson and colleagues.[19] This represented a shift from the traditional open surgical technique for obtaining tissue specimens. Early experiences with percutaneous RMB were marred by poor diagnostic yields (nondiagnostic rate 31% and false negative rate 25%), various complications, and reports of tumor tract seeding.[20,21] As such, RMB was reserved for a limited number of indications such as the diagnosis of metastatic disease, ruling out infection, or malignancies of nonrenal origin such as lymphoma.[22] Indeed, this paradigm is reflected in earlier iterations of the clinical practice guidelines.[23] Despite advances in biopsy technique, the limited role of RMB has persisted within the urological community. A recent study showed that only 8% of urologists perform the biopsy in more than 20% of their SRM patients and 73% of urologists rarely or never perform the biopsy.[24] Among the latter, the reason for the rare or never SRM biopsy approach included concerns that biopsy would: not alter management (80%), provide a false negative (60%), provide a false positive (10%), result in complications (20%), or seed the biopsy needle tract with

malignant cells (8%).[25] RMBs that allow clinicians to risk stratify patients continue to be employed at a low rate and thus pretreatment RMB remains controversial.[26] The recent resurgence of interest in RMB as reflected in recent clinical practice guidelines, is due to our increased understanding of the oncologic potential of varying histological subtypes, increased detection of smaller tumors with increased likelihood of benign histology and the emergence of more conservative treatment modalities such as TA and AS.

Limitations of Current Imaging

The mainstay modality for detecting and monitoring renal masses has been cross-sectional imaging and there has been a significant investigation into whether imaging can be used as a diagnostic tool for both renal cysts and SRMs. Renal cysts are increasingly common and present in approximately 27% percent of women and 34% of men as shown in a study population of 2063 adults ranging in age from 20 to >70 years old.[27] Morton Bosniak[28] created an effectively computed tomography (CT)-based classification system to differentiate malignant from benign cysts, which has since undergone several iterations and validations including the addition of the Bosniak IIF cyst designation.[29,30] In addition, a proposed update in 2019 encourages the use of imaging modalities other than limited ultrasound (US) and CT.[31] With regard to renal masses there are now over 40 described histological subtypes;[32] however, it is generally accepted that 70% of malignant lesions are clear cell renal cell carcinoma (ccRCC), 15% papillary RCC, and 5% are chromophobe RCC with the remaining malignant subtypes being rarer. There is ongoing improvement in imaging assessments and technology to differentiate malignant from benign masses, as well as between the histological subtypes to improve patient risk stratification. Lee-Felker and colleagues[33] performed a retrospective cohort study of 156 patients with solid renal masses with a median size of 3 cm to assess qualitative and quantitative features of preoperative CT scans and found that attenuation profiles allowed the radiologists to differentiate ccRCC from other solid masses (lipid-poor angiomyolipoma and oncocytoma) with a sensitivity of 70% and specificity of 98%. A second study assessing 58 patients with solid renal masses, the majority of which were T1a, assessed the relative enhancement on MRI to differentiate ccRCC masses from masses diagnosed as papillary, chromophobe, and oncocytoma with that conclusion that MRI did aid in differentiating ccRCC from the other histologic subtypes with a sensitivity of

90% and specificity of 90%.[34] Although much work discerning ccRCC from other renal masses has been encouraging, Hindman and colleagues35 assessed the MRI image properties to determine how well signal intensity index or tumor-to-spleen signal intensity ratio could distinguish ccRCC from lipid-poor angiomyolipoma in a retrospective cohort study of 108 patients with pathologically diagnosed masses and found no difference in MRI parameters when comparing the two groups. Papillary renal cell carcinoma (pRCC) has also been an area of imaging interest. In a study retrospectively evaluating quantitative and qualitative MRI signal intensity parameters and comparing them to pathologic features in 49 RCC tumors to identify the characteristic of pRCC compared with ccRCC masses, the authors found that, among other features, a T2 signal intensity ratio of <0.66 had a specificity of 100% and sensitivity of 54% for papillary RCC. Notably in the conclusion, the authors mention that RMB is warranted if imaging features cannot be used to differentiate between subtypes.[36] Much focus has been placed on CT and MRI; however, US is also being used to characterize renal masses with the advantages of being a contrast-free and ability to be used during procedures, such as biopsy.[37] Radiologic studies are a critical tool in the management of renal masses and there is much effort to improve their diagnostic capability, but radiologic studies alone cannot be relied upon at this time.

Indications for Renal Mass Biopsy

As noted above, the historical indications for RMB were limited to the evaluation of metastatic disease, ruling out infection and malignancies of hematologic origin. However, with recent evidence regarding favorable outcomes of more conservative modalities such as TA and AS, there has been an evolution in the practice guidelines regarding RMB.[38,39] Most recommendations, however, are still informed by low-level evidence and expert opinion suggesting the need for high-quality studies to inform guideline statements. The recently updated 2021 American Urological Association (AUA) guideline for the management of renal masses emphasizes the accuracy and safety of RMB and recommends RMB before ablative therapies and as an option for risk stratification before initiation of AS.[13] However, the AUA considers biopsy of an SRM exempt in younger and elderly patients, who due to their "unwillingness to accept the uncertainties of biopsy" or due to advanced age, would likely pursue surgical or conservative treatment, respectively, regardless of biopsy results. Similarly, the National

Comprehensive Cancer Network (NCCN) in 2021, the EUA 2022, and the most recent iteration of the American Society of Clinical Oncology (ASCO) 2017 guidelines generally only recommend RMB in cases where biopsy may alter management but strongly recommend RMB before ablative therapy.[15,40,41] The NCCN guidelines recommend biopsy before initiation of AS, whereas ASCO considers this an option. Most guidelines agree, that RMB should be offered in select cases if the origin of the mass is suspected to be hematologic, metastatic, inflammatory, or infectious in nature, and before initiation of systemic therapy. It should be noted that biopsy recommendations from all guideline sources are made with low-level data and largely represent expert opinion. With respect to systemic therapy, advancements in the treatment of advanced renal cell carcinoma such as immune checkpoint inhibitors and in combination with novel tyrosine kinase inhibitors, there is an increasing role of RMB to identify tumor histology in advanced RCC before systemic therapy and in determining eligibility for clinical trials.[42,43]

Accuracy and Diagnostic Outcomes

The true utility of RMB as a diagnostic test lies in its ability to differentiate benign from malignant lesions. Counseling patients on the role of RMB in the management of SRMs is challenging due to concerns regarding nondiagnostic rates, negative predictive values (NPVs), and grade discordance.[44] RMB continues to be a highly sensitive and specific diagnostic test. A recent bivariate meta-analysis of seven studies performed by the AUA guideline committee in 2021 regarding diagnosis using core RMB compared with surgical pathology, revealed a sensitivity of 96.7%, specificity of 94.4%, and a positive predictive value (PPV) of 98.8%.[13] Histologic subtype determination also remains highly accurate within contemporary series.[45] One of the concerns regarding RMB is the NPV. In a systematic review by Patel and colleagues,[45] the NPV of RMB was approximately 63%, suggesting that approximately 37% of patients with a negative biopsy may harbor a malignant tumor. However, more recent metanalyses such as the one carried out in the 2021 AUA guideline committee for the management of SRMs note a more favorable NPV of 80%.[13] Another area of concern for RMB is its initial biopsy nondiagnostic rate of 14%.[13] Indeed, among patients with an initial nondiagnostic biopsy, a repeat biopsy resulted in a 94% histological diagnosis.[46] In another study by Okhunov and colleagues,[47] patients with cT1a SRM undergoing US-guided biopsy in a urology office setting showed an overall diagnostic rate of 80% on the initial biopsy, which similarly improved to 93% on subsequent repeat biopsy. Unlike RMB's diagnostic accuracy, the ability of RMB to identify tumor grade is highly variable with concordance rates between tumor grades on biopsy to surgical pathology being approximately 62% (interquartile range 52.1% to 72.1%).[48] Others have reported a Fuhrman upgrading rate of 16% (low grade [1 or 2] to high grade [3 or 4]) from biopsy to surgical pathology.[45] This remains a significant limitation of RMB and is pertinent in differentiating higher-grade tumors with increased metastatic potential. Methods to improve the accuracy of histologic grade include the use of core biopsies as opposed to fine needle aspiration (FNA), the use of novel targeting modalities such as optical coherence tomography (OCT) and robotic platforms, and the use of novel molecular marker profiling.[49–51]

Renal Mass Biopsy Technique

RMB is generally performed in an outpatient setting under local anesthesia and sedation. Although traditionally performed by an interventional radiologist (IR), a recent prospective study evaluating a multidisciplinary approach including urologist and gastroenterologist performed RMB has shown excellent outcomes.[52] This study showed that urologists who performed US-guided RMB under local anesthesia provided a diagnostic rate of 80%, with 57% of patients going on AS and an overall benign surgery rate of only 3%. In addition to better patient comfort and decreased facility costs, the mean time from diagnosis to definitive management was only 34 days.[53] US or CT image guidance is typically used for RMB, and tissues can be sampled with either FNA or core needle biopsy.[54] Core needle biopsy with at least two to three cores is preferred for adequate diagnostic yield as opposed to FNA. In a recent systematic review, the core biopsy was found to have a sensitivity of 97.5% as compared with 62.5% in FNA.[55] Tumors that are inaccessible with conventional techniques due to their anterior or medial locations can be approached through the stomach or duodenum with a novel gastrointestinal endoscopic ultrasound approach with satisfactory yield.[52]

Safety of Renal Mass Biopsy

RMB is generally considered a safe diagnostic procedure with complication rates ranging from 1.4% to 4.7% and a major complication rate of 0.46%.[56] In a systematic review by Patel and colleagues,[45] the rate of complications including hematoma, macroscopic hematuria, and clinically

significant pain following RMB were only 4.9%, 1.0%, and 1.2%, respectively. The risk of significant hemorrhage requiring transfusion (0.7%) and complications greater than Clavien grade 2 remains low (<0.5%) in the reported series.[48] In the hands of experienced practitioners, these complications can further be decreased as reported by Okhunov and colleagues[47] among 72 SRM biopsies, no patient experienced procedural or post-procedural-related complications using an office-based, US-guided RMB technique under no sedation. It is generally recommended that anticoagulant and antiplatelet medications be held before RMB to reduce the risk of bleeding complications.[57] In addition, the risk of biopsy tract seeding with modern techniques is exceptionally rare with only a few case reports presented in the current literature.[58,59]

Clinical Implications

With the increased detection of SRMs, the number of surgically resected benign renal masses in the United States has increased by 82% between 2000 and 2009.[5] Despite this, RMB continues to be severely underutilized.[4,24,60] Surgical extirpation of benign masses is not trivial as the overall risk for death from comorbidities such as CKD and cardiovascular risk can be exacerbated by surgical management. Comorbidity competing risk of death has been evaluated in a retrospective SEER database study of 6665 patients who underwent surgical management for SRM by comparing their risk of kidney cancer-specific death with risk of death by competing comorbidities. The study concluded that, overall, patients have a lower risk of cancer-specific death compared with death from competing comorbidities depending on their comorbidity score (probabilities of cancer-specific death vs competing causes; 3 years (4.7% vs 10.9%), 5 years (7.5% vs 20.1%), and 10 years (11.9% vs 44.4%)).[61] The baseline competing comorbidities of patients are not the only risks patients may encounter as current surgical management strategies can affect factors related to longevity, such as renal function. Patel and colleagues[62] performed a meta-analysis to quantify renal dysfunction caused by various urologic interventions. This study evaluated 58 studies from 1997 to 2015 that reported functional renal outcomes of estimated glomerular filtration rate (eGFR), CKD, and acute kidney injury (AKI) in the setting of RN, PN, TA, and AS. The authors found that RN compared with PN had a larger reduction in eGFR, greater risk of CKD stage 3 or worse, and higher risk of AKI in T1a tumors. Of those 58 studies, only two studies evaluated AS. The first showed that in 537 patients 75 years old or older with renal masses ≤7 cm, there was a significant decrease in eGFR for urologic interventions compared with AS (RN 34%, vs PN 18% vs AS 0%) and that the decrease in eGFR was associated increased cardiovascular mortality, that accounted for 29% of deaths compared with cancer progression which accounted for only 4% of deaths. Newly diagnosed CKD was more common among patients that received RN (47%) and PN (25%) compared with AS (5%) and the incidence of cardiovascular death at 5 years was 15% for patients with stage 3 CKD or greater compared with 6% for patients without stage 3 CKD or greater.[63] The second study comparing outcomes of management following RN, PN, TA, and AS showed a greater decrease in eGFR for RN compared with AS (change in eGFR RN vs AS; −9.2 mL/min/1.73 m^2 vs −0.5 mL/min/1.73 m^2).[64] AS for SRMs with delayed intervention continues to be a safe option for well-selected patients. A multi-institutional study that prospectively compared 497 patients with renal masses ≤4.0 cm from 2009-2014 who chose either AS or primary intervention and found similar overall survival at 2 years that worsened for patients that chose AS at 5 years (AS vs PI; 2 years 96% vs 98%, 5 years 75% vs 92%, log rank, p = 0.06) but cancer-specific survival (CSS) was similar (AS vs PI; 5 years 100% vs 99%, p = 0.3) owing to the demographics of the AS cohort being older, had a worse Eastern Cooperative Oncology group score, more comorbidities, and smaller or multiple tumors.[38] As such, RMB may serve as a clinical tool by which patients can be risk stratified to more conservative management such as TA and AS. Indeed, a recent prospective multicenter trial showed an eightfold reduction in surgical extirpation of benign SRMs in patients who underwent a pretreatment biopsy (3% vs 23%).[47] Patients who underwent RMB were 6.7 times less likely to have a benign diagnosis at final pathology compared with patients who did not receive a biopsy. In addition, patients who underwent RMB were more likely to opt for AS (30%) based on their biopsy results. This is similar to another study by the above authors reporting 57% of patients who received RMB in an office setting went on to be managed with AS.[52] In addition, Dave and colleagues[65] reported a fourfold decrease in the likelihood of benign pathology after surgery in patients who had routine pretreatment RMB.

Another area where RMB may play a clinical role is before or during ablative therapy. TA has emerged as a viable option for SRMs especially those <3 cm in size. Recent metanalyses have shown comparable oncological outcomes of TA compared with PN (CSS; PN 100% vs TA 92%)

albeit with a slightly higher risk of local recurrence (risk ratio [RR] 0.55 confidence interval [CI] 0.33 to 0.91 in favor of PN).[66] TA by virtue of its nature causes tissue destruction precluding histological analysis; therefore, RMB before TA can guide management. For example, if benign histology then a patient may choose to forgo treatment and begin AS or if malignant histology then biopsy results may guide the intensity of surveillance or options for retreatment and/or systemic therapy if the disease recurs locally or at a distant site, respectively. In addition, there is emerging evidence regarding the efficacy of TA in various histologic RCC subtypes that may inform the intensity of thermal ablative treatment. Lay and colleagues[67] showed in 229 patients undergoing TA less favorable outcomes for ccRCC as opposed to papillary RCC due to differences in tumor vascularity. In patients with concurrent nonrenal malignancies, a positive RMB confirming metastatic disease to the kidney may also completely alter their management.

Finally, RMB may play a clinical role in patients with multiple or bilateral tumors such as patients with hereditary syndromes (eg, hereditary papillary RCC with type 1 pRCC and oncocytoma), or in patients with solitary or transplant kidneys to guide nephron sparing management options.

FUTURE DIRECTIONS

The ultimate utility of RMB lies in its ability to distinguish between benign and malignant renal masses that cannot be characterized by imaging alone. By allowing clinicians to adequately risk stratify patients, the morbidity and mortality associated with surgical management can be avoided. The current limitations of RMB including technical limitations, tumor heterogeneity, and histologic grade discordance hinder widespread adoption. However, as described above with refinement in technique and experience, the diagnostic accuracy and utility of RMB have been shown to be beneficial. Across the horizon, there are multiple advancements that are emerging to address these limitations. More recently, novel technologies have been used for image guidance in RMB. Liu and colleagues[68] evaluated Raman spectroscopy for differentiating ccRCC from oncocytoma in 63 patients who underwent partial/RN. A Raman spectroscope measures scattered photons after the area of interest is illuminated with a light beam. The authors reported an accuracy of 100% with a sensitivity of 91.8% and a specificity of 71.1% in differentiating ccRCC from oncocytoma. In addition, the technology was also able to distinguish between different RCC histologic subtypes with an accuracy of 93.4%. Similarly, OCT has been used to augment RMB. OCT relies on a beam of light with a single wavelength (coherent) which when passes through tissue is reflected and causes interference within the coherent light to create a phase difference. Wagstaff and colleagues[69] first evaluated the use of OCT in 40 renal mass biopsies. They reported a sensitivity of 86% and specificity of 75% in differentiating oncocytoma from RCC. Fiberoptic laser confocal microscopy for real-time optical diagnostic biopsy has also been developed.[70] Robotic technologies that are mainstream in the surgical management of kidney cancer are now being evaluated in robotic-assisted renal biopsy.[71] Noninvasive *liquid* biopsies have been developed to profile molecular and genomic markers of circulating tumor cells within the blood.[72,73] There is an increased interest in the identification of novel molecular and genomic markers that can improve the performance of RMB and predict the oncologic potential of tumors and differentiate benign from malignant disease. For example, a recent study showed that higher expression of hypoxia-inducible factor (HIF)-1α and carbonic anhydrase-9 (CA IX) were associated with higher-stage tumors, increased risk of recurrence, and tumor progression.[74] Similarly, immunohistochemistry has also been evolving. A study evaluating known tumor prognostic factors such as tumor grade, necrosis, and sarcomatoid/rhabdoid features with BRCA1-associated protein-1 (BAP1) status concluded that the presence of BAP1 on immunohistochemistry significantly correlated with higher pathologic stage.[50] DNA-methylation an early process in carcinogenesis has also been used as an assay to augment RMB. Using DNA-methylation probes, Chopra and colleagues[75] were able to predict malignancy and histologic subtype in 272 RMB specimens. Overall, in the age-increased detection of SRM numerous new imaging and targeting modalities plus the detection of novel molecular and genomic markers with liquid biopsies represents a new and exciting frontier in the management of SRMs.

SUMMARY

The incidence and prevalence of SRMs continues to rise and with increased detection comes increases in surgical management, although the probability of an SRM being benign is upward of 30%. An extirpative treatment first diagnose-later strategy persists and clinical tools for risk stratification such as RMB remain severely underutilized. The overtreatment of SRMs has multiple detrimental effects including surgical complications, psychosocial stress, financial loss, and reduced renal function leading to downstream effects such as the need for dialysis and cardiovascular disease. RMB is a safe and effective tool that is highly accurate in the diagnosis SRMs and can guide management. A collaborative multidisciplinary approach between specialties can improve the outcomes of RMB and lead to increased utilization of conservative management options such as . The current paradigm regarding RMB as promulgated by the current clinical guidelines is informed by low-level evidence or expert opinion and needs to be bolstered with high-quality studies. Pretreatment RMB for all renal masses should eventually become mainstream, especially with the development of new technologies and the adoption of novel genomic and molecular markers for the detection of kidney cancer, ushering in an age of individualized management of SRMs.

CLINICS CARE POINTS

- Renal mass biopsy should be routinely discussed and offered to patients with small renal masses (<4 cm) prior to management.

- A shared decision-making approach should be utilized after discussing the risks and benefits of RMB.

- At least 2-3 cores should be obtained for an adequate sampling of the mass. Fine needle aspiration (FNA) has been shown to be inferior to core biopsy.

- In general, cystic masses should not be biopsied unless there is a soft tissue component in order to reduce the risk of seeding and inadequate/non-diagnostic biopsy.

- Anti-coagulation and anti-platelet medications should be stopped prior to biopsy to reduce the risk of bleeding complications.

- Patients with a non-diagnostic biopsy should be offered repeat biopsy after discussing the risks and benefits of repeat RMB.

- RMB should be performed prior to or during tumor ablative therapies for risk stratification and pathologic diagnosis.

- RMB should be performed in patients suspected of having non renal pathology such as lymphoma, metastasis form non renal primary and infection.

- RMB should be performed in suspected metastatic renal cell carcinoma for risk stratification and assessing candidacy for systemic treatments and/or clinical trials.

REFERENCES

1. Capitanio U, Montorsi F. Renal cancer. Lancet 2016; 387(10021):894–906.
2. Turner RM 2nd, Morgan TM, Jacobs BL. Epidemiology of the small renal mass and the treatment disconnect phenomenon. Urol Clin North Am 2017;44(2):147–54.
3. Yang G, Villalta JD, Meng MV, et al. Evolving practice patterns for the management of small renal masses in the USA. BJU Int 2012;110(8):1156–61.
4. Patel AK, Lane BR, Chintalapati P, et al. Utilization of renal mass biopsy for T1 renal lesions across Michigan: results from MUSIC-KIDNEY, a statewide quality improvement collaborative. Eur Urol Open Sci 2021;30:37–43.
5. Johnson DC, Vukina J, Smith AB, et al. Preoperatively misclassified, surgically removed benign renal masses: a systematic review of surgical series and United States population level burden estimate. J Urol 2015;193(1):30–5.
6. Kutikov A, Fossett LK, Ramchandani P, et al. Incidence of benign pathologic findings at partial nephrectomy for solitary renal mass presumed to be renal cell carcinoma on preoperative imaging. Urology 2006;68(4):737–40.
7. Lee SH, Park SU, Rha KH, et al. Trends in the incidence of benign pathological lesions at partial nephrectomy for presumed renal cell carcinoma in renal masses on preoperative computed tomography imaging: a single institute experience with 290 consecutive patients. Int J Urol 2010;17(6):512–6.
8. Duchene DA, Lotan Y, Cadeddu JA, et al. Histopathology of surgically managed renal tumors: analysis of a contemporary series. Urology 2003;62(5):827–30.
9. Frank I, Blute ML, Cheville JC, et al. Solid renal tumors: an analysis of pathological features related to tumor size. J Urol 2003;170(6 Pt 1):2217–20.
10. Bhindi B, Thompson RH, Lohse CM, et al. The Probability of Aggressive Versus Indolent Histology Based on Renal Tumor Size: Implications for Surveillance and Treatment. Eur Urol 2018;74(4):489–97.
11. Rothman J, Egleston B, Wong YN, et al. Histopathological characteristics of localized renal cell carcinoma correlate with tumor size: a SEER analysis. J Urol 2009;181(1):29–33.
12. Palumbo C, Pecoraro A, Knipper S, et al. Contemporary Age-adjusted Incidence and Mortality Rates of Renal Cell Carcinoma: Analysis According to Gender, Race, Stage, Grade, and Histology. Eur Urol Focus 2021;7(3):644–52.
13. Campbell SC, Clark PE, Chang SS, et al. Renal Mass and Localized Renal Cancer: Evaluation, Management, and Follow-Up: AUA Guideline: Part I. J Urol 2021;206(2):199–208.
14. Nguyen MM, Gill IS, Ellison LM. The evolving presentation of renal carcinoma in the United States: trends from the Surveillance, Epidemiology, and End Results program. J Urol 2006;176(6 Pt 1):2397–400 [discussion: 2400].
15. Ljungberg B, Albiges L, Abu-Ghanem Y, et al. European Association of Urology Guidelines on Renal Cell Carcinoma: The 2022 Update. Eur Urol 2022;82(4):399–410.
16. Richard PO, Violette PD, Bhindi B, et al. Canadian Urological Association guideline: Management of small renal masses -. Full-text. Can Urol Assoc J 2022;16(2):E61–75.
17. Kunkle DA, Egleston BL, Uzzo RG. Excise, ablate or observe: the small renal mass dilemma–a meta-analysis and review. J Urol 2008;179(4):1227–33 [discussion: 1233-4].
18. Volpe A, Cadeddu JA, Cestari A, et al. Contemporary management of small renal masses. Eur Urol 2011;60(3):501–15.
19. Iversen P, Brun C. Aspiration biopsy of the kidney. Am J Med 1951;11(3):324–30.
20. Dechet CB, Zincke H, Sebo TJ, et al. Prospective analysis of computerized tomography and needle biopsy with permanent sectioning to determine the nature of solid renal masses in adults. J Urol 2003;169(1):71–4.
21. Herts BR, Baker ME. The current role of percutaneous biopsy in the evaluation of renal masses. Semin Urol Oncol 1995;13(4):254–61.
22. Silverman SG, Gan YU, Mortele KJ, et al. Renal masses in the adult patient: the role of percutaneous biopsy. Radiology 2006;240(1):6–22.
23. Mickisch G, Carballido J, Hellsten S, et al. Guidelines on renal cell cancer. Eur Urol 2001;40(3):252–5.
24. Khan AA, Shergill IS, Quereshi S, et al. Percutaneous needle biopsy for indeterminate renal masses: a national survey of UK consultant urologists. BMC Urol 2007;7(10).
25. Barwari K, de la Rosette JJ, Laguna MP. The penetration of renal mass biopsy in daily practice: a survey among urologists. J Endourol 2012;26(6):737–47.
26. Patel RM, Safiullah S, Okhunov Z, et al. Pretreatment Diagnosis of the Small Renal Mass: Status of Renal Biopsy in the United States of America. J Endourol 2018;32(9):884–90.
27. Mensel B, Kühn JP, Kracht F, et al. Prevalence of renal cysts and association with risk factors in a general population: an MRI-based study. Abdom Radiol (NY) 2018;43(11):3068–74.
28. Bosniak MA. The current radiological approach to renal cysts. Radiology 1986;158(1):1–10.
29. O'Malley RL, Godoy G, Hecht EM, et al. Bosniak Category IIF Designation and Surgery for Complex Renal Cysts. Journal of Urology 2009;182(3):1091–5.
30. Gabr AH, Gdor Y, Roberts WW, et al. Radiographic surveillance of minimally and moderately complex renal cysts. BJU International 2009;103(8):1116–9.

31. Silverman SG, Pedrosa I, Ellis JH, et al. Bosniak Classification of Cystic Renal Masses, Version 2019: An Update Proposal and Needs Assessment. Radiology 2019;292(2):475–88.

32. Moch H, Cubilla AL, Humphrey PA, et al. The 2016 WHO Classification of Tumours of the Urinary System and Male Genital Organs—Part A: Renal, Penile, and Testicular Tumours. European Urology 2016;70(1):93–105.

33. Lee-Felker SA, Felker ER, Tan N, et al. Qualitative and Quantitative MDCT Features for Differentiating Clear Cell Renal Cell Carcinoma From Other Solid Renal Cortical Masses. American Journal of Roentgenology 2014;203(5):W516–24.

34. Young JR, Coy H, Kim HJ, et al. Performance of Relative Enhancement on Multiphasic MRI for the Differentiation of Clear Cell Renal Cell Carcinoma (RCC) From Papillary and Chromophobe RCC Subtypes and Oncocytoma. AJR Am J Roentgenol 2017;208(4):812–9.

35. Hindman N, Ngo L, Genega EM, et al. Angiomyolipoma with minimal fat: can it be differentiated from clear cell renal cell carcinoma by using standard MR techniques? Radiology 2012;265(2):468–77.

36. Oliva MR, Glickman JN, Zou KH, et al. Renal Cell Carcinoma: T1 and T2 Signal Intensity Characteristics of Papillary and Clear Cell Types Correlated with Pathology. American Journal of Roentgenology 2009;192(6):1524–30.

37. King KG, Gulati M, Malhi H, et al. Quantitative assessment of solid renal masses by contrast-enhanced ultrasound with time-intensity curves: how we do it. Abdom Imaging 2015;40(7):2461–71.

38. Pierorazio PM, Johnson MH, Ball MW, et al. Five-year analysis of a multi-institutional prospective clinical trial of delayed intervention and surveillance for small renal masses: the DISSRM registry. Eur Urol 2015;68(3):408–15.

39. Pierorazio PM, Johnson MH, Patel HD, et al. Management of Renal Masses and Localized Renal Cancer: Systematic Review and Meta-Analysis. J Urol 2016;196(4):989–99.

40. National Comprehensive Cancer Network. Kidney Cancer (Version 1.2021). https://www.nccn.org/professionals/physician_gls/pdf/kidney.pdf. Accessed July 01, 2021.

41. Finelli A, Ismaila N, Bro B, et al. Management of Small Renal Masses: American Society of Clinical Oncology Clinical Practice Guideline. J Clin Oncol 2017;35(6):668–80.

42. Motzer RJ, Tannir NM, McDermott DF, et al. Nivolumab plus Ipilimumab versus Sunitinib in Advanced Renal-Cell Carcinoma. N Engl J Med 2018;378(14):1277–90.

43. Rini BI, Plimack ER, Stus V, et al. Pembrolizumab plus Axitinib versus Sunitinib for Advanced Renal-Cell Carcinoma. N Engl J Med 2019;380(12):1116–27.

44. Campbell SC, Novick AC, Herts B, et al. Prospective evaluation of fine needle aspiration of small, solid renal masses: accuracy and morbidity. Urology 1997;50(1):25–9.

45. Patel HD, Johnson MH, Pierorazio PM, et al. Diagnostic Accuracy and Risks of Biopsy in the Diagnosis of a Renal Mass Suspicious for Localized Renal Cell Carcinoma. Systematic Review of the Literature. J Urol 2016;195(5):1340–7.

46. Leveridge MJ, Finelli A, Kachura JR, et al. Outcomes of small renal mass needle core biopsy, nondiagnostic percutaneous biopsy, and the role of repeat biopsy. Eur Urol 2011;60(3):578–854.

47. Okhunov Z, Gorin MA, Jefferson FA, et al. Can preoperative renal mass biopsy change clinical practice and reduce surgical intervention for small renal masses? Urol Oncol 2021;39(10):735.

48. Marconi L, Dabestani S, Lam TB, et al. Systematic Review and Meta-analysis of Diagnostic Accuracy of Percutaneous Renal Tumour Biopsy. Eur Urol 2016;69(4):660–73.

49. Schmidbauer J, Remzi M, Memarsadeghi M, et al. Diagnostic accuracy of computed tomography-guided percutaneous biopsy of renal masses. Eur Urol 2008;53(5):1003–11.

50. Kapur P, Setoodeh S, Araj E, et al. Improving Renal Tumor Biopsy Prognostication With BAP1 Analyses. Arch Pathol Lab Med 2022;146(2):154–65.

51. Aminsharifi A, Polascik TJ. Renal mass biopsy: future trends and developments. In: Leveillee RJ, Jorda M, editors. Renal mass biopsy: indications, risks, technical aspects and future trends. Cham: Springer International Publishing; 2020. p. 195–207.

52. Jiang P, Arada RB, Okhunov Z, et al. Multidisciplinary Approach and Outcomes of Pretreatment Small (cT1a) Renal Mass Biopsy: Single-Center Experience. J Endourol 2022;36(5):703–11.

53. Dutta R, Okhunov Z, Vernez SL, et al. Cost Comparisons Between Different Techniques of Percutaneous Renal Biopsy for Small Renal Masses. J Endourol 2016;30(Suppl 1):S28–33.

54. Menhadji AD, Nguyen V, Okhunov Z, et al. Technique for office-based, ultrasonography-guided percutaneous biopsy of renal cortical neoplasms using a novel transducer for facilitated ultrasound targeting. BJU Int 2016;117(6):948–53.

55. Patel HD, Druskin SC, Rowe SP, et al. Surgical histopathology for suspected oncocytoma on renal mass biopsy: a systematic review and meta-analysis. BJU Int 2017;119(5):661–6.

56. Volpe A, Mattar K, Finelli A, et al. Contemporary results of percutaneous biopsy of 100 small renal masses: a single center experience. J Urol 2008;180(6):2333–7.

57. Brachemi S, Bollee G. Renal biopsy practice: what is the gold standard? World J Nephrol 2014;3(4):287–94.

58. Sainani NI, Tatli S, Anthony SG, et al. Successful percutaneous radiologic management of renal cell carcinoma tumor seeding caused by percutaneous biopsy performed before ablation. J Vasc Interv Radiol 2013;24(9):1404–8.

59. Andersen MF, Norus TP. Tumor Seeding With Renal Cell Carcinoma After Renal Biopsy. Urol Case Rep 2016;9(43–4).

60. Breau RH, Crispen PL, Jenkins SM, et al. Treatment of patients with small renal masses: a survey of the American Urological Association. J Urol 2011; 185(2):407–13.

61. Kutikov A, Egleston BL, Canter D, et al. Competing risks of death in patients with localized renal cell carcinoma: a comorbidity based model. J Urol 2012; 188(6):2077–83.

62. Patel HD, Pierorazio PM, Johnson MH, et al. Renal Functional Outcomes after Surgery, Ablation, and Active Surveillance of Localized Renal Tumors: A Systematic Review and Meta-Analysis. Clin J Am Soc Nephrol 2017;12(7):1057–69.

63. Lane BR, Abouassaly R, Gao T, et al. Active treatment of localized renal tumors may not impact overall survival in patients aged 75 years or older. Cancer 2010;116(13):3119–26.

64. Danzig MR, Ghandour RA, Chang P, et al. Active Surveillance is Superior to Radical Nephrectomy and Equivalent to Partial Nephrectomy for Preserving Renal Function in Patients with Small Renal Masses: Results from the DISSRM Registry. J Urol 2015;194(4):903–9.

65. Dave CN, Seifman B, Chennamsetty A, et al. Office-based Ultrasound-guided Renal Core Biopsy Is Safe and Efficacious in the Management of Small Renal Masses. Urology 2017;102:26–30.

66. Pierorazio PM, Johnson MH, Patel HD, et al. Management of Renal Masses and Localized Renal Cancer, 2016, Rockville (MD):Agency for Healthcare Research and Quality (US); 2016 Feb. Report No.: 16-EHC001-EF.

67. Lay AH, Faddegon S, Olweny EO, et al. Oncologic Efficacy of Radio Frequency Ablation for Small Renal Masses: Clear Cell vs Papillary Subtype. J Urol 2015;194(3):653–7.

68. Liu Y, Du Z, Zhang J, et al. Renal mass biopsy using Raman spectroscopy identifies malignant and benign renal tumors: potential for pre-operative diagnosis. Oncotarget 2017;8(22):36012–9.

69. Wagstaff PGK, Ingels A, de Bruin DM, et al. Percutaneous Needle Based Optical Coherence Tomography for the Differentiation of Renal Masses: a Pilot Cohort. J Urol 2016;195(5):1578–85.

70. Su LM, Kuo J, Allan RW, et al. Fiber-Optic Confocal Laser Endomicroscopy of Small Renal Masses: Toward Real-Time Optical Diagnostic Biopsy. J Urol 2016;195(2):486–92.

71. Bruyere F, Ayoub J, Arbeille P. Use of a telerobotic arm to perform ultrasound guidance during renal biopsy in transplant recipients: a preliminary study. J Endourol 2011;25(2):231–4.

72. Farber NJ, Kim CJ, Modi PK, et al. Renal cell carcinoma: the search for a reliable biomarker. Transl Cancer Res 2017;6(3):620–32.

73. Lakshminarayanan H, Rutishauser D, Schraml P, et al. Liquid Biopsies in Renal Cell Carcinoma-Recent Advances and Promising New Technologies for the Early Detection of Metastatic Disease. Front Oncol 2020;10(582843).

74. Papworth K, Sandlund J, Grankvist K, et al. Soluble carbonic anhydrase IX is not an independent prognostic factor in human renal cell carcinoma. Anticancer Res 2010;30(7):2953–7.

75. Chopra S, Liu J, Alemozaffar M, et al. Improving needle biopsy accuracy in small renal mass using tumor-specific DNA methylation markers. Oncotarget 2017;8(3):5439–48.

Cystic Renal Masses
Old and New Paradigms

Majed Alrumayyan, MD, Lucshman Raveendran, MD, MSc, Keith A. Lawson, MD, PhD,
Antonio Finelli, MD, MSc*

KEYWORDS

- Complex renal cysts • Bosniak • Renal biopsy • Renal cyst • Active surveillance • Surgery
- Small renal mass • Cystic renal masses

KEY POINTS

- Cystic renal masses are defined as masses containing less than 25% enhancing component. They are classified according to the Bosniak system, following characterization with cross-sectional, contrast-enhanced imaging.
- Biopsy of cystic renal masses should be performed only if the results would change patient management and when technically feasible (typically >1 cm solid component).
- Active surveillance is a feasible management option for Bosniak III and IV cysts, given their indolent nature relative to solid renal masses. However, given the limited long-term data, active surveillance should currently be reserved for patients who are not surgical candidates.

BACKGROUND

Cystic renal masses describe a spectrum of lesions with benign and/or malignant features. About 5% to 15% of renal tumors have a cystic component. The definition of a "cystic" renal mass is based on radiographic and/or pathologic findings. The cystic component of these masses ranges from 75% to 90%, with the updated Bosniak classification defining a cystic renal mass as containing less than 25% of enhancing tissue. A point of major discussion surrounding cystic renal masses is defining those lesions that are benign and those that require follow-up and treatment. Carefully delineating the characteristics of cystic renal masses has major implications for health systems including avoiding unnecessary cost, improving early detection and management, and reducing patient treatment morbidity. This article provides a contemporary update on the best practices and areas of controversy in cystic renal masses.

RADIOGRAPHIC DIAGNOSIS

The incidental radiographic identification of cystic renal masses has increased in parallel with solid renal masses, with clinical management largely dictated by radiologic features as defined by the Bosniak classification system first proposed by Morton Bosniak more than 30 years ago (**Table 1**).[7] It is currently validated for use in computed tomography (CT) and MRI.[1] Categories I and II are considered benign and do not require follow-up.[1] Category IIF requires follow-up and category III and IV are often malignant and undergo treatment.[1] In 2019, the Bosniak system underwent several updates that included separate criteria for MRI and CT.[7] Furthermore, greater clarity was given to described key features of cysts, with the goal of improving interrater reliability.[1] Thin-walled is now defined as less than 2 mm, minimally thick 3 mm, and thick greater than 4 mm. "Many" septations is defined as greater than or equal to four.[7]

Division of Urology, Department of Surgery, Princess Margaret Cancer Centre, University Health Network, Toronto, Ontario, Canada
* Corresponding author. Division of Urology, Department of Surgery, Princess Margaret Cancer Centre, University Health Network, 6-925, 700 University Avenue, Toronto, Ontario M5G 1X6, Canada.
E-mail address: Antonio.finelli@uhn.ca

Urol Clin N Am 50 (2023) 227–238
https://doi.org/10.1016/j.ucl.2023.01.003

Table 1
Bosniak classification

Bosniak Classification	Description	Malignant Potential	Recommended Management
I	They are thin-walled and nonenhancing, with -9 to 20 HU attenuation on unenhanced computed tomography, strong hyperintensity on T2-weighted MRI sequence, and hypodense on T1-weighted images.[1,2]	Extremely unlikely.[3]	No follow-up.[4]
II	Thin-walled with few, thin septa, which are minimally enhancing. Complicated renal cysts stemming from proteinaceous (20–40 HU, anechoic) or hemorrhagic (40–50 HU, complex) content <3 cm are included in this category.[1,2]	Pooled malignant rate <10%.[3,5,6]	No follow-up.[4]
IIF	Bosniak IIF cysts may have minimal thickening of their wall or septa with multiple septations. Those with perceptible enhancement of multiple septa and cysts >3 cm are included in this category. These lesions are heterogeneously hypertintense on T1-weighted imaging.[1,2]	Category IIF renal cysts are benign 75%–95% of the time.[3,5,6]	Imaging follow-up is required for surveillance. No specific consensus on sequence of follow-up.[4]
III	Lesions that have irregularly thick wall and septa, irregular enhancement.[1,2]	These lesions carry a 50% risk of malignant diagnosis on pathology.[3,5,6]	Definitive management or strict follow-up.[4]
IV	Enhancing nodularity.[1,2]	>85%.[3,5]	Definitive management.[4]

Greater specificity was given to differentiate a nodule from irregular thickening or confluent septa.[1] Nodules are defined as focal enhancing convex protrusions of any size that have acute margins with the wall or septa, or focal enhancing convex protrusions greater than or equal to 4 mm that have obtuse margins with the wall or septa.[1] The differentiation between "irregular thickening" (Bosniak III) and "nodule" (Bosniak IV) is intended to reduce the percentage of Bosniak IV masses that are benign.[1] Another major change has been the shift from measured to perceived enhancement, with quantitative thresholds for enhancement no longer recommended (eg, >20 Hounsfield units (HU), or >15% signal intensity on MRI). Enhancement may be permitted in Bosniak class I and II; however, depending on the precise features of the lesion that enhance (septa, nodules) the lesion may be staged higher. This classification scheme is intended for patients in general and not for those with an inherited renal cell carcinoma (RCC) syndrome.

Notably, the updated Bosniak classification suggests avoiding the terms "complicated" or "complex" cyst, given the lack of standardized definition of these terms.[1,8] As mentioned, cystic renal masses are those containing less than 25% enhancing tissue. The risk of malignancy according to the Bosniak 2019 version classification is 10% in Bosniak IIF, 50% to 60% in Bosniak III, and 85% in Bosniak IV. Similar rates of malignancy were described in a meta-analysis that showed

6% to 18% malignancy rate in Bosniak IIF, 51% to 55% in Bosniak III, and 89% to 91% in Bosniak IV cysts.[5]

In regard to first-line imaging modality as per the American College of Radiology for the evaluation of renal masses, CT is recommended.[9] Phases should include unenhanced, corticomedullary, and nephrogenic phases. Crucial to the evaluation of renal masses is the comparison of attenuation values in unenhanced and enhanced phases. Enhancing areas help differentiate solid components from hemorrhage or debris. Enhancement of at least 15 to 20 HU warrants further follow-up.[10] Dual-energy CT allows for more precise evaluation of heterogeneity within a lesion, because it uses two separate X-ray photon energy spectra, which are used to reconstruct detailed images.[11] Material decomposition refers to mapping or removing substances of known attenuation characteristics, such as iodine, calcium, or uric acid.[12] Pseudoenhancement may occur in small, more endophytic lesions that sit close to enhancing renal parenchyma. Reconstruction with better correction of beam hardening and iodine overlay images can mitigate the effects of pseudoenhancement.[13]

Ultrasound imaging in the diagnosis and surveillance of cystic renal masses is attractive because of the lack of radiation, accessibility, and low cost. However, several limitations must be acknowledged including the inability to reliably evaluate enhancement of septations, which may cause cystic renal masses to appear more complex on simple grey-scale ultrasound than CT or MRI.[14] Limitations may be partially mitigated by color/-power Doppler techniques. Contrast-enhanced ultrasound uses a small amount of contrast within gas-filled microbubbles to more precisely evaluate indeterminate cystic renal lesions by visualizing real-time blood flow.[15,16] This modality may be useful in those with renal insufficiency or allergy to contrast material. Disadvantages include operator dependency, large body habitus, and limitations in deep tumors.

MRI offers the ability to evaluate the contents of a cystic renal lesion more carefully with higher contrast resolution.[17] It is indicated in those with contraindications to CT (eg, patients with allergy to iodinated contrast agent) or to further interrogate equivocal findings on CT. For example, MRI can more clearly define septa that are difficult to appreciate on CT imaging.[18] Disadvantages include cost, limited accessibility, and poor image quality in those unable to suspend their respirations. Use of breath-holding MRI techniques, subtraction MRI with the use of gadolinium, and higher

resolution 3-T magnets can improve image quality.[19–21]

Renal mass biopsy (RMB) offers a histopathologic diagnosis that is critical in determining optimal next steps in managing a renal mass. RMB has been shown to facilitate active surveillance strategies for small renal masses and lead to cost savings for health systems.[22–24] Currently, the European Urology Association guidelines do not recommend RMB for cystic renal masses because of their low diagnostic yield, unless there is a clearly targetable solid component.[25]

In the American Urologic Association guidelines, RMB is recommended when the patient prefers active surveillance and if the risk-benefit analysis is equivocal. In the Canadian Urologic Association and European Urology Association guidelines, RMB is recommended if the results might change management. The diagnostic rate of RMB successfully targeting the mass ranges from 78% to 92%.[26,27] RMB of cystic masses was reported in several studies to have lower yield of diagnosis compared with small renal masses (sensitivity in small renal masses reaches up to 99% compared with a range of 33%–83% for cystic masses). If the solid part of the cystic mass can be targeted, the sensitivity increases to get an informative tissue pathology report. The difference in follow-up between small renal masses and cystic masses is that cystic masses can grow in size but with no morphologic changes that is described in the Bosniak classification, and in this case, it is considered to be stable with no indication to intervene.[28] A large retrospective study showed that the most common malignant pathology was clear cell RCC (ccRCC).[29] Another study by Sefik and colleagues showed that nodular Bosniak cysts had a higher chance to be malignant compared with nonnodular cysts.[30] Lastly, dissimilar to solid small renal masses, benign histologies, such as oncocytoma and fat poor angiomyolipoma, which can lead to treatment avoidance, are not in the differential diagnosis for cystic renal masses. Thus, the role of RMB is limited and not generally recommended.

PATHOLOGIC DIAGNOSIS AND OUTCOMES

Cystic renal masses may reflect distinct entities with inherent cystic architecture or other more common renal masses with cystic degeneration and necrosis of the primary solid component of the lesion (**Table 2**). Cystic changes can occur across various subtypes of RCC including clear cell, papillary, and chromophobe RCC. There also exists a more indolent subtype of cystic renal epithelial tumor called multilocular cystic renal

Table 2
Clinicopathologic characteristics of cystic renal masses

Lesion	Pathologic Characteristics	Imaging Characteristics	Outcomes
ccRCC (predominantly cystic)	Cited in recent literature as those ccRCC masses with at least 50% cystic component[31]	Mixed solid and cystic components on CT/MRI	Variable but overall improved survival and metastatic profile compared with conventional ccRCC[31]
Clear cell papillary RCC	Gross Well-circumscribed, encapculated, confined to the renal parenchyma without perinephric/vascular invasion or necrosis[32] Microscopic Low-grade nuclei (ISUP 1 or 2)[32] Clear cells arranged in tubules and papillae with linear alignment[32]	Imaging characteristics are highly variable, ranging from categories IIF to IV renal cysts	CCP RCC demonstrates excellent cancer-specific survival (100% at 10- and 20-y mark)[33]
Multilocular cystic renal neoplasm of low malignant potential	Gross Unilateral, typically <5 cm Cysts of various sizes with clear or hemorrhagic debris No significant nodularity[34,35] Microscopic ISUP grade 1–2 nuclear atypica Thin fibrous septa No expansile growth of tumor cells or nodules[34]	Imaging characteristics are highly variable, ranging from categories IIF to IV renal cysts	Excellent prognosis with no recurrences or metastases[36]
Mixed epithelial and stromal tumor	Gross Solitary with a mixture of solid and cystic areas Can protrude into the renal hilum[34] Cystic nephromas Minimal to no cystic components[34] Microscopic[16] Stromal cells typically positive for ER/ PR Stomal cells and epithelium with a wide spectrum of features Cystic nephromas Multilocular cysts lined by flat to cuboidal epithelium and	CT: Cystic with heterogeneous and delayed contrast enhancement of septations and solid components; most classified into Bosniak category III or IV[37] MRI: Cystic areas, T1 hypointensity and T2 hyperintensity; solid areas, T1 hyperintensity and T2 hypointensity[38] Cystic nephromas: US: anechoic with thin septations and rare calcifications, no vascularity CT: well circumscribed with multiple	Relatively benign Can undergo rare malignant transformation[,36]

(continued on next page)

Table 2
(continued)

Lesion	Pathologic Characteristics	Imaging Characteristics	Outcomes
	separated by fibrous septae[36]	septations and subtle enhancement[38]	
Tubulocystic RCC	Gross Well circumscribed tumor with spongy bubble wrap appearance[39] Microscopic[39] Cystic and tubular architecture; no solid areas, hemorrhage or necrosis Composed of tubules and cysts lined by a single layer of cells with prominent nucleoli (equivalent to ISUP/WHO grade 3) and abundant eosinophilic cytoplasm	MRI superior to CT; characterized by multilocular cystic lesions, Bosniak classification II-IV, with hypovascular septa[40] US pattern may exhibit high echogenicity and posterior acoustic enhancement[41]	Relatively indolent with <10% cases showing disease progression, local recurrence, or metastasis to bone, liver, and lymph nodes[39]
Acquired cystic disease-associated RCC	Gross Can be multifocal and bilateral[42] Microscopic Characterized by a "sieve-like" pattern and may contain oxalate crystal deposits Primarily ISUP grade 3 nuclei[42]	Mix radiologic presentation; can appear solid, cystic, or mixed[43]	Similar prognosis to ccRCC with exception of reduced risk of delayed recurrence[44,45]

Abbreviations: CCP, Clear cell papillary; ER, estrogen receptor; ISUP, International Society of Urological Pathology; PR, progesterone receptor; WHO, World Health Organization.

neoplasm of low malignant potential (MCNLMP), previously multilocular cystic RCC.

Multilocular cystic renal adenocarcinomas were first introduced in 1982 and were adopted as a subtype of ccRCC by the World Health Organization in 2004.[46] In 2012, The Vancouver International Society of Urological Pathology modification recommended referring to these lesions as MCNLMP.[47] It is a distinct subtype of RCC that carries an overall favorable prognosis.[48] It is linked with chromosome 3p deletions in 74% of cases and VHL mutations in 25%.[49] MCNLMP has been reported to comprise 1% to 2% of all renal tumors and about 10% of cystic tumors, although the true incidence could be higher because Bosniak I and II cysts usually do not undergo resection or follow-up.[50,51] Imaging characteristics are highly variable, ranging from categories IIF to IV renal cysts, and as such

these lesions are generally resected. Previous case series have demonstrated excellent disease-free survival with no recurrence at 5 years.[48,52,53] Cancer-specific survival is high regardless of grade, when diagnosed via strict criteria, as demonstrated in more recent case series.[48,52]

A recent systematic review of Bosniak II-IV cysts (n = 3000 total with n = 970 resections of Bosniak IIF-IV cysts) reported malignancy in 51% and 86% of resected Bosniak III and IV cysts, respectively. Of the 373 malignant cysts, there was minimal recurrence (1.35%) and metastasis (1%).[5] Based on these numbers, it was estimated that 1.9 Bosniak III cysts are needed to be treated to have one malignant diagnosis, but 140 Bosniak III cysts are needed to be treated to avoid one metastasis.[5] Two recent pathologic correlation studies of resected Bosniak IIF-IV cysts (270 in total) identified greater than 80% as being malignant.[5,44] The most common malignant tumors were ccRCC, papillary RCC type 1, papillary RCC type 2, with about 10% being MCNLMP.[5,44] Despite the high proportion of malignant characterization in these cohorts, long-term follow-up was extremely favorable, demonstrating only one cancer-specific death.[5,44]

The histopathology of MCNLMP shares parallels with conventional ccRCC with cystic changes, and as such these lesions are considered as existing along a spectrum of pathologic diagnosis. Post-nephrectomy analysis of long-term cystic ccRCC outcomes is favorable.[5,44,53–55] Those lesions with at least a 50% cystic component had a progression-free survival of 97.1% over 5 years, and a cohort with higher cystic cutoff component of greater than 75% had an overall survival of 100% at 10 years.[31,33,56] MCNLMP in these cohorts consistently demonstrate excellent prognosis, with no metastasis or disease-specific death noted in more than 200 patients.[31,33] Overall, cystic RCC behaves better than noncystic RCC, suggesting a spectrum with MCNLMP being at the most indolent end.

Another subtype of ccRCC are clear cell papillary RCCs, first described in those with acquired cystic renal disease and malignant transformation, now recognized as a spontaneous RCC entity.[47] They may present similarly to MCNLMP but have a characteristic cell nuclear arrangement and immunophenotype.[47] Pathologic analysis of cystic renal mass nephrectomies suggest that they may make up approximately 4% to 6% of overall masses fitting under the umbrella of ccRCC with cystic features.[33] Data from more than 300 cases of clear cell papillary RCCs have identified one case of metastasis leading to death with the lesion having undergone sarcomatoid change.[57]

Papillary and chromophobe RCC with cystic changes are potential findings on pathologic assessment of cystic renal masses undergoing resection. Papillary RCC is inherently less enhancing than ccRCC on imaging and is subject to pseudocystic changes, such as necrosis and hemorrhage.[58,59] A study of 138 papillary RCC lesions, correlating their radiologic and histopathologic outcomes, found that approximately 30% of these lesions presented with cystic features.[60] Of these, only two patients with cystic presentation had progression after surgery.[60] It is unclear if the cystic features found in these masses correlate with favorable prognosis as seen in cystic ccRCC, or if the solid components of the lesions are indolent by nature. Other cystic non-ccRCCs include acquired cystic disease–associated RCC, tubulocystic RCC, and fumarate hydratase–deficient RCC.

Mixed epithelial and stromal tumors appear as complex multiloculate cysts.[61] They are confined to the kidney and are sometimes seen bulging into the renal hilum.[62] These tumors are predominantly found in perimenopausal women.[61] They are well-defined, multiloculated cysts with mixed solid and cystic components.[61] A subset of mixed epithelial and stromal tumors are cystic nephromas that present as well-circumscribed, multicystic tumors with no apparent solid component.[61,63]

There are no randomized trials or long-term studies describing the natural history of malignant cystic renal masses. A study conducted by Chandrasekar and colleagues[44] included more than 300 patients showing that half of the IIF cysts eventually were classified as III, but Bosniak III cysts were rarely reclassified over time to category IV cysts. The increase in the fluid component and overall size of the cystic mass is not considered progression as long as the solid/nodular component remains stable. In this series more than 80% of the patients were followed with active surveillance and no surgical intervention.[44]

Active surveillance has been established as an accepted management strategy for small renal masses, but is not well described in cystic masses. During surveillance, the patients are usually followed with imaging and delayed intervention depending on the growth of the mass and patient preference. Surveillance of Bosniak III and IV should not be similar given the difference in the progression percentage and prevalence of cancer in each. A study by Tse and colleagues[64] that included 112 patients with Bosniak III and IV renal cysts showed that the linear growth rate for patients with Bosniak III cysts was 0 mm per year, whereas Bosniak IV cysts had an average growth rate of 2.2 mm per year. The study also showed that 24% of Bosniak III were upgraded to IV and 9% were downgraded from Bosniak IV to III. Solid renal masses have similar growth rates to Bosniak IV cysts, which is 2.5 mm per year. Another study showed that patients with small solid renal masses with high likelihood of clear cell histology showed a growth rate of 1.5 mm per year.[65] A large cohort of patients with small solid RCC proven by RMB were treated by active surveillance. The average rate of growth in that cohort was 8% per year (0.19 cm/y at 3 years follow-up) and was higher in ccRCC compared with other subtypes. It was also found that ccRCC had the highest progression and possible metastasis rate.[66]

Another study showed that the rate of growth of solid renal masses is higher in masses larger than 2 cm.[67] It was also reported that Bosniak IV cysts larger than 4 cm have a higher growth rate compared with lower categories. According to the guidelines for solid renal masses, large or fast-growing lesions usually show more aggressive nature of disease and pathology. Cystic masses are different because the nonenhancing part of the mass might grow, which does not change the risk of progression. Also, in cystic masses measuring the small enhancing part is challenging and can be missed. A study assessing progression for cystic renal masses showed that the median progression for Bosniak IV cysts was 710 days. Overtreating cystic masses was described in several studies. Half of Bosniak III cysts that were surgically resected showed benign pathology and those showing malignant pathology had low-grade cancer and low risk of metastasis.[67–69]

Multiple studies of small renal masses have demonstrated the relationship between size and risk of malignancy. In cystic masses, this relationship may be different because a retrospective study showed that small Bosniak III cysts were found to be malignant (although the size was smaller than 4 cm); however, they showed no progression/metastasis with follow-up of 3 years and also showed low grade of RCC. A clinical prediction model for Bosniak III cysts showed that small renal Bosniak III cysts can have a high rate of malignancy.[70]

Active surveillance in renal cystic masses, although not described as well as for for small renal masses, has been recommended for Bosniak IIF cysts given that most are benign (10% chance of malignancy). Bosniak IIF cysts mostly remain stable in size and may contract during follow-up. Active surveillance was also described for Bosniak III and IV renal cysts and showed that more than half of the patients had stability in size and/or experienced downgrading.[29] Multiple retrospective studies showed low risk of metastasis with cystic renal masses that have been followed.[5,6,69,71] A retrospective study that included more than 1000 patients followed for median of 65 months showed no progression in Bosniak III cysts masses.[72] Follow-up using imaging is similar to small renal masses, except for Bosniak IIF cysts, where the gap after the first follow-up can be yearly.[73] With the latest Bosniak 2019 classification MRI and CT achieve the same grading, but a study concluded that it was preferable to continue on the same imaging modality (CT or MRI) to have better comparison of images.[26,74,75] A cost-effective analysis study comparing active surveillance to nephron-sparing surgery in Bosniak IIF and III cysts showed that active surveillance is more effective given that the risk of progression and metastasis is low in IIF and III cysts.[73]

A study of long-term outcomes of renal cysts, which included Bosniak III and IV cysts, showed that both were associated with excellent disease-free survival; 92% at 5 years of follow-up. These percentages were within the ranges reported from other studies, which were between 83% and 98% after 5 years of follow-up.[54,73,76,77] Mortality was also reported in multiple retrospective studies and showed very low rates when patients with syndromes, such as von Hippel-Lindau, were excluded.[44,73]

Canadian urologists were surveyed to assess their approach in managing cystic renal masses.[78] One-third of Canadian urologists who responded to the survey managed half of Bosniak III cysts with active surveillance. Around 60% of urologists avoided active surveillance in Bosniak IV cysts with the reason being a lack of evidence for active surveillance and no clear guidelines on how to follow patients. Characteristics of the cysts also affected the decision of the physicians including the size and location of the tumor.[78]

The Canadian Urologic Association published guidelines for managing cystic renal lesions in 2017.[4] Bosniak I and II renal cysts do not need any follow-up because there is no risk of malignancy. For Bosniak IIF renal cysts, follow-up is recommended given that there is risk of malignancy and the suggested management is follow-up every 6 months in the first year and then yearly for 5 years, if no sign of progression is seen. Given the risk of malignancy for Bosniak III and IV cysts, surgical resection, including partial nephrectomy if feasible, is recommended. At that time there were no well-designed studies on active surveillance or thermal ablation. Thus, the Canadian guidelines suggested surveillance only for patients who are not candidates for surgery because of comorbidities and/or limited life expectancy. The role of RMB in the Canadian guidelines was suggested for Bosniak IV cysts in patients at high risk of perioperative morbidity or mortality. RMB was not suggested for Bosniak III cysts given the lack of solid elements and lower yield.[4]

In regards to the American Urologic Association guidelines published in 2021, active surveillance was listed as an option for small renal masses less than 2 cm, but it can also be offered for patients with Bosniak III and IV cysts for whom the risk and benefits analysis for treatment is equivocal. The guideline also suggests RMB of the solid component to identify the pathology with the intention to treat if progression was noted. Follow-up every 3 to 6 months with imaging to rule out progression was also recommended.[79]

FUTURE DIRECTIONS

There has been mounting evidence to suggest overdiagnosis and treatment of many incidentally detected tumors, including small renal masses and cystic renal masses. Guidelines continue to suggest treatment of Bosniak IV and most Bosniak III cysts. This is based on the higher likelihood of malignancy in these lesions but not necessarily metastatic potential. Based on retrospective and prospective series, many clinicians have adopted a more conservative approach to Bosniak III and IV cysts. Although a randomized controlled trial would be ideal, lack of clinical equipoise and long-term follow-up may preclude such studies from ever being conducted. In the absence of such efforts, one is left with weaker, albeit important data, to guide management.

Imaging is the cornerstone of cystic renal mass management. The Bosniak system is an excellent categorization based on clear imaging features that is reliable and generalizable. Cysts are common and thus, can pose a burden to health care systems. Artificial intelligence (AI) in medicine is rapidly evolving to develop algorithms that can aid health care practitioners in the diagnosis and treatment of multiple diseases. Radiomics is part of AI and through machine and deep learning has many applications to improving the management of cystic renal masses. Applying radiomics to detect and classify renal cysts without the need for review by a physician or radiologist could address this issue. This would be of particular benefit to Bosniak I and II cysts. In general, the Bosniak system has served well, particularly with categories I through III. The challenge with Bosniak IV cysts lies in the metastatic potential of the solid component. Furthermore, there is also a risk of necrotic solid tumor being misclassified as Bosniak IV cysts. Improved ability to discern necrotic tumors and dissemination of such knowledge is needed to ensure that patients are not undertreated because necrotic solid tumors have significantly higher metastatic potential. Emerging carbonic anhydrase 9–based PET scans using TLX250-CDx may aid in better resolving such lesions and warrant further investigation, particularly given the more limited role of RMB for cystic masses.[80]

The genomics of cystic renal masses may shed light on malignant and metastatic potential. Although large-scale genomics studies on solid renal masses have revealed several alterations with significant prognostic utility across the histologic spectrum of RCC,[81–83] data contextualizing these results to cystic renal masses are lacking. Given the aforementioned limited role of RMB for cystic renal masses, we anticipate liquid biopsy–based genomic biomarkers to provide the most translatable data to guide treatment decisions in this space and should be prioritized in future clinical trial settings.[84] Ultimately, a deeper understanding of the biology of cystic renal masses will best enable the ability to offer precision medicine approaches for patients that maximize efficacy while minimizing morbidity.

SUMMARY

Cystic renal masses are common and often incidentally detected. Many are benign, but the more complex lesions, especially those with solid components, have a high rate of malignancy. Diagnosis by imaging and classification with the Bosniak system have informed the management of such masses. CT scan has been the gold standard to characterize the features of the cysts in terms of the solid component and also the features of the cyst itself. RMB is not routinely recommended because of the high rate of malignancy in the solid/cystic lesions coupled with the higher nondiagnostic rate. Pathology of resected masses has shown multiple malignant subtypes including ccRCC (most common) and non-ccRCC in addition to other benign subtypes.

Surgical removal has been the standard of care, but ablation and surveillance are gaining traction. The natural history of cystic renal masses is similar to small solid renal masses, but the difference is that cysts may be greater than 4 cm with a discrete smaller solid component. The solid nodule may remain stable for years with increase only in the fluid part of the cyst. Active surveillance has been established well in solid renal masses and can also be applied in cystic RCC given the low risk of progression and metastasis that has been described. Multiple guidelines have been published to unify the approach toward all types of cysts and establish best practices for managing patients with cystic renal masses. Moving forward, it is anticipated that ongoing advancements in AI-driven radiomics coupled with novel liquid biopsy–based genetic biomarkers will continue to improve the ability to discern those patients requiring surgical intervention from those that can be safely managed with active surveillance.

CLINICS CARE POINTS

- The 2019 Bosniak classification system adds greater nuance and specificity to the evaluation of cystic renal masses - care should be taken by clinicians to adhere carefully to this updated framework.

- CT scan is the recommended first line imaging modality in the evaluation of renal masses. Contrast-enhanced ultrasound (CEUS) and MRI allow clinicians to effectively evaluate equivocal findings on CT imaging. CEUS is an effective modality to evaluate renal masses in those at risk of axial imaging with contrast.

- Renal mass biopsy is less effective in yielding tissue diagnosis in cystic renal masses, unless there is a clearly targetable solid component which can be operator and institution dependent. Tissue diagnosis can assist in determining possible active surveillance strategies.

- Adopting an active surveillance approach is a viable strategy for stratifying risk and determining optimal timing of management in cystic renal masses * Active surveillance of Bosniak IIF and III lesions is reasonable, given malignant rate of 10% and 50%, respectively, with the known low risk of progression and metastasis. * Bosniak IV cysts demonstrate growth rates similar to other clear cell RCC series and active surveillance can be an option in stable in size masses.

- Future directions in cystic renal masses include increasing uptake of active surveillance of Bosniak III and IV cysts, integration between radiomics and artificial intelligence to evaluate cystic lesions, and genomics to characterize the biology and malignant potential.

DISCLOSURE

The authors have no relevant conflict of interests to disclose.

ACKNOWLEDGMENTS

The authors thank Maria Komisarenko, Xiaoyu Zhang, and Dr Lisa Martin for their assistance with literature review and edits to this manuscript. Dr A. Finelli's research is supported by the Princess Margaret Cancer Foundation and the Anna-Liisa Farquharson Chair in Kidney Cancer Research.

REFERENCES

1. Silverman SG, Pedrosa I, Ellis JH, et al. Bosniak classification of cystic renal masses, version 2019: an update proposal and needs assessment. Radiology 2019;292(2):475–88.
2. Krishna S, Schieda N, Pedrosa I, et al. Update on MRI of cystic renal masses including Bosniak Version 2019. J Magn Reson Imaging 2021;54(2): 341–56.
3. Sevcenco S, Spick C, Helbich TH, et al. Malignancy rates and diagnostic performance of the Bosniak classification for the diagnosis of cystic renal lesions in computed tomography: a systematic review and meta-analysis. Eur Radiol 2016;27(6):2239–47.
4. Richard PO, Violette PD, Jewett MAS, et al. CUA guideline on the management of cystic renal lesions. Can Urol Assoc J 2017;11(3–4):66.
5. Schoots IG, Zaccai K, Hunink MG, et al. Bosniak Classification for Complex Renal Cysts reevaluated: a systematic review. J Urol 2017;198(1):12–21.
6. Smith AD, Remer EM, Cox KL, et al. Bosniak category IIF and III cystic renal lesions: outcomes and associations. Radiology 2012;262(1):152–60.
7. Bosniak MA. The current radiological approach to renal cysts. Radiology 1986;158(1):1–10.
8. Hartman DS, Choyke PL, Hartman MS. From the RSNA Refresher Courses: a practical approach to the cystic renal mass. Radiographics 2004; 24(suppl_1):S101–15.
9. Heilbrun ME, Remer EM, Casalino DD, et al. ACR Appropriateness Criteria Indeterminate Renal Mass. J Am Coll Radiol 2015;12(4):333–41.
10. Chawla SN, Crispen PL, Hanlon AL, et al. The natural history of observed enhancing renal masses: meta-analysis and review of the world literature. J Urol 2006;175(2):425–31.
11. Kaza RK, Platt JF, Cohan RH, et al. Dual-energy CT with single- and dual-source scanners: current applications in evaluating the genitourinary tract. Radiographics 2012;32(2):353–69.
12. Maki DD, Birnbaum BA, Chakraborty DP, et al. Renal cyst pseudoenhancement: beam-hardening effects on CT numbers. Radiology 1999;213(2):468–72.
13. Tappouni R, Kissane J, Sarwani N, et al. Pseudoenhancement of renal cysts: influence of lesion size, lesion location, slice thickness, and number of MDCT detectors. AJR Am J Roentgenol 2012; 198(1):133–7.
14. Siddaiah M, Krishna S, McInnes MDF, et al. Is ultrasound useful for further evaluation of homogeneously hyperattenuating renal lesions detected on CT? AJR Am J Roentgenol 2017;209(3):604–10.
15. Park BK, Kim B, Kim SH, et al. Assessment of cystic renal masses based on Bosniak classification: comparison of CT and contrast-enhanced US. Eur J Radiol 2007;61(2):310–4.
16. Herms E, Weirich G, Maurer T, et al. Ultrasound-based "CEUS-Bosniak" classification for cystic renal lesions: an 8-year clinical experience. World J Urol 2022. https://doi.org/10.1007/s00345-022-04094-0 [published online August 20.
17. Israel GM, Hindman N, Bosniak MA. Evaluation of cystic renal masses: comparison of CT and MR

imaging by using the Bosniak classification system. Radiology 2004;231(2):365–71.

18. Ferreira AM, Reis RB, Kajiwara PP, et al. MRI evaluation of complex renal cysts using the Bosniak classification: a comparison to CT. Abdom Radiol 2016; 41(10):2011–9.

19. Ramamurthy NK, Moosavi B, McInnes MDF, et al. Multiparametric MRI of solid renal masses: pearls and pitfalls. Clin Radiol 2015;70(3):304–16.

20. Wang H, Cheng L, Zhang X, et al. Renal cell carcinoma: diffusion-weighted MR imaging for subtype differentiation at 3.0 T. Radiology 2010;257(1): 135–43.

21. Rosenkrantz AB, Wehrli NE, Mussi TC, et al. Complex cystic renal masses: comparison of cyst complexity and Bosniak classification between 1.5T and 3T MRI. Eur J Radiol 2014;83(3):503–8.

22. Volpe A, Finelli A, Gill IS, et al. Rationale for percutaneous biopsy and histologic characterisation of renal tumours. Eur Urol 2012;62(3):491–504.

23. Herrera-Caceres JO, Finelli A, Jewett MAS. Renal tumor biopsy: indicators, technique, safety, accuracy results, and impact on treatment decision management. World J Urol 2018;37(3):437–43.

24. Richard PO, Jewett MAS, Bhatt JR, et al. Renal tumor biopsy for small renal masses: a single-center 13-year experience. Eur Urol 2015;68(6):1007–13.

25. Ljungberg B, Albiges L, Abu-Ghanem Y, et al. European Association of Urology Guidelines on Renal Cell Carcinoma: the 2019 update. Eur Urol 2019; 75(5):799–810.

26. Ma LX, Craig KM, Mosquera JM, et al. Contemporary results and clinical utility of renal mass biopsies in the setting of ablative therapy: a single center experience. Cancer Treat Res Commun 2020;25:100209.

27. Volpe A, Mattar K, Finelli A, et al. Contemporary results of percutaneous biopsy of 100 small renal masses: a single center experience. J Urol 2008; 180(6):2333–7.

28. Marconi L, Dabestani S, Lam TB, et al. Systematic review and meta-analysis of diagnostic accuracy of percutaneous renal tumour biopsy. Eur Urol 2016;69(4):660–73.

29. Luomala L, Rautiola J, Järvinen P, et al. Active surveillance versus initial surgery in the long-term management of Bosniak IIF–IV cystic renal masses. Sci Rep 2022;12(1).

30. Sefik E, Bozkurt IH, Adibelli ZH, et al. The histopathologic correlation of Bosniak 3 cyst subclassification. Urology 2019;129:126–31.

31. Westerman ME, Cheville JC, Lohse CM, et al. Long-term outcomes of patients with low grade cystic renal epithelial neoplasms. Urology 2019;133:145–50.

32. Williamson SR, Eble JN, Cheng L, et al. Clear cell papillary renal cell carcinoma: differential diagnosis and extended immunohistochemical profile. Mod Pathol 2013;26(5):697–708.

33. Zhou H, Zheng S, Truong LD, et al. Clear cell papillary renal cell carcinoma is the fourth most common histologic type of renal cell carcinoma in 290 consecutive nephrectomies for renal cell carcinoma. Hum Pathol 2014;45(1):59–64.

34. Epstein J, Netto GJ. Differential diagnoses in surgical pathology: genitourinary system. Philadelphia, PA: Lippincott Williams & Wilkins; 2021.

35. Murad T, Komaiko W, Oyasu R, et al. Multilocular cystic renal cell carcinoma. Am J Clin Pathol 1991; 95(5):633–7.

36. Montironi R, Mazzucchelli R, Lopez-Beltran A, et al. Cystic nephroma and mixed epithelial and stromal tumour of the kidney: opposite ends of the spectrum of the same entity? Eur Urol 2008;54(6):1237–46.

37. Sahni VA, Mortele KJ, Glickman J, et al. Mixed epithelial and stromal tumour of the kidney: imaging features. BJU Int 2010;105(7):932–9.

38. Adsay NV, Eble JN, Srigley JR, et al. Mixed epithelial and stromal tumor of the kidney. Am J Surg Pathol 2000;24(7):958–70.

39. Amin MB, MacLennan GT, Gupta R, et al. Tubulocystic carcinoma of the kidney: clinicopathologic analysis of 31 cases of a distinctive rare subtype of renal cell carcinoma. Am J Surg Pathol 2009;33(3): 384–92.

40. Honda Y, Nakamura Y, Goto K, et al. Tubulocystic renal cell carcinoma: a review of literature focused on radiological findings for differential diagnosis. Abdom Radiol 2018;43(7):1540–5.

41. Cornelis F, Hélénon O, Correas JM, et al. Tubulocystic renal cell carcinoma: a new radiological entity. Eur Radiol 2015;26(4):1108–15.

42. Kuroda N, Ohe C, Mikami S, et al. Review of acquired cystic disease-associated renal cell carcinoma with focus on pathobiological aspects. Histol Histopathol 2011;26(9):1215–8.

43. Berkenblit R, Ricci Z, Kanmaniraja D, et al. CT features of acquired cystic kidney disease-associated renal cell carcinoma. Clin Imaging 2022;83:83–6.

44. Chandrasekar T, Ahmad AE, Fadaak K, et al. Natural history of complex renal cysts: clinical evidence supporting active surveillance. J Urol 2018;199(3): 633–40.

45. Kondo T, Sassa N, Yamada H, et al. Comparable survival outcome between acquired cystic disease associated renal cell carcinoma and clear cell carcinoma in patients with end-stage renal disease: a multi-institutional central pathology study. Pathology 2021;53(6):720–7.

46. Halat SK, MacLennan GT. Multilocular cystic renal cell carcinoma. J Urol 2007;177(1):343.

47. Srigley JR, Delahunt B, Eble JN, et al. The International Society of Urological Pathology (ISUP) Vancouver Classification of Renal Neoplasia. Am J Surg Pathol 2013;37(10):1469–89.

48. Suzigan S, López-Beltrán A, Montironi R, et al. Multi-locular cystic renal cell carcinoma. Am J Clin Pathol 2006;125(2):217–22.

49. Rechsteiner MP, von Teichman A, Nowicka A, et al. VHL gene mutations and their effects on hypoxia inducible factor HIF: identification of potential driver and passenger mutations. Cancer Res 2011;71(16): 5500–11.

50. Nassir A, Jollimore J, Gupta R, et al. Multilocular cystic renal cell carcinoma: a series of 12 cases and review of the literature. Urology 2002;60(3): 421–7.

51. Wahal SP, Mardi K. Multilocular cystic renal cell carcinoma: a rare entity with review of literature. J Lab Physicians 2014;6(01):050–2.

52. Bhatt JR, Jewett MAS, Richard PO, et al. Multilocular cystic renal cell carcinoma: pathological T staging makes no difference to favorable outcomes and should be reclassified. J Urol 2016;196(5):1350–5.

53. Webster WS, Thompson RH, Cheville JC, et al. Surgical resection provides excellent outcomes for patients with cystic clear cell renal cell carcinoma. Urology 2007;70(5):900–4.

54. Boissier R, Ouzaid I, Nouhud FX, et al. Long-term oncological outcomes of cystic renal cell carcinoma according to the Bosniak classification. Int Urol Nephrol 2019;51(6):951–8.

55. Kashan M, Ghanaat M, Hötker AM, et al. Cystic renal cell carcinoma: a report on outcomes of surgery and active surveillance in patients retrospectively identified on pretreatment imaging. J Urol 2018;200(2): 275–82.

56. Tretiakova M, Mehta V, Kocherginsky M, et al. Predominantly cystic clear cell renal cell carcinoma and multilocular cystic renal neoplasm of low malignant potential form a low-grade spectrum. Virchows Arch 2018;473(1):85–93.

57. Diolombi ML, Cheng L, Argani P, et al. Do clear cell papillary renal cell carcinomas have malignant potential? Am J Surg Pathol 2015;39(12):1621–34.

58. Couvidat C, Eiss D, Verkarre V, et al. Renal papillary carcinoma: CT and MRI features. Diagn Interv Imaging 2014;95(11):1055–63.

59. Egbert ND, Caoili EM, Cohan RH, et al. Differentiation of papillary renal cell carcinoma subtypes on CT and MRI. AJR Am J Roentgenol 2013;201(2): 347–55.

60. Procházková K, Mírka H, Trávníček I, et al. Cystic appearance on imaging methods (Bosniak III-IV) in histologically confirmed papillary renal cell carcinoma is mainly characteristic of papillary renal cell carcinoma type 1 and might predict a relatively indolent behavior of papillary renal cell carcinoma. Urol Int 2018;101(4):409–16.

61. Lane BR, Campbell SC, Remer EM, et al. Adult cystic nephroma and mixed epithelial and stromal tumor of the kidney: clinical, radiographic, and pathologic characteristics. Urology 2008;71(6):1142–8.

62. Chu LC, Hruban RH, Horton KM, et al. Mixed epithelial and stromal tumor of the kidney: radiologic-pathologic correlation. Radiographics 2010;30(6): 1541–51.

63. Caliò A, Eble JN, Grignon DJ, et al. Cystic nephroma in adults. Am J Surg Pathol 2016;40(12):1591–600.

64. Tse JR, Shen J, Shen L, et al. Bosniak Classification of Cystic Renal Masses Version 2019: comparison of categorization using CT and MRI. AJR Am J Roentgenol 2021;216(2):412–20.

65. Rasmussen RG, Xi Y, Sibley RC, et al. Association of clear cell likelihood score on MRI and growth kinetics of small solid renal masses on active surveillance. AJR Am J Roentgenol 2022;218(1):101–10.

66. Finelli A, Cheung DC, Al-Matar A, et al. Small renal mass surveillance: histology-specific growth rates in a biopsy-characterized cohort. Eur Urol 2020; 78(3):460–7.

67. Mason RJ, Abdolell M, Trottier G, et al. Growth kinetics of renal masses: analysis of a prospective cohort of patients undergoing active surveillance. Eur Urol 2011;59(5):863–7.

68. Crispen PL, Viterbo R, Boorjian SA, et al. Natural history, growth kinetics, and outcomes of untreated clinically localized renal tumors under active surveillance. Cancer 2009;115(13):2844–52.

69. Bhindi B, Thompson RH, Lohse CM, et al. The probability of aggressive versus indolent histology based on renal tumor size: implications for surveillance and treatment. Eur Urol 2018;74(4):489–97.

70. Goenka AH, Remer EM, Smith AD, et al. Development of a clinical prediction model for assessment of malignancy risk in Bosniak III renal lesions. Urology 2013;82(3):630–5.

71. Mousessian PN, Yamauchi FI, Mussi TC, et al. Malignancy rate, histologic grade, and progression of Bosniak category III and IV complex renal cystic lesions. AJR Am J Roentgenol 2017;209(6):1285–90.

72. Smith AD, Allen BC, Sanyal R, et al. Outcomes and complications related to the management of Bosniak cystic renal lesions. AJR Am J Roentgenol 2015; 204(5):W550–6.

73. Smith AD, Carson JD, Sirous R, et al. Active surveillance versus nephron-sparing surgery for a Bosniak IIF or III renal cyst: a cost-effectiveness analysis. AJR Am J Roentgenol 2019;212(4):830–8.

74. Miskin N, Qin L, Matalon SA, et al. Stratification of cystic renal masses into benign and potentially malignant: applying machine learning to the Bosniak classification. Abdom Radiol 2020;46(1):311–8.

75. Choyke PL. The Bosniak classification gets even better. Radiology 2020;297(3):606–7.

76. Winters BR, Gore JL, Holt SK, et al. Cystic renal cell carcinoma carries an excellent prognosis regardless of tumor size. Urol Oncol 2015;33(12):505. e9-e13.

77. Donin NM, Mohan S, Pham H, et al. Clinicopathologic outcomes of cystic renal cell carcinoma. Clin Genitourin Cancer 2015;13(1):67–70.

78. Couture F, Finelli A, Tétu A, et al. Management of complex renal cysts in Canada: results of a survey study. BMC Urol 2020;20(1). https://doi.org/10.1186/s12894-020-00614-5.

79. Campbell SC, Uzzo RG, Karam JA, et al. Renal mass and localized renal cancer: evaluation, management, and follow-up: AUA Guideline: Part II. J Urol 2021;206(2):209–18.

80. 89Zr-TLX250 for PET/CT Imaging of ccRCC – ZIRCON Study. Clinical Trials.gov identifier: NCT03849118. Available at: https://clinicaltrials.gov/ct2/show/NCT03849118. Updated November 10, 2022. Accessed November 28, 2022.

81. Ricketts CJ, De Cubas AA, Fan H, et al. The Cancer Genome Atlas Comprehensive Molecular Characterization of Renal Cell Carcinoma. Cell Rep 2018; 23(1):313–26. e5.

82. Turajlic S, Xu H, Litchfield K, et al. Tracking cancer evolution reveals constrained routes to metastases: TRACERx Renal. Cell 2018;173(3):581–94. e12.

83. Turajlic S, Xu H, Litchfield K, et al. Deterministic evolutionary trajectories influence primary tumor growth: TRACERx Renal. Cell 2018;173(3): 595–610. e11.

84. Nuzzo PV, Berchuck JE, Korthauer K, et al. Detection of renal cell carcinoma using plasma and urine cell-free DNA methylomes. Nat Med 2020;26(7): 1041–3.

Long-Term Renal Function Following Renal Cancer Surgery
Historical Perspectives, Current Status, and Future Considerations

Andrew M. Wood, MD, MS*, Tarik Benidir, MD, MSc,
Rebecca A. Campbell, MD, Nityam Rathi, BS, Robert Abouassaly, MD,
Christopher J. Weight, MD, Steven C. Campbell, MD, PhD

KEYWORDS

- Radical nephrectomy • Partial nephrectomy • Kidney function • Cancer surgery • Kidney Cancer

KEY POINTS

- PN is now preferred for most patients with localized renal masses due to better functional outcomes, although whether this translates to better overall survival in patients with a normal contralateral kidney remains controversial.
- Parenchymal volume preserved is the primary determinant of functional recovery after PN.
- Ischemia time correlates with functional recovery although primarily as a confounder. Most nephrons recover from prolonged cold ischemia or limited durations (<25-30 minutes) warm ischemia.
- The reconstructive phase of PN is most important with respect to nephron-mass preservation and functional recovery.
- Controversies remain, including appropriate patient selection for zero-ischemia PN and the duration of warm ischemia at which irreversible ischemic injury begins to occur.

SUBCHAPTER 1: INTRODUCTION AND DEFINITIONS

According to the American Cancer Society, kidney cancer remains the seventh most common solid organ malignancy, and accounts for the 10th most deaths nationwide.[1] Fortunately, advances in cross-sectional imaging have resulted in a clinical environment in which over two-thirds of cases are diagnosed while still localized.[2] Historically, radical nephrectomy (RN) was regarded as the reference standard for the treatment of patients with localized kidney cancer, whereas partial nephrectomy (PN) was traditionally reserved for patients for whom RN would result in imminent dialysis. At the turn of the millennium however, an increased appreciation of the importance of chronic kidney disease (CKD) on long-term survival and health outcomes prompted urologists to rethink the importance of nephron-sparing surgery.

A landmark study published in the *New England Journal of Medicine* in 2004 highlighted the effects of mild/moderate CKD on long-term health outcomes. Evaluating more than a million patients in a population-based study, the authors reported an association between an increasing degree of CKD and increased rates of cardiovascular events, hospitalization, and mortality.[3] This naturally led some to question the importance of CKD following renal cancer surgery. In 2004, Huang reported that the rate of new-onset CKD within 3 years after

Glickman Urological and Kidney Institute, Cleveland Clinic Foundation, Q Building - Glickman Tower, 2050 East 96th Street, Cleveland, OH 44195, USA
* Corresponding author.
E-mail address: wooda10@ccf.org

Urol Clin N Am 50 (2023) 239–259
https://doi.org/10.1016/j.ucl.2023.01.004

extirpative surgery was over threefold higher following RN (65%) than PN (20%), and other studies confirmed these findings.[4,5]

As awareness has increased regarding the importance of avoiding CKD, both short- and long-term renal function preservation have become increasingly important goals for Urologists. Combined with a realization that for most small renal masses (SRMs) PN provides equivalent oncologic outcomes to RN, nephron-sparing approaches have become the mainstay of SRM management. Recognizing this change within the field, the last two iterations of the American Urologic Association's guidelines on localized renal cancer have focused on the importance of preservation of renal function, estimation of preoperative glomerular filtration rate (GFR)/CKD stage, and restriction of RN to patients meeting strict criteria for which RN is likely more beneficial.[6,7] In addition to decisions about PN/RN, recent research has focused on other techniques to preserve both short- and long-term renal function following PN. Factors such as type and duration of ischemia, degree of parenchymal-volume-loss, renorrhaphy technique, and method of resection all play a role in determining functional outcomes after renal cancer surgery. In discussing how each of these factors impacts renal function, it is important to define parameters for how renal function changes over time after surgery (**Table 1**).

Immediately following PN, kidney function is almost always affected, at least to some degree, by acute kidney injury (AKI). By definition, AKI is a transitory decline in renal function resulting from temporary insult(s) to nephrons. In the case of AKI after PN, insults such as warm or cold ischemia, abdominal insufflation, or intraoperative fluid shifts can result in transitory increases in serum creatinine levels for a few to several days after surgery. After AKI has resolved, renal function improves before stabilizing at the new-baseline GFR (NBGFR). Most studies have defined NBGFR as the GFR measured 1 to 12 months after surgery, providing a full 30 days for the preserved nephrons to recover. There is strong evidence that renal function remains stable during this time period in most patients.[8–10] Finally, long-term GFR (LTGFR) indicates renal function measured 3 to 20 years after surgery and is determined by a combination of the effects of renal cancer surgery and long-term exposure of the remaining nephrons to medical comorbidities, along with natural decline related to aging, which averages approximately 0.8 mL/min/1.73 m^2 per year after age 40.[11]

Despite the increased academic attention to the patterns and predictors of renal function following surgery, significant questions remain about best practices in the field. First, the concept that improved renal function after PN necessarily results in improved overall-survival remains in dispute.[12,13] Relatedly, the hypothesis that CKD primarily due to surgical intervention has the same implications as CKD due to medical comorbidities has come into question.[8,14] In addition, substantial evidence is emerging that duration of warm ischemia during PN may be less influential on NBGFR than previously thought.[15,16] These controversies can affect both preoperative and intraoperative management and deserve careful consideration by any Urologist performing surgery for localized kidney cancer. In this article, we review past and current evidence regarding these controversies, and provide an update on recent advances in the field.

SUBCHAPTER 2: PARTIAL VERSUS RADICAL NEPHRECTOMY

Before the 1990s, nephron-sparing surgery was employed selectively by the Urology community primarily for imperative indications. Concerns over PN centered around two major issues: lack of confidence regarding cancer control, and uncertainty regarding increased perioperative complication rates (mostly bleeding) and ambiguous management strategies for those complications. Attitudes began to shift in the early 2000s when multiple studies were published demonstrating impressive recurrence-free survival rates with PN in appropriately selected patients.[17,18] Combined with increased surgeon experience with PN and the realization of acceptably low complication rates even in patients with cT2 renal masses,[19] PN began to achieve greater acceptance. In 2009, the AUA guidelines codified this shift by defining PN as the reference standard for T1a renal masses.[20] Since then, various academic centers have continued to expand the utilization of PN into larger and more complex renal masses while still maintaining low perioperative complications and strong oncologic outcomes.[19,21] Despite this paradigm shift, a fundamental question remains. In a healthy patient with a normal contralateral kidney, does a nephron-sparing approach really result in improved overall survival?

With the field transitioning toward PN, a flurry of retrospective studies were published demonstrating improved renal functional outcomes, equivalent oncologic outcomes, and improved overall survival with PN versus RN (**Table 2**). However, given the substantial residual comfort with RN and remaining anxiety over the appropriateness of PN, comparative studies during this time were almost perfectly set up for significant

Table 1
Definitions related to functional recovery after kidney cancer surgery

Term	Definition
Baseline GFR	Renal function before any procedure for kidney cancer. Primarily determined by age and medical comorbidities.
Acute kidney injury (AKI)	Functional decline in the early days following PN/RN. Defined by serum creatinine levels because GFR cannot be determined until steady state is realized, typically several days later.
New baseline GFR (NBGFR)	GFR 1 to 12 mo following PN/RN, after AKI has resolved. Renal function tends to remain stable throughout this time period.
Long-term GFR (LTGFR)	Determined by NBGFR after PN/RN plus changes in function over time secondary to patient comorbidities, other surgeries or insults, and the aging process.

selection bias. The problems with these observational studies are best demonstrated by the meta-analysis published by Kim and colleagues.[22] Synthesizing over 40,000 patients from 36 retrospective studies, Kim demonstrated an impressive 19% relative risk reduction in all-cause mortality for those undergoing PN versus RN. Most telling however was that they also demonstrated a 29% improvement in cancer-specific mortality for those undergoing PN. Given the inherent differences between PN and RN, with RN more closely approximating the classic tenets of surgical oncology, the only plausible explanation for improved oncologic outcomes with PN was substantial and systemic selection bias inherent in the included studies. During the same time period, several studies were published that attempted to use statistical techniques to correct for inherent selection bias. Using propensity scores to account for measurable and identifiable sources of bias, these studies again demonstrated improved overall survival with PN.[23,24] However, unmeasured selection bias remained a concern.

In this setting, a randomized controlled trial (RCT) is required, and there was such a trial in this domain, namely EORTC-30904, published in 2011 and updated in 2014.[26,27] The inclusion criteria of the study included a single, localized tumor ≤5 cm with a normal contralateral kidney. Patients were randomized 1:1 to PN or RN. Surprisingly, despite the expected improvement in functional outcomes, PN did not demonstrate improved 10-year overall survival (81% for RN vs 76% for PN). Follow-up analysis 3 years later again did not demonstrate an overall-survival advantage for PN.[26] Despite methodological flaws including

being underpowered secondary to poor accrual and allowing crossover between treatment arms (15% of PN subjects had RN), the results of EORTC-30904 reopened the debate regarding PN versus RN. A school of thought began to emerge that CKD caused primarily by surgery (CKD-S) might be less impactful on survival than CKD caused by medical comorbidities (CKD-M) or a combination of comorbidities and surgery (CKD-M/S).

Lane and colleagues[28] attempted to address this question with a large retrospective study comparing patients with preexisting CKD who underwent renal surgery (CKD-M/S) to those with postoperative CKD resulting from surgery alone (CKD-S). These groups were compared with a third group who did not develop CKD even after surgery. Renal function was compared between these three groups longitudinally (median follow-up 6.6 years). Notably, annual GFR decline was substantially increased for CKD-M/S versus CKD-S (4.7% vs 0.7%, $P < .05$), and this was linked to survival, as an average annual decline greater than 4.0% was associated with a 43% increase in all-cause mortality. In the follow-up study 2 years later, the CKD-M/S group had the highest rates of both nonrenal cancer-related mortality and all-cause mortality on multivariate analysis.[8] These studies helped to clarify the role that the etiology of CKD plays in long-term survival outcomes. Patients with medical comorbidities that have impacted their GFR before surgery will continue to experience the deleterious effects of these comorbidities, their GFR will continue to fall, and they will experience compromised cardiovascular health and reduced survival. In contrast,

Table 2
Select studies regarding partial versus radical nephrectomy

Study	Design	Outcomes	Findings	Limitations/Perspective
Retrospective studies comparing PN versus RN				
Kim et al,[22] 2012	Meta-analysis of 36 studies	ACM, CSM, CKD	PN associated with 19% relative risk reduction for ACM, 29% reduction for CSM, 61% reduction for CKD incidence	It is very likely that improved CSM in PN cohort represents selection bias
Tan et al,[23] 2012	SEER-Medicare study of patients with cT1a renal tumors, instrumental variable approach	OS CSS	Improved OS with PN. No difference in CSS between PN and RN	Instrumental variable approach, population database study means it is not possible to fully control for confounders
Weight et al,[24] 2010	Retrospective study using propensity scoring to account for bias in cT1b patients	OS, CSS, cardiac specific survival	PN and RN had equivalent CSS (94% vs 89%). Postop CKD, often related to RN, was an independent predictor of OS and cardiac-specific survival	Retrospective, single-center, propensity scoring cannot account for unrecognized confounders
Gershman et al,[25] 2018	Retrospective review of PN or RN in >2400 patients with cT1 renal masses using propensity scoring	ACM, CSM, OCM, drop in GFR >10%, incidence of GFR <45	RN associated with increased risk of CKD10% (HR 2.07 to 2.21; $P <.001$) and CKD<45 (HR 2.70 to 2.99; $P < .001$). No difference in OCM, CSM, ACM	Retrospective, single-center study
Randomized trial comparing PN versus RN				
Van Poppel et al,[26] 2011; Scosyrev et al,[27] 2013 (EORTC 30904)	Randomized trial of PN vs RN for <5 cm renal masses with normal contralateral kidney	OS, CKD	10 y OS favors RN vs PN (81% vs 75%, HR 1.5, $P = .03$) Median follow-up of 6.7 y RN vs PN, eGFR<60: 86% vs 64% RN vs PN, eGFR <30:10% vs 6.3% RN vs PN, eGFR <15: 1.5% vs1.6%	Underpowered secondary to poor accrual. Significant percent of PN arm crossed over to RN (15%). Despite limitations, called into question survival advantage from PN.

Impact of CKD due to surgical nephron loss (CKD-S) vs medical nephron loss (CKD-M)

Study	Description	Outcomes	Results	Perspective
Lane et al,[28] 2013	Large cohort study of RN and PN	Annual renal function decline, ACM	Annual renal function decline was 4.7% for CKD-M and 0.7% for CKD-S. Annual renal function decline >4% is associated with a 43% increase in mortality ($P <$ .0001).	Single tertiary center, retrospective study. Perspective: CKD-M with decreased survival and less stable renal function. CKD-S decline of function is similar to the normal aging process.
Capitanio et al,[29] 2015	Multicenter series of 1189 patients undergoing RN and PN	CKD and OCM	PN is associated with a lower risk of CKD, but no significant difference in other-cause mortality (HR 0.8, CI 0.67 to 1.40)	Retrospective study. Perspective: Improved renal function preservation for PN but again no survival benefit
Lane et al,[8] 2015	Large cohort study of RN and PN with longer-term follow-up	NBGFR, ACM, nonrenal cancer mortality	CKD-M/S is associated with increased GFR decline, all-cause mortality, and nonrenal cancer mortality. CKD-S survival and stability of renal function similar to no CKD cohort	Tertiary center retrospective study, Perspective: CKD-S has Improved prognosis vs CKD M/S especially if new baseline GFR is >45 mL/min/1.73 m²

Collaborative review of literature comparing PN vs RN

Study	Description	Outcomes	Results	Perspective
Kim et al,[5] 2017	Critical review of the literature comparing PN and RN outcomes for complex tumors	Risks and benefits of PN over RN	For anatomically complex tumors, PN preserves more renal parenchyma, although it has increased perioperative risk. RCT needed to draw definitive conclusions.	Analysis of retrospective studies with selection bias and a single flawed randomized clinical trial. Perspective: Available literature is unable to establish the superiority of PN over RN

Abbreviations: ACM, all-cause mortality; CKD, chronic kidney disease; CKD-M, chronic kidney disease due to medical diseases; CKD-S, chronic kidney disease primarily due to surgical removal of nephrons; CSS, cancer-specific mortality; CSS, cancer-specific survival; eGFR, estimated glomerular filtration rate; GFR, glomerular filtration rate; HR, hazard ratio; MFS, metastasis-free survival; NBGFR, new baseline glomerular filtration rate; OCM, other cause mortality; OS, overall survival; PN, partial nephrectomy; RN, radical nephrectomy; SEER, surveillance, epidemiology, and end results.

for patients with CKD-S the primary driver for developing CKD was the renal surgery, which is most often a one-time event, so their GFR can stabilize and long-term survival is typically not impacted.

As it was appreciated that the interplay between renal cancer surgery, functional outcomes, and overall survival was less clear than previously assumed, multiple studies have recently attempted to create models to predict overall and non-renal cancer-related survival.[29–31] Zabell and colleagues[30] analyzed over 4000 patients undergoing renal cancer surgery with 10-year median follow-up to predict 10-year non-renal cancer-related mortality. Factors such as age, sex, comorbidities, preoperative GFR, and NBGFR were incorporated, yet the analysis was agnostic to management with PN versus RN. Preoperative GFR strongly reflects general health, as shown by the population-based studies discussed earlier, and it, along with age, were the strongest predictors of non-renal cancer-related mortality, whereas NBGFR failed to correlate on multivariable analysis. The models demonstrated that there was relatively little absolute difference in 10-year overall survival (1% to 3%) between patients experiencing 10% loss of renal function with surgery (prototypical PN) versus those experiencing 40% loss of function (prototypical RN). A subsequent multicenter study of patients without preoperative CKD by Capitanio and colleagues[29] demonstrated that despite decreased rates of new-onset CKD in patients undergoing PN, there was no difference in other cause mortality at 10 to 15 years follow-up, and other recent studies have also supported this.

The clearest explanation for these findings is that preoperative GFR strongly reflects health status, and there is a level of NBGFR above which the deleterious effects of CKD on overall survival are less significant. For example, if a healthy patient with preoperative GFR of 80 mL/min/1.73 m^2 undergoes PN (predicted NBGFR 70 to 75 mL/min/1.73 m^2), it is unlikely that there will be a substantial survival benefit over the same patient managed with RN (predicted NBGFR 45 to 55 mL/min/1.73 m^2). Contrast this with a patient with a preoperative GFR of 50 mL/min/1.73 m^2, where the difference in NBGFR between the two procedures (predicted GFRs of approximately 45 vs 30 mL/min/1.73 m^2) is more likely to impact survival. Further evidence of a threshold for NBGFR at which survival is likely affected was provided by a recent study by Wu and colleagues[31] on CKD-S patients. Wu and colleagues found that CKD-S patients with NBGFR less than 45 mL/min/1.73 m^2 had significantly reduced overall survival versus those with NBGFR of 45 to 60 mL/min/

1.73 m^2. In addition, the survival of the latter group was nearly identical to those with no CKD after surgery. These studies suggest that prioritization of NSS is most important in patients with preexisting CKD or when the NBGFR would fall below 45 mL/min/1.73 m^2 following RN.

To summarize, recommendations about RN/PN in patients with a normal contralateral kidney and minimal comorbidities remain uncertain. PN optimizes renal function, but the impact of this on overall survival remains unclear. The only prospective RCT to address this issue did not demonstrate an overall survival benefit for PN, whereas most retrospective studies that show a benefit for PN are plagued by selection biases. The most recent AUA guidelines addressed this by defining which patients should be prioritized for RN, as follows.[7] RN should be considered whenever the tumor demonstrates increased oncologic potential based on increased tumor size, imaging findings (infiltrative or locally advanced features), or high-risk histology (if renal-mass-biopsy has been obtained). In the setting of increased oncologic potential, RN is then preferred if all of the following criteria are met: (1) high tumor complexity making PN challenging even in experienced hands, (2) no preexisting CKD/proteinuria, and (3) there is a normal contralateral kidney and NBGFR will likely be > 45 mL/min/1.73 m^2 even if RN is performed. If all three of these criteria are not met, PN should be considered unless there are overriding concerns about the safety or oncologic efficacy of PN.[7]

SUBCHAPTER 3: DETERMINANTS OF GLOMERULAR-FILTRATION-RATE AFTER PARTIAL NEPHRECTOMY: ISCHEMIA AND PARENCHYMAL VOLUME LOSS

Choice of RN versus PN is hardly the only factor impacting functional recovery after extirpative surgery for renal cancer. Before discussing additional factors in detail it is important to reiterate that the most impactful determinant of long-term function after surgery for kidney cancer is the preoperative-GFR (Fig. 1). Among the many conditions that contribute to preoperative CKD, the most commonly encountered include diabetes mellitus (DM), hypertension (HTN), and advanced age.[32] In addition to these common conditions, Urologists should also be aware of the importance of proteinuria as it relates to functional outcomes. Several studies have demonstrated that higher levels of proteinuria are associated with progressive increases in all-cause mortality, progression of CKD, and ESRD, all independent of GFR.[33] Recognizing this, the AUA Guidelines now recommend clinicians assign a CKD stage to all patients

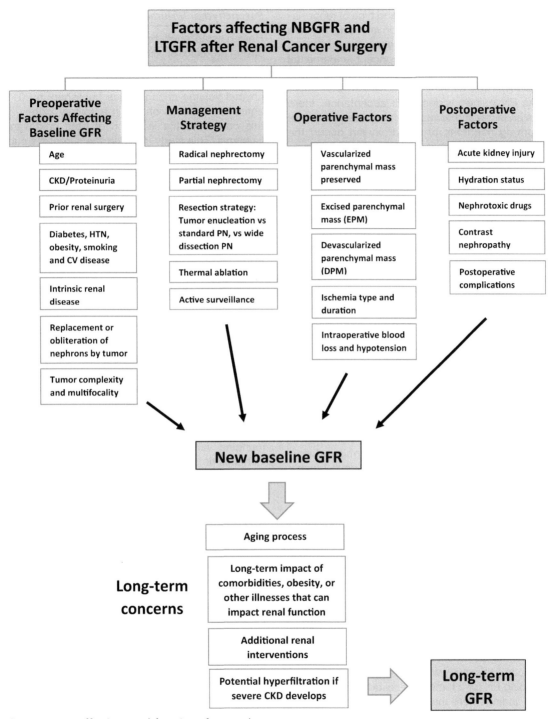

Fig. 1. Factors affecting renal function after renal cancer surgery.

as a part of the initial evaluation.[7] Unfortunately, although preoperative factors are recognized as vitally important for long-term functional outcomes, they are generally non-modifiable. Because of this, a greater portion of academic interest in recent years has centered on surgical considerations that may minimize nephron loss. As already discussed, PN clearly results in superior nephron preservation over RN; however, functional recovery after PN can be variable. In the remainder of this subchapter, we will focus on how surgical strategies such as duration/type of ischemia, resection strategy, and type of renorrhaphy can impact functional recovery after PN. We will discuss these strategies within the context of parenchymal volume loss, a concept fundamental to our current understanding of functional recovery after PN.

As PN gained widespread acceptance, there was an increased focus on the consequences of depriving nephrons of blood/oxygen during the hilar clamping phase of PN. Typically, hilar clamping can be performed in one of two ways: with or without hypothermia. For cold ischemia, hypothermic conditions are usually accomplished through the application of ice slush before/during the occlusion of arterial inflow. This results in decreased cellular metabolism and has been proven to have a protective effect. Indeed, multiple studies involving PN and renal transplantation have demonstrated that functional recovery after cold ischemia is impressively robust even as durations of ischemia extend beyond several hours.[34–37] A recent analysis by Dong and colleagues[35] of 400 patients undergoing PN demonstrated that median GFR recovered to 99% of that predicted by parenchymal volume preservation when hypothermia was used. Despite substantial evidence of a strong and consistent protective effect with hypothermia, there remains strong interest regarding the impact of warm ischemia during PN. This has been driven in part by the logistical difficulty in achieving hypothermia during minimally-invasive procedures that have quickly become the norm.

Unfortunately, functional recovery after warm ischemia seems to be more variable and somewhat less complete, although the clinical relevance of this is often inconsequential. Several early retrospective studies demonstrated what appeared to be a conceptually obvious association: the longer the renal hilum was clamped under warm ischemia conditions, the higher the risk of postoperative CKD.[38–41] A particularly influential study published on this topic in European Urology in 2010 contributed to this perspective. Titled "Every minute counts when the renal hilum is clamped," this study was restricted to patients undergoing PN for a tumor in a solitary kidney.[42] The main findings were that every additional minute of warm ischemia correlated with a 5% increase in the incidence of AKI, and a 6% increase in the incidence of *de novo* stage 4 CKD. Given the robust sample size ($n = 360$) and intellectually compelling findings, this study became widely disseminated. What we have discovered over the intervening years, however, is a striking example of age-old wisdom: correlation does not necessarily imply causation (**Table 3**).

Parenchymal Volume Preservation

Having established that warm ischemia time was a strong predictor of NBGFR after PN, attention then turned to other possible predictors. The first rigorous multicenter study to examine parenchymal volume changes was published in 2011, again with a focus on PN in a solitary kidney, in this case with the inclusion of both cold/warm ischemia. This study included the surgeon's subjective post-procedural estimation of the percent of parenchymal volume preserved, and when this was incorporated into the analysis, warm ischemia time lost all statistical significance, and the percent parenchymal volume preserved proved to be the most important factor predicting postoperative renal function.[34] Follow-up studies used manually drawn segmentation of pre/postoperative (3 to 12 months later) cross-sectional imaging to directly measure the degree of preservation of vascularized parenchyma volume, which again confirmed these findings.[44,53,54] More recently, measurement of parenchymal volumes has been aided by software, enabling more rapid and accurate calculation of parenchymal volume preservation, and an even stronger relationship between this factor and the percent GFR preserved was reported.[55,56] Central to the mistaken assignment of ischemia time as the prime determinant of function after PN was the seemingly ever-present issue of confounding variables. In all of the above studies, ischemia time significantly correlated with postoperative function as long as parenchymal volume changes were excluded from the analysis. However, PN procedures that require longer ischemia time typically involve larger, more complex, centrally located tumors, and these are exactly the cases where preservation of vascularized parenchymal mass will be reduced. Contrast this with a small, peripheral, well-encapsulated tumor that will require minimal ischemia time and likely can be resected with minimal parenchymal volume loss. With the discovery of the confounding relationship between ischemia time and parenchymal volume preservation, attention turned to the question of what, if any, independent impact warm ischemia time had on post-PN functional outcomes. More importantly, at what duration of warm ischemia does this impact begin to be felt? Fortunately, the previously mentioned study by Dong[35] published in 2018 also examined the effect of warm ischemia on functional outcomes. Importantly, this series included a substantial number of patients managed with warm ischemia ($n = 250$) and a greater proportion with more prolonged durations of warm ischemia (including some with >35 min), which made it ideal for

Table 3
Select studies regarding functional recovery after partial nephrectomy

Study	Design	Outcomes	Findings	Limitations/Perspective
Studies regarding importance of ischemia vs parenchymal volume preservation				
Thompson et al,[42] 2010	Retrospective review of 362 patients with solitary kidneys undergoing PN with warm ischemia	ARF, acute-onset GFR <15, new-onset stage IV CKD	Risk of new-onset stage IV CKD increased by 6% with each additional minute of WIT. Risk of AKI increased by 5% with each additional minute of WIT	Parenchymal mass preservation was not included in the analysis. Perspective: Conclusions about the importance of WIT are likely misleading because PMP not included
Lane et al,[34] 2011	Multicenter study of PN patients with solitary kidney (n = 660). Both warm and cold ischemia included.	AKI CKD	Preoperative GFR and % parenchyma preserved are associated with the incidence of AKI and CKD. Ischemia time is not a significant predictor	Retrospective study with a subjective estimation of PMP. Perspective: Preop GFR and PMP are the strongest predictors of functional outcomes after PN. Most nephrons recover from warm ischemia of limited duration.
Mir et al,[43] 2014	Retrospective analysis of 155 patients undergoing PN with renal volume/split function estimation by CT scan and MAG3 Scan (estimate split function)	Percent GFR saved, percent parenchymal volume saved	The median percent GFR saved in the operated kidney was 80% and the median parenchymal volume saved was 83%. The overall median rate of recovery from ischemia was 95% when corrected for PMP.	Retrospective studies are limited to patients with requisite imaging and other data necessary for detailed functional analyses. Perspective: Preoperative GFR (quality of nephrons) and percent parenchyma
Ginzburg et al,[44] 2015	Analysis of 179 patients with bilateral kidneys undergoing PN. CT estimated parenchymal volume preservation	Percent GFR preservation immediately post-op and 6 mo later	Immediately post-PN, WIT, not residual parenchymal volume, was associated with % GFR preservation. However, 6 mo post-PN, preop GFR, and % residual parenchymal volume, but not WIT, demonstrated	preserved (quantity of remaining nephrons) are the strongest predictors of NBGFR. Recovery from cold ischemia is very reliable even with prolonged cold ischemia. Recovery from warm ischemia is also robust out to

(continued on next page)

Table 3
(continued)

Study	Design	Outcomes	Findings	Limitations/Perspective
			significant association with % GFR preservation.	35 min (>90% when normalized by parenchymal mass preserved). The impact of longer durations of warm ischemia needs further study
Dong et al,[45] 2017	Review of 168 patients who underwent PN with necessary pre- and postop CT scans to measure parenchymal mass and MAG3 scan if contralateral kidney	Total parenchymal mass lost, EPM, DPM, GFR preservation in ipsilateral kidney	Median EPM and DPM: 9 and 16 cm³, respectively. Total parenchymal mass loss and DPM were associated strongly with GFR preservation in the operated kidney. EPM only weakly associated with functional outcomes.	Retrospective study limited to patients with necessary imaging for detailed functional analysis. Perspective: DPM seems to be the primary contributor to parenchymal mass lost, with almost twice the impact of EPM.
Impact of cold and warm ischemia and medical comorbidities, within context of parenchymal volume changes				
Dong et al,[35] 2018	Review of 401 patients managed with PN with necessary studies for analysis of function and nephron mass preserved within the kidney exposed to ischemia.	% nephron mass preserved, % function preserved, recovery from ischemia (normalizes for mass preservation)	% GFR preserved strongly correlated with nephron mass preserved. Recovery from ischemia was significantly higher for hypothermia (99% vs 92%; $P < .001$). Recovery from ischemia associated with ischemia time ($P < .05$). However, each added 10 min WIT was associated with only a 2.5% decline in recovery	Retrospective, limited to patients with necessary imaging for detailed functional analysis. Perspective: Confirms the importance of parenchymal mass preservation. When correcting for parenchymal mass preservation, WIT is still a predictor of postop functional outcomes, but this impact is limited to a 2.5% decline in recovery per 10 min of WIT.
Isharwal et als,[46] 2018	Review of 405 patients undergoing PN with necessary imaging studies to evaluate parenchymal mass	% preserved ipsilateral GFR	Median preserved ipsilateral glomerular filtration rate was 79%. Preserved parenchymal mass and ischemia type and duration	Retrospective, limited to patients with necessary imaging for detailed functional analysis. Perspective: Recovery after

	with a focus on effect of medical comorbidities		were significantly associated with functional recovery (all $P < .001$). On MV analysis none of the analyzed comorbidities were associated with functional recovery.	PN depends primarily on parenchymal mass preservation and ischemia characteristics. Comorbidities may impact function leading into surgery and/or influence long-term functional stability, but do not typically impact NBGFR after-PN
Review articles regarding zero or minimally ischemic PN				
Greco et al,[15] 2019	Meta-analysis of 152 studies examining cold, warm, and zero ischemia PN	EBL, postop complications, positive margins, local recurrences, estimated GFR change	There were no differences in intraoperative, cancer-related, or renal functional outcomes between warm, cold, and zero ischemia PN.	Overall low level of evidence, most studies retrospective, with high-risk selection bias, and heterogeneity within included studies. Perspective: Low-quality evidence and confounding variables make it impossible to recommend any single technique for managing the hilum during PN
Cacciamani et al,[47] 2019	Meta-analysis of 19 qualified studies comparing zero or minimal ischemia PN techniques to clamped PN	EBL, LOS, transfusions, complications, margin status, short- and long-term renal functional outcomes	Off-clamp or minimally ischemic techniques had higher EBL, but transfusion rates were similar. Functional outcomes were superior in the off-clamp and minimally ischemic group compared with the on-clamp.	Retrospective studies, significant risk of selection bias, and unrecognized confounding variables are all concerns. No measures of parenchymal mass loss. Perspective: Difficult to draw conclusions without data about parenchymal volume changes
Randomized trials of on-clamp vs off-clamp PN				
Anderson et al,[48] 2019	Prospective, RCT of 80 patients undergoing robotic PN. Randomized 1:1 to renal artery clamping vs no clamping.	OR time, EBL, postop complications, +margins, GFR at 3 mo postop	No difference in EBL, postop complications, and positive margin rate. At 3-mo follow-up, no differences in change in postoperative GFR between both groups.	Generalizability limited by small tumor size and brief duration of warm ischemia in the on-clamp cohort (19 min). Perspective: further evidence

(continued on next page)

Table 3
(*continued*)

Study	Design	Outcomes	Findings	Limitations/Perspective
				that WIT of limited duration has a limited effect on functional outcomes.
Antonelli et al,[49] 2022	Multicenter RCT (*n* = 324 patients) with normal baseline GFR, two kidneys undergoing PN with and without hilar clamping.	Primary endpoint: 6-mo AV-GFR. Multiple secondary functional endpoints too.	No difference between the two groups with regard to any of the primary or secondary function-related endpoints.	Limited WIT had minimal impact on functional outcomes after PN. Further complicating comparison and demonstrating the potential difficulty of off-clamp PN was a 43% crossover (to on-clamp) in the off-clamp cohort

Predictors and impact of acute kidney injury

Study	Design	Outcomes	Findings	Limitations/Perspective
Zhang et al,[50] 2016	Retrospective, *n* = 83 with solitary kidneys managed with PN. AKI is defined by standard criteria or proposed criteria (comparison to projected postop Cr based on parenchymal mass reduction).	Functional Recovery is defined as % function preserved/% mass saved.	Grade 2/3 AKI occurred in 23 patients by standard and 16 patients by proposed criteria. On MV analysis, only ischemia time was associated with AKI occurrence (*P* = .016). Median recovery from ischemia was 99%/95%/90%/88% for grades 0/1/2/3 AKI, respectively	Generalizability is hampered by several factors: Small patient cohort limited by availability of necessary studies, single-center retrospective study, only patients with solitary kidney included.
Zabell et al,[51] 2018	90 patients w/solitary kidneys managed by PN. Functional data at 4 time points: preop SCR, peak postop SCR, new baseline SCR 3 to 12 mo postop and long-term SCR >12 mo postop.	Adjusted AKI: ratio of peak postop SCR to projected postop SCR adjusted for parenchymal mass loss. Long-term change in function: final GFR/NBGR	Adjusted AKI occurred in 42%, including grade 1 in 20 (22%) and grade 2/3 in 18 (20%). UV analysis: degree of adjusted AKI did not correlate with long-term GFR change. MV analysis: adjusted AKI did not associate with a long-term functional change. DM and warm ischemia are modestly associated with a long-term functional decline.	Single tertiary care center, retrospective, limited sample size of 90 patients due to the exclusion of patients with a contralateral kidney, only patients with solitary kidney.

| Bravi et al,[52] 2019 | Retrospective analysis of 1893 patients treated by PN for a single cT1 N0 M0 renal mass to determine importance of AKI on functional recovery after PN | (1) recovery of at least 90% of baseline GFR 1 yr after PN, (2) % change of 1-y GFR vs baseline GFR, and (3) CKD upstaging | 20% incidence of AKI after PN. The rate of recovering 90% of baseline GFR was lower in the AKI group (30% vs 61%), whereas the proportion of patients with CKD upstaging was significantly higher (51% vs 23%; both P <.0001). MV analysis: AKI associated with worse function 1 yr after PN for all 3 outcomes (P <.0001). | Duration of functional follow-up was limited to 1 y. Renal parenchymal mass loss was not considered in determining AKI. This likely overestimates both AKI incidence and subsequent effect on NBGFR. |

Abbreviations: AKI, acute kidney injury; AV-GFR, absolute variation in glomerular filtration rate; AV-SRF, absolute variation in ipsilateral split renal function; CKD, chronic kidney disease; DPM, devascularized parenchymal mass; EBL, estimated blood loss; EPM, excised parenchymal mass; GFR, glomerular filtration rate; HR, hazard ratio; LOS, length of stay; MV, multivariate; NBGFR, new baseline glomerular filtration rate; PMP, parenchymal mass preserved; PN, partial nephrectomy; RCT, randomized controlled trial; RN, radical nephrectomy; RV-GFR, >25 relative, variation in glomerular filtration rate over 25%; SCR, serum creatinine; UV, univariate; WIT, warm ischemia time.

examining the potential contributions of warm ischemia. On multivariate analysis, parenchymal volume preservation remained the predominant predictor of functional recovery; however, warm ischemia time also remained statistically significant. The impact of ischemia time, however, had a relatively marginal effect on NBGFR. On average, the median recovery after warm ischemia was 92% of what would be expected by parenchymal volume changes, and it was estimated that each successive 10-min interval of warm ischemia only decreased the functional recovery by an additional 2.5%. The duration of warm ischemia at which renal function begins to decline more precipitously has yet to be defined and indeed there are reports in the literature of meaningful renal recovery after 90+ min of warm ischemia.[57] Great progress has been made in this field over the past decade, although there are still many ongoing controversies (see KEY POINTS).

Acute Kidney Injury

As evidence mounted that warm ischemia time had a relatively minor impact on NBGFR, certain groups began examining another indicator of post-PN renal dysfunction, AKI (see **Table 3**). In the context of PN, early increases in serum creatinine, which define the incidence and degree of AKI (see **Table 1**), can be due to several factors including ischemia, loss of nephron mass, and perioperative events (eg, hypovolemia). In the general population, AKI due to medical etiologies such as congestive heart failure, can predispose patients to CKD because most such patients will experience recurrent episodes of heart failure, and eventually this will irreversibly harm the kidneys.[58] However, does AKI after surgery, such as after PN, also eventually lead to CKD? As discussed below, this may not be the case because most such patients recover from AKI and the inciting event is almost never repeated.

To determine the role of ischemia and parenchymal volume loss on AKI and to assess the impact on functional recovery, Zhang and colleagues[50] evaluated a cohort of 83 patients undergoing clamped PN with a solitary kidney. Overall, 54% of patients experienced some degree of AKI when classified in the usual manner. However, when parenchymal volume loss was taken into account, only 46% of patients experienced AKI, and the incidence of severe AKI was reduced. On multivariable analysis, only the duration of ischemia, whether warm or cold, was associated with AKI incidence. Degree of AKI was a significant predictor of NBGFR; however, this relationship accounted for only a small degree of the overall

change in GFR following PN. The median recoveries after grade 1, 2, and 3 AKI were 95%, 90%, and 88% of that expected based on parenchymal volume preservation, respectively. In summary, despite a clear relationship between ischemia time and AKI, the vast majority of kidneys eventually recovered to within about 90% of the functional level predicted by parenchymal volume preservation.[59]

Some have suggested that AKI might result in a frail kidney, and although it may recover to a reasonable NBGFR, it may be more prone to GFR decline as time passes. In a report by Bravi,[52] presence of AKI was associated with reduced renal function and increased CKD 1 year after PN, with worse results correlating with a longer duration of AKI. Although provocative and supported by a large sample size, parenchymal volume changes were not accounted for and thus it is difficult to draw conclusions from this study. Loss of parenchymal volume contributes to increased serum creatinine after PN and thus to AKI, and to reduced renal function long-term, and thus to CKD, and if not accounted for it is difficult to assess the true impact of ischemia. Around the same time, a competing study restricted to patients with a solitary kidney was published by Zabell.[51] The authors adjusted for parenchymal volume loss to assess the true impact of ischemia, and found no association between the degree of AKI and LTGFR change (defined as the last known GFR normalized by NBGFR). Despite contemporary methodology, this and other studies suffer from limited numbers of subjects with long-term functional outcome data. As a result, the impact of post-PN AKI on LTGFR trends remains controversial (see KEY POINTS).

Zero or Minimal Ischemia Partial Nephrectomy

Although ischemia seems to be of secondary importance with respect to functional recovery after PN, it is modifiable and many centers have developed zero or minimally ischemic approaches to optimize functional outcomes. One of the first series to document successful off-clamp PN was published by Gill and colleagues.[60] Using pharmacologically induced hypotension during tumor resection, they completed 15 minimally invasive cases without hilar clamping. No patients required blood transfusion and the median change in discharge GFR as compared with preoperative levels was zero. Subsequent reports demonstrated that intraoperative hypotension was not necessary to achieve consistent results, and by 2015 a systematic review was published in European Urology synthesizing data from over 50 studies (see **Table 3**).[61] In general, off-clamp PN was used primarily for patients with peripheral tumors, whereas selectively/minimally ischemic techniques were used for hilar/medially located tumors. There was a small but significant increase in intraoperative blood loss and transfusion rates compared with on-clamp PN. Surgical margins were almost uniformly negative, and NBGFR levels ranged from 85% to 96% of preoperative levels. Although these results were encouraging, the authors properly concluded that "these techniques are technically demanding, with potential for increased blood loss, and require considerable experience with PN."

In 2019, a systematic review and meta-analysis was published by Cacciamani and colleagues[47] including studies that compared on-clamp PN to early unclamping, selective clamping, or completely off-clamp PN. Patients undergoing zero or minimally-ischemic PN demonstrated higher estimated blood loss (EBL) compared with on-clamp PN; however, transfusion rates were similar. There were no significant differences in complication rates or positive-margin rates, and functional outcomes "appeared superior in the off-clamp and super-selective clamp groups compared with the on-clamp PN cohort." However, selection bias was a major concern in these studies and the functional outcomes with the reduced-ischemia approaches are at most only marginally improved when compared with traditional clamped PN, which sets the bar very high because it typically saves 90% of the global GFR.

The selection bias and data heterogeneity concerns raised by these retrospective studies resulted in more recent efforts to study the question of off versus on-clamp PN in a prospective randomized manner. Fortunately, two randomized trials have recently been published that bring additional clarity to the matter. The first trial randomized 80 patients with two kidneys and an average tumor size of 3.0 cm to on-clamp versus off-clamp PN.[48] There were no differences noted between the two groups in EBL, transfusion rates, complication rates, and positive-margin rates. Most importantly, there were no significant differences in functional recovery between the two groups. The generalizability of the conclusions from this study was limited by the overall small tumor size and brief duration of warm ischemia in the on-clamp cohort (median = 19 min).

The second randomized trial to explore this issue, the CLOCK trial from Italy, randomized 324 patients to on-clamp vs off-clamp PN. All patients had a normal renal function, a functional contralateral kidney, and RENAL nephrometry score ≤10.[49] The median tumor size was again less than 3.0 cm and the median RENAL scores were 6 and 7 in the off-clamp and on-clamp cohorts, respectively. The primary endpoint was an absolute change in GFR at 6 months and secondary functional endpoints were also explored. Similar to the previous trial, there were again no differences in any of the primary or secondary functional endpoints between the on-clamp and off-clamp PN groups. Also similar to the prior trial, the median ischemia time in the on-clamp group was only 14 min. As we know that recovery from warm ischemia less than 25 to 30 min in duration is generally strong,[35] it is not surprising that no differences in functional outcomes were observed in these studies. Also worth discussing is that the CLOCK trial intentionally involved only the most experienced robotic surgeon at each center. Despite this, 43% of the patients in the off-clamp group eventually ended up on-clamp for some duration during their surgery. By far the most commonly cited reason for conversion was concern about "excessive bleeding." Given the overall small size of the tumors and the advanced expertise of the surgeons involved, a 40+% conversion rate calls into question the generalizability of off-clamp PN for the vast majority of Urologic surgeons.

In summary, minimal and zero-ischemia techniques for PN appear to be safe and effective and can, in theory, optimize renal functional outcomes. However, they can be challenging, with high conversion rates reported even in experienced hands. In addition, the types of tumors (ie, small, peripheral) for which off-clamp PN is often undertaken can be resected with short warm ischemia time that is unlikely to result in significant nephron loss in the first place. There is likely a subset of the patient who can benefit from reduced ischemia techniques (eg, patients with severe CKD), but this is not well defined (see KEY POINTS).

Excised and Devascularized Parenchymal Mass

With the realization that preservation of vascularized nephron mass is the most important factor for functional recovery after PN came to an additional interest in exactly how parenchyma is lost during PN. There are two distinct ways that functioning renal parenchyma can be lost during PN: (1) excised parenchymal mass (EPM) that is physically removed alongside the tumor and (2) devascularized parenchymal mass (DPM) that remains *in vivo*, but becomes devascularized secondary to thermal energy and/or during the process of capsular closure and renal reconstruction.

In the last decade, much research focus has been placed on resection strategy (see **Fig. 1**), with either standard PN or tumor-enucleation (TE) (**Fig. 2**). A large retrospective analysis by Dong compared TE ($n = 71$) to standard PN ($n = 373$).[62] Tumors in the TE group were slightly smaller (3.0 cm vs 3.3 cm), but otherwise the two groups were similar. Importantly, both preserved vascularized parenchymal volume and NBGFR were superior for TE, with no differences in positive-margin rate. A systematic review and meta-analysis published by Xu in 2019 examined 13 studies comparing TE and standard PN including more than 4800 patients.[63] There were no significant differences between the cohorts in terms of warm ischemia time, positive-margin rates, or recurrence rates. TE demonstrated fewer complications, a smaller decrease in eGFR, less EBL, and a shorter operative time. Although many of these benefits may be related to selection biases within the included studies, there are sufficient data at this point to suggest that TE in appropriately selected patients results in improved functional recovery without significant compromise in cancer control.

Another operative consideration studied recently is the question of renorrhaphy technique after resection. A robust renorrhaphy protects against intraoperative and postoperative hemorrhage and urine leak; however, it can also result in increased DPM. To investigate this possibility, Dong examined both EPM and DPM in 168 patients undergoing PN.[45] On average, the magnitude of DPM was approximately twice that of EPM, thus accounting for the lion's share of the total loss of parenchymal mass. Furthermore, DPM strongly associated with reduced NBGFR in the operated kidney. This study and others raised the question of whether less aggressive renorrhaphy techniques might minimize devascularization and improve functional outcomes. A systematic review and meta-analysis by Bertolo addressed this by combining data from six retrospective PN studies containing information about renorrhaphy techniques.[64] Although there was no difference between interrupted and running closure, patients who received a single rather than double-layer renorrhaphy had a reduced decline in postoperative GFR (3.2 mL/min vs 6.1 mL/min). Other studies suggest that renorrhaphy of any type may not be needed in some PN cases and this would further reduce DPM.

In summary, the current literature suggests that optimizing parenchymal volume preservation is far more important to functional recovery after PN than minimizing ischemia. EPM tends to be low in this era given preference for minimal margin PN or TE. The reconstructive phase of PN, with efforts to minimize DPM, is key to optimal functional recovery after PN. Precise placement of sutures into the parenchyma to ligate any transected vessels, with avoidance of collateral vessels going to uninvolved parts of the kidney, and careful and judicious capsular closure, are all important to minimize DPM and optimize NBGFR.

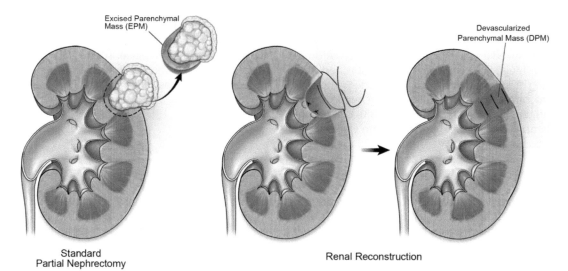

Fig. 2. Excised parenchymal mass (EPM) versus devascularized parenchymal mass (DPM). EPM can be reduced by minimal margin PN or tumor enucleation. DPM can be minimized by precise reconstruction of the kidney, which seems to be the most important step for optimizing functional outcomes after PN. (*From* Dong W, Wu J, Suk-Ouichai C, et al. Devascularized parenchymal mass associated with partial nephrectomy: predictive factors and impact on functional recovery. J Urol. 2017;198(4):787-794.)

SUBCHAPTER 4: PREDICTING NEW-BASELINE GLOMERULAR FILTRATION RATE AFTER RADICAL NEPHRECTOMY AND PARTIAL NEPHRECTOMY

RN remains an important consideration for tumors with increased oncologic potential and high tumor complexity, particularly when there is a healthy-appearing contralateral kidney that can provide NBGFR greater than 45 mL/min/1.73 m[2].[7] Thus, accurate prediction of NBGFR after RN/PN has relevant implications for management, particularly in challenging cases where RN and PN each offer unique advantages. For predicting NBGFR after RN, recent studies have shown that preoperative global-GFR, split renal function (SRF), and renal functional compensation (RFC) are fundamentally important.[65] In fact, a simple model based on these three factors demonstrated significantly improved accuracy for predicting NBGFR after RN than complex, multivariate algorithms developed for this purpose.[66] RFC has ranged from 1.20 to 1.30 in adults in various studies, with an average of 1.25, so this can be used as an estimate for RFC. Hence, the conceptually simple formula: $NBGFR_{post-RN} = preoperative\ global\ GFR \times SRF_{contralateral} \times 1.25$. Although SRF has traditionally been obtained from nuclear renal scans (NRS), it can now be obtained at point of care using 3D-imaging software that performs parenchymal volume analysis (PVA) on routine preoperative CT/MRI (**Fig. 3**).[59] SRF derived from PVA has been shown to be more accurate than SRF derived from NRS, and ultimately leads to more accurate prediction of NBGFR after RN.[67]

For PN, several methods for predicting parenchymal volume preservation, and by extension NBGFR, have been proposed, including those that rely on contact-surface-area or direct measurement of the rim of tissue likely to be lost during PN.[68] The latter was done by manual segmentation of preoperative imaging studies, which is subjective and labor intensive.[69,70] These methods provide strong predictions of functional outcomes after PN with high correlation coefficients between predicted/observed NBGFR ($r = 0.91$). However, a much simpler way to estimate NBGFR after PN has recently been proposed. Tanaka and colleagues[55] found that if the median percent global-GFR preserved in a large series of PN cases, which was 0.89, was applied as follows: $NBGFR_{post-PN} = 0.89 \times preoperative\ global\ GFR$, this proved to be just as accurate ($r = 0.91$) as the more sophisticated approaches. Rathi and colleagues[71] also compared this straightforward approach to several published multivariate algorithms derived from large databases, and the minimalistic approach again proved to be equivalent or better than the alternatives. Strong anchoring by preoperative GFR and the fact that, on average, only a small amount of function (10% to 11%) is lost with the typical PN likely accounts for these observations. In summary, these studies suggest that conceptually simple approaches for predicting NBGFR after PN/RN provide high accuracy and can be readily implemented in clinical settings to facilitate patient counseling/management.

SUBCHAPTER 5: ONGOING CONTROVERSIES AND FUTURE DIRECTIONS

Although we have learned much about functional outcomes following PN or RN, many areas of inquiry remain controversial. For the debate about PN versus RN in patients with a normal contralateral kidney, the data suggesting that overall survival may be equivalent with the two management strategies is fairly robust, with a median follow-up of 9 to 10 years. However, further follow-up would be helpful and may be particularly relevant for counseling younger patients with prolonged life expectancy. RCTs are also greatly

A 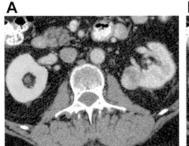 **B** 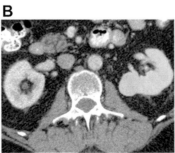 **C**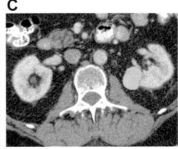

Fig. 3. Parenchymal volume analysis (PVA). Using parenchymal volume analysis software (PVA), renal parenchyma and tumor volumes can now be more easily and objectively measured. (*A*) Contralateral kidney (tumor-free). (*B*) Ipsilateral kidney and tumor. (*C*) Tumor alone. The relative parenchymal volumes on each side correlate strongly with function and provide a more accurate estimation of split renal function than nuclear renal scans.

needed in this domain to provide a higher level of evidence to facilitate more informed patient counseling.

Regarding functional recovery after PN specifically, ongoing controversies are mostly centered on the impact of warm ischemia and the point at which irreversible ischemic-injury begins. Patient-related factors that might increase the risk of AKI or incomplete recovery from ischemia remain uncertain, and long-term outcomes for kidneys exposed to ischemia or AKI would also benefit from further study. Are such kidneys more vulnerable to functional erosion as some have suggested?

Zero-ischemia PN was described over a decade ago, but we still do not know which patients should be prioritized for this. In patients with preoperative stage 4 CKD or a solitary kidney with stage 3 to 4 CKD, avoidance of AKI and even marginally improved functional recovery might be clinically relevant. The alternative argument is that in these circumstances optimal preservation of parenchymal volume is absolutely vital, and so a bloodless field for tumor enucleation and careful minimalist reconstruction might be more important. Clearly, further studies are needed in these patient populations.

With respect to the preservation of nephron mass during PN, the use of indocyanine-green dye or 3D-printed models derived from preoperative cross-sectional imaging has shown promise to identify collateral vessels in the vicinity of the tumor that ideally would be preserved.[72–75] Further study of these approaches incorporating 3- to 12-month follow-up of functional outcomes should be considered.

CLINICS CARE POINTS

- Partial nephrectomy clearly results in improved long term renal function. How this translates to overall survival is less clear.

- Prioritization of PN appears to be most important in those for whom radical nephrectomy would likely result in new baseline GFR (NBGFR) <45 ml/min/1.73m2.

- While warm ischemia time may have a minor secondary effect, the primary driver of NBGFR after surgery is the amount of parenchymal mass preserved.

- AKI after surgery is associated with ischemia time, however the translation of degree of AKI into functional recovery to NBGFR is minimal.

- Evidence regarding renal function benefit of so called "Zero-Ischemia" PN is inconsistent at best and the indications for this procedure remain unclear.

- Approximately 1/3 of parenchymal mass lost during PN surgery comes from resection, the remaining 2/3 comes from devascularization during reconstruction.

- Minimizing loss of parenchymal mass during resection and reconstruction is the most important controllable aspect of long-term post-operative renal function preservation.

DISCLOSURE

The Authors have nothing to disclose.

REFERENCES

1. Siegel RL, Miller KD, Fuchs HE, et al. Cancer statistics, 2022. CA Cancer J Clin 2022;72(1):7–33.
2. Siegel RL, Miller KD, Jemal A. Cancer statistics, 2020. CA Cancer J Clin 2020;70(1):7–30.
3. Go AS, Chertow GM, Fan D, et al. Chronic kidney disease and the risks of death, cardiovascular events, and hospitalization. N Engl J Med 2004; 351(13):1296–305.
4. Huang WC, Levey AS, Serio AM, et al. Chronic kidney disease after nephrectomy in patients with renal cortical tumours: a retrospective cohort study. Lancet Oncol 2006;7(9):735–40.
5. Kim SP, Campbell SC, Gill I, et al. Collaborative review of risk benefit trade-offs between partial and radical nephrectomy in the management of anatomically complex renal masses. Eur Urol 2017;72(1):64–75.
6. Campbell S, Uzzo RG, Allaf ME, et al. Renal mass and localized renal cancer: AUA guideline. J Urol 2017;198:520–9.
7. Campell SC, Clark PE, Chang SS, et al. Renal mass and localized renal cancer: evaluation, management, and follow-up: aua guideline parts I and II. J Urol 2021;206:199.
8. Lane BR, Demirjian S, Derweesh IH, et al. Survival and functional stability in chronic kidney disease due to surgical removal of nephrons: importance of the new baseline glomerular filtration rate. Eur Urol 2015;68:996–1003.
9. Mason R, Kapoor A, Liu Z, et al. The natural history of renal function after surgical management of renal cell carcinoma: results from the Canadian Kidney Cancer Information System. Urol Oncol 2016;34: 486.e1.
10. Lane BR, Babineau DC, Poggio ED, et al. Factors predicting renal functional outcome after partial nephrectomy. J Urol 2008;180:2363–9.
11. Van der Burgh AC, Rizopoulos D, Ikram MA, et al. Determinants of the evolution of kidney function with age. Kidney Int Rep 2021;6(12):3054–63.

12. Weight CJ, Miller DC, Campbell SC, et al. The management of a clinical t1b renal tumor in the presence of a normal contralateral kidney. J Urol 2013;189(4): 1198–202.

13. Van Poppel H, Da Pozzo L, Albrecht W, et al. A prospective, randomised EORTC intergroup phase 3 study comparing the oncologic outcome of elective nephron-sparing surgery and radical nephrectomy for low-stage renal cell carcinoma. Eur Urol 2011; 59(4):543–52.

14. Gor R, Uzzo R, Li T, et al. Surgical chronic kidney disease appears to be a distinct subtype of chronic kidney disease based on mortality risks following renal surgery. J Urol 2015;193:e975–6.

15. Greco F, Autorino R, Altieri V, et al. Ischemia techniques in nephron-sparing surgery: a systematic review and meta-analysis of surgical, oncological, and functional outcomes. Eur Urol 2019;75:477–9.

16. Ginsburg KB, Schober JP, Kutikov A. Ischemia time has little influenceon renal function following partial nephrectomy: is it time for urology to stop the ticktock dance? Eur Urol 2022;81:501–2.

17. Russo P, Goetzl M, Simmons R, et al. Partial nephrectomy: the rationale for expanding the indications. Ann Surg Oncol 2002;9(7):680–7.

18. Leibovich BC, Blute M, Cheville JC, et al. Nephron sparing surgery for appropriately selected renal cell carcinoma between 4 and 7 cm results in outcome similar to radical nephrectomy. J Urol 2004;171(3):1066–70.

19. Breau RH, Crispen PL, Jimenez RE, et al. Outcome of stage T2 or greater renal cell cancer treated with partial nephrectomy. J Urol 2010;183(3):903–8.

20. Campbell SC, Novick AC, Belldegrun A, et al. Guideline for management of the clinical T1 renal mass. J Urol 2009;182(4):1271–9.

21. Karellas ME, O'Brien MF, Jang TL, et al. Partial nephrectomy for selected renal cortical tumours of ≥7 cm. BJU Int 2010;106(10):1484–7.

22. Kim SP, Thompson RH, Boorjian SA, et al. Comparative effectiveness for survival and renal function of partial and radical nephrectomy for localized renal tumors: a systematic review and meta-analysis. J Urol 2012;188(1):51–7.

23. Tan H-J, Norton EC, Ye Z, et al. Long-term survival following partial vs radical nephrectomy among older patients with early-stage kidney cancer. JAMA 2012;307(15):1629–35.

24. Weight CJ, Larson BT, Fergany AF, et al. Nephrectomy induced chronic renal insufficiency is associated with increased risk of cardiovascular death and death from any cause in patients with localized cT1b renal masses. J Urol 2010;183(4): 1317–23.

25. Gershman B, Thompson RH, Boorjian SA, et al. Radical versus partial nephrectomy for cT1 renal cell carcinoma. Eur Urol 2018;74(6):825–32.

26. Van Poppel H, Da Pozzo L, Albrecht W, et al. A prospective, randomised EORTC intergroup phase 3 study comparing the oncologic outcome of elective nephron-sparing surgery and radical nephrectomy for low-stage renal cell carcinoma. Eur Urol 2011;59(4):543–52.

27. Scosyrev E, Messing EM, Sylvester R, et al. Renal function after nephron-sparing surgery versus radical nephrectomy: results from EORTC randomized trial 30904. Eur Urol 2014;65(2):372–7.

28. Lane BR, Campbell SC, Demirjian S, et al. Surgically induced chronic kidney disease may be associated with a lower risk of progression and mortality than medical chronic kidney disease. J Urol 2013; 189(5):1649–55.

29. Capitanio U, Terrone C, Antonelli A, et al. MP44-04 nephron-sparing surgery protects from chronic kidney disease relative to radical nephrectomy but does not impact on other-causes mortality: long-term (more than 10 years) survival and functional outcomes in patients with a T1A-T1B renal mass. J Urol 2015;193(4):e527.

30. Zabell J, Demirjian S, Campbell SC. MP59-15 long-term outcomes after renal cancer surgery: predictors of chronic kidney disease and non-renal cancer mortality. J Urol 2017;197(4):e786–7.

31. Wu J, Suk-Ouichai C, Dong W, et al. Analysis of survival for patients with chronic kidney disease primarily related to renal cancer surgery. BJU Int 2018; 121(1):93–100.

32. Erfanpoor S, Etemad K, Kazempour S, et al. Diabetes, hypertension, and incidence of chronic kidney disease: is there any multiplicative or additive interaction? Int J Endocrinol Metab 2020;19(1): e101061.

33. Levey AS, de Jong PE, Coresh J, et al. The definition, classification, and prognosis of chronic kidney disease: a KDIGO Controversies Conference report. Kidney Int 2011;80(1):17–28.

34. Lane BR, Russo P, Uzzo RG, et al. Analysis of cold vs. warm ischemia during partial nephrectomy in 660 solitary kidneys reveals predominant role of non-modifiable factors in determining ultimate renal function. J Urol 2011;185:421–7.

35. Dong W, Wu J, Suk-Ouichai C, et al. Ischemia and functional recovery from partial nephrectomy: refined perspectives. Eur Urol Focus 2018;4:572–8.

36. Funahashi Y, Yoshino Y, Sassa N, et al. Comparison of warm and cold ischemia on renal function after partial nephrectomy. Urology 2014;84:1408–12.

37. Mir MC, Ercole C, Takagi T, et al. Decline in renal function after partial nephrectomy: etiology and prevention. J Urol 2015;193(6):1889–98.

38. Thompson RH, Frank I, Lohse CM, et al. The impact of ischemia time during open nephron sparing surgery on solitary kidneys: a multiinstitutional study. J Urol 2007;177:471–6.

39. Porpiglia F, Renard J, Billia M, et al. Is renal warm ischemia over 30 minutes during laparoscopic partial nephrectomy possible? One-year results of a prospective study. Eur Urol 2007;52:1170–8.

40. Porpiglia F, Fiori C, Bertolo R, et al. Long-term functional evaluation of the treated kidney in a prospective series of patients who underwent laparoscopic partial nephrectomy for small renal tumors. Eur Urol 2012;62:130–5.

41. Yasuyuki K, Yukio U, Masanori S, et al. Evaluation of renal function after laparoscopic partial nephrectomy with renal scintigraphy using 99mtechnetium mercaptoacetyltriglycine. Int J Urol 2006;13:1371–4.

42. Thompson RH, Lane BR, Lohse CM, et al. Every minute counts when the renal hilum is clamped during partial nephrectomy. Eur Urol 2010;58:340–5.

43. Mir MC, Takagi T, Campbell RA, et al. Poorly functioning kidneys recover from ischemia after partial nephrectomy as well as strongly functioning kidneys. J Urol 2014;192(3):665–70.

44. Ginzburg S, Uzzo R, Walton J, et al. Residual parenchymal volume, not warm ischemia time, predicts ultimate renal functional outcomes in patients undergoing partial nephrectomy. Urology 2015;86:300–5.

45. Dong W, Wu J, Suk-Ouichai C, et al. Devascularized parenchymal mass associated with partial nephrectomy: predictive factors and impact on functional recovery. J Urol 2017;198(4):787–94.

46. Isharwal S, Wang A, Ye W, et al. Impact of comorbidities on functional recovery from partial nephrectomy. J Urology 2018;199(6):1433–9.

47. Cacciamani GE, Medina LG, Gill TS, et al. Impact of renal hilar control on outcomes of robotic partial nephrectomy: systematic review and cumulative meta-analysis. Eur Urol Focus 2019;5:619–35.

48. Anderson BG, Potretzke AM, Du K, et al. Comparing off-clamp and on-clamp robot-assisted partial nephrectomy: a prospective randomized trial. Urology 2019;126:102–9.

49. Antonelli A, Cindolo L, Sandri M, et al. Is off-clamp robot-assisted partial nephrectomy beneficial for renal function? data from the CLOCK trial. BJU Int 2022;129:217–24.

50. Zhang Z, Zhao J, Dong W, et al. Acute kidney injury after partial nephrectomy: role of parenchymal mass reduction and ischemia and impact on subsequent functional recovery. Eur Urol 2016;69(4):745–52.

51. Zabell J, Isharwal S, Dong W, et al. Acute kidney injury after partial nephrectomy of solitary kidneys: impact on long-term stability of renal function. J Urol 2018;200(6):1295–301.

52. Bravi CA, Vertosick E, Benfante N, et al. Impact of acute kidney injury and its duration on long-term renal function after partial nephrectomy. Eur Urol 2019;76(3):398–403.

53. Mir MC, Campbell RA, Sharma N, et al. Parenchymal volume preservation and ischemia during partial nephrectomy: functional and volumetric analysis. Urology 2013;82:263–8.

54. Mibu H, Tanaka N, Hosokawa Y, et al. Estimated functional renal parenchymal volume predicts the split renal function following renal surgery. World J Urol 2015;33:1571–7.

55. Tanaka H, Wang Y, Suk-Ouichai C, et al. Can we predict functional outcomes after partial nephrectomy? J Urol 2019;201(4):693–701.

56. Wu J, Suk-Ouichai C, Dong W, et al. Vascularized parenchymal mass preserved with partial nephrectomy: functional impact and predictive factors. Eur Urol Oncol 2019;2(1):97–103.

57. Campbell RA, Dewitt-Foy ME, Tanaka H, et al. Functional recovery from prolonged warm ischemia: compelling case scenarios. Urology 2019;132:22–7.

58. Zabell JR, Wu J, Suk-Ouichai C, et al. Renal ischemia and functional outcomes following partial nephrectomy. Urol Clin North Am 2017;44(2):243–55.

59. Ye Y, Tanaka H, Wang Y, et al. Split renal function in patients with renal masses: utility of parenchymal volume analysis vs nuclear renal scans. BJU Int 2020;125(5):686–94.

60. Gill IS, Eisenberg MS, Aron M, et al. "Zero ischemia" partial nephrectomy: novel laparoscopic and robotic technique. Eur Urol 2011;59:128–34.

61. Simone G, Gill IS, Mottrie A, et al. Indications, techniques, outcomes, and limitations for minimally ischemic and off-clamp partial nephrectomy: a systematic review of the literature. Eur Urol 2015;68:632–40.

62. Dong W, Gupta GN, Blackwell RH, et al. Functional comparison of renal tumor enucleation versus standard partial nephrectomy. Eur Urol Focus 2017;3(4–5):437–43.

63. Xu C, Lin C, Xu Z, et al. Tumor enucleation vs. partial nephrectomy for t1 renal cell carcinoma: a systematic review and meta-analysis. Front Oncol 2019;9:473.

64. Bertolo R, Campi R, Mir MC, et al. Systematic review and pooled analysis of the impact of renorrhaphy techniques on renal functional outcome after partial nephrectomy. Eur Urol Oncol 2019;2(5):572–5.

65. Rathi N, Palacios DA, Abramczyk E, et al. Predicting GFR after radical nephrectomy: the importance of split renal function. World J Urol 2022;40(4):1011–8.

66. Rathi N, Yasuda Y, Palacios DA, et al. Split renal function is fundamentally important for predicting functional recovery after radical nephrectomy. Eur Urol Open Sci 2022;40:112–6.

67. Rathi N, Yasuda Y, Attawettayanon W, et al. Optimizing prediction of new-baseline glomerular filtration rate after radical nephrectomy: are algorithms really necessary? Int Urol Nephrol 2022;54(10):2537–45.

68. Campbell SC, Campbell JA, Munoz-Lopez C, et al. Every decade counts: a narrative review of

functional recovery after partial nephrectomy. BJU Int 2023;131(2):165–72.

69. Hsieh PF, Wang YD, Huang CP, et al. A mathematical method to calculate tumor contact surface area: an effective parameter to predict renal function after partial nephrectomy. J Urol 2016;196(1):33–40.

70. Suk-Ouichai C, Wu J, Dong W, et al. Tumor contact surface area as a predictor of functional outcomes after standard partial nephrectomy: utility and limitations. Urology 2018;116:106–13.

71. Rathi N, Attawettayanon W, Tanaka H, et al. Prediction of new baseline glomerular filtration rate (nbgfr) after partial nephrectomy for localized renal cell carcinoma. poster presented at: 2022 society of urologic oncology annual meeting dates: November 30, 2022- December 2, 2022; December, 2022; San Diego, CA.

72. Gadus L, Kocarek J, Chmelik F, et al. Robotic partial nephrectomy with indocyanine green fluorescence navigation. Contrast Media Mol Imaging 2020;1-8: 1–8.

73. Shirk JD, Thiel DD, Wallen EM, et al. Effect of 3-dimensional virtual reality models for surgical planning of robotic-assisted partial nephrectomy on surgical outcomes: a randomized clinical trial. JAMA Netw Open 2019;2(9):e1911598.

74. Kobayashi S, Cho B, Mutaguchi J, et al. Surgical navigation improves renal parenchyma volume preservation in robot-assisted partial nephrectomy: a propensity score matched comparative analysis. J Urol 2020;204(1):149–56.

75. Amparore D, Pecoraro A, Checcucci E, et al. Three-dimensional virtual models' assistance during minimally invasive partial nephrectomy minimizes the impairment of kidney function. Eur Urol Oncol 2022;5(1):104–8.

Surgical Management of Renal Cell Carcinoma with Inferior Vena Cava Tumor Thrombus

Shawn Dason, MD[a], Jahan Mohebali, MD, MPH[b], Michael L. Blute Sr., MD[c], Keyan Salari, MD, PhD[c,d],*

KEYWORDS

• Kidney cancer • Inferior vena cava • Tumor thrombectomy

KEY POINTS

• Renal cell carcinoma can invade contiguous veins, such as the renal vein and the inferior vena cava, a phenomenon referred to as tumor thrombus.
• Surgical resection of non-metastatic RCC with tumor thrombus may provide long-term cure in more than half of patients. Cytoreductive nephrectomy and tumor thrombectomy may also be important in the management of metastatic RCC.
• Tumor thrombus extent is described by the Mayo classification which ranges from level 0 (renal vein) to level 4 (supradiaphragmatic IVC).
• Comprehensive preoperative workup and multidisciplinary care are essential to optimizing surgical outcomes in nephrectomy and IVC tumor thrombectomy.
• The surgical approach to IVC tumor thrombectomy is comprehensively described in this review.

INTRODUCTION

In the United States, an estimated 79,000 cases and 13,920 deaths will be attributable to kidney cancer in 2022.[1] Most kidney cancers are primary renal cell carcinomas (RCC) of clear cell histology.[2] RCC is unique in its tendency to invade into contiguous veins—a phenomenon termed venous tumor thrombus. Tumor thrombus is distinct from the bland thrombus formed from coagulated blood more commonly encountered in venous thromboembolic disease. Patients with RCC with tumor thrombus are also at risk of bland thrombus formation,[3] often possessing all 3 components of Virchow's triad—a low flow state resulting from venous occlusion, a prothrombotic state associated with advanced malignancy, and an abnormal vascular surface on the tumor thrombus. Management of RCC with venous involvement requires consideration of both bland and tumor thrombus burden.[4]

Surgical resection is indicated for most patients with RCC and an inferior vena cava (IVC) thrombus in the absence of metastatic disease. Resection also has an important role in selected patients with metastatic disease. In this review, the authors discuss the comprehensive management of the patient with RCC with IVC tumor thrombus.

ANATOMY

The IVC forms from confluence of the right and left common iliac veins that return blood from the lower

a Department of Urology, Ohio State University, 915 Olentangy River Road, Ste 3100, Columbus, OH 43212, USA; b Division of Vascular and Endovascular Surgery, Massachusetts General Hospital, Harvard Medical School, 55 Fruit Street, Boston, MA 02114, USA; c Department of Urology, Massachusetts General Hospital, Harvard Medical School, 55 Fruit Street, Boston, MA 02114, USA; d Broad Institute of MIT and Harvard, 415 Main Street, Cambridge, MA 02142, USA
* Corresponding author. Department of Urology, Massachusetts General Hospital, 55 Fruit Street, GRB-1106H, Boston, MA 02114.
E-mail address: ksalari@mgh.harvard.edu

Urol Clin N Am 50 (2023) 261–284
https://doi.org/10.1016/j.ucl.2023.01.007
0094-0143/23/© 2023 Elsevier Inc. All rights reserved.

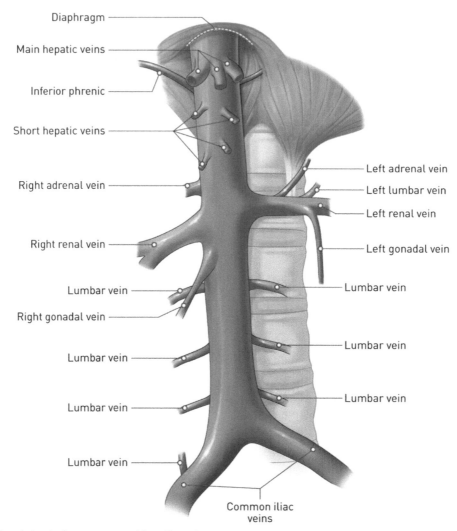

Fig. 1. The abdominal vena cava and its tributaries.

extremities and pelvis (**Fig. 1**). A variable number of lumbar veins drain into the infrarenal vena cava along with the right gonadal vein.[5] In cases of obstruction, these lumbar branches are often the first to form collateral drainage pathways via communications to the paraspinal plexus as well as the azygous and hemiazygos veins, which ultimately drain into the superior vena cava. At the renal level, anatomic variants are common—namely, right accessory renal veins (16.6%) along with left retroaortic (3%), left circum-aortic (3.5%), and left accessory (2.1%) renal veins.[6] The right adrenal vein drains into the posterolateral vena cava above the right renal vein.[7]

Short hepatic veins—highly variable in number and size—drain the caudate hepatic lobe into the anterior suprarenal cava.[8] The main hepatic veins and phrenic veins then drain into the IVC just below the diaphragm.[9] The supradiaphragmatic IVC enters the pericardium before draining into the right atrium. The IVC has no further tributaries between the diaphragm and right atrium other than phrenic veins in some patients.[9,10]

Surgical anatomy is distorted in RCC with an IVC thrombus due to tumor-related neovascularization; mass effect from bulky renal, nodal, and/or IVC tumor; and collateralization that results from venous obstruction.

CYTOREDUCTIVE NEPHRECTOMY

Cytoreductive nephrectomy (CN) has an essential role in metastatic RCC. CN has been associated with a survival benefit with modern systemic therapy regimens.[11,12] Nonetheless, indications for cytoreductive nephrectomy are unclearly defined, and there are patients who will not benefit from CN.[13]

The use of International Metastatic RCC Database Consortium (IMDC) risk stratification alone is not indicated to decide on CN in a patient with IVC thrombus.

Contemporary indications for cytoreductive nephrectomy include the following:

- Limited metastatic disease that can be controlled completely with metastasis-directed therapy (MDT) following CN
- Limited metastatic disease that can be observed without systemic therapy following CN ± MDT
- Significant local symptoms that require hospitalization and prevent receipt of systemic therapy
- 1 IMDC risk factor with most of the tumor burden located in the kidney[14]

Additional relative indications for CN in the patient with an IVC thrombus include the following:

- An inability to anticoagulate an IVC thrombus patient requiring therapeutic anticoagulation due to significant hematuria
- A thrombus close to the hepatic veins or diaphragm where progression may significantly increase surgical complexity
- A friable-appearing thrombus that may be of high risk for embolization
- A thrombus causing obstructive venous sequelae or at risk of causing obstructive sequelae

Although we perform CN more commonly when a patient has an IVC thrombus, careful consideration should be given to upfront systemic therapy. Relative indications for upfront systemic therapy include the following:

- Significant extrarenal disease
- Excessive surgical morbidity
- Poor performance status unrelated to IVC thrombus
- Patient preference

Additional factors that predict poor prognosis following CN and IVC thrombectomy include sarcomatoid histology, poor risk group, supradiaphragmatic thrombus, and systemic symptoms.[15]

PREOPERATIVE EVALUATION

The preoperative evaluation in a patient undergoing IVC thrombectomy has several essential components described later. There is no checklist that will be applicable to every patient and institution. Indications for hospital admission include facilitating a timely preoperative workup, need for heparin drip, significant symptoms, or for monitoring of thrombi at high risk of complications. Hospital admission can sometimes be counterproductive if (1) transfer to a specialized center is more appropriate to facilitate care or (2) an operation is not planned, and inpatient status will prevent coverage of systemic therapy (as is generally the case in the United States).

Staging

Staging involves cross-sectional imaging of the chest, abdomen, and pelvis.[16] Neurologic symptoms indicate brain imaging and bony symptoms, elevated alkaline phosphatase, or hypercalcemia prompt bone imaging.[16] The diagnosis of metastatic disease is important in the shared decision-making to proceed with IVC thrombectomy.

Inferior Vena Cava Thrombus Assessment

Imaging to assess IVC thrombus extent is critical for preoperative planning. The Mayo classification is used to describe RCC IVC thrombi (**Fig. 2**). Because thrombus progression can be rapid, imaging should be done as close to planned surgery as possible (ideally within 48 hours); this is particularly important for the surgical team that requires special preparation to mobilize the liver, reconstruct the IVC, or handle a supradiaphragmatic thrombus.

IVC thrombi are heterogeneous, and the imaging necessary to understand a particular case may vary. Computed tomography (CT) is often the initial imaging modality available in a patient with RCC and IVC thrombus. The venous phase of a CT scan is quite accurate in predicting tumor thrombus level[17–19] and very intuitive for a surgeon to correlate to surgical anatomy. Modern CT technology has overcome some historical limitations in identifying tumor thrombus.[20] A CT arteriogram with 1 mm cuts can be helpful in planning complex cases, particularly amid significant tumor bulk and neovascularization. In some cases, precise thrombus delineation can be difficult because of artifact from altered venous flow or enhancing tumor thrombus. Although patients with RCC frequently have coexistent chronic kidney disease, the benefits of contrast CT may outweigh the relatively low risks of contrast-induced nephropathy, estimated to be 0%, 0% to 2%, and 0% to 17% with a glomerular filtration rate of greater than 45, 30 to 44, and less than 30, respectively.[21]

Contrast-enhanced MRI is used adjunctively to CT and can often provide the best anatomic delineation of the IVC thrombus. It is critical when ordering an MRI for a patient with known IVC thrombus that the indication is communicated to the radiologist, because a standard renal mass MRI may not be protocoled to visualize thrombus well or extend

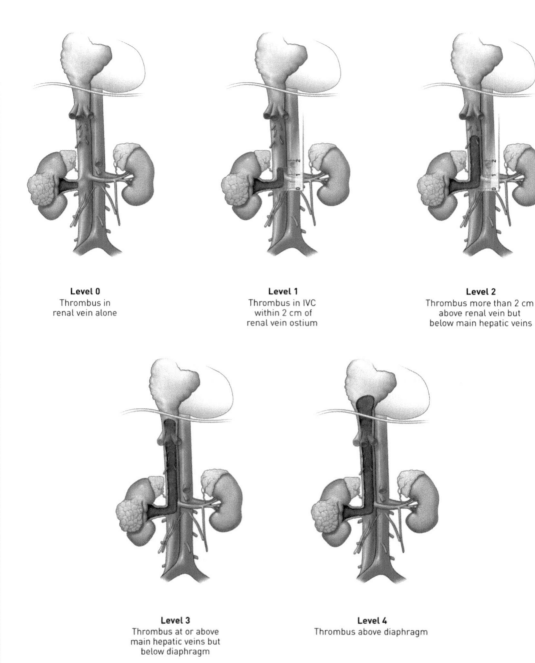

Level 0
Thrombus in
renal vein alone

Level 1
Thrombus in IVC
within 2 cm of
renal vein ostium

Level 2
Thrombus more than 2 cm
above renal vein but
below main hepatic veins

Level 3
Thrombus at or above
main hepatic veins but
below diaphragm

Level 4
Thrombus above diaphragm

Fig. 2. The Mayo classification for tumor thrombus extent in renal cell carcinoma.

cephalad enough. In addition to assessing tumor thrombus level, MRI can distinguish bland from tumor thrombus[22] and assess IVC wall invasion.[23,24] Modern gadolinium contrast has a nephrogenic systemic fibrosis risk less than 0.07% in patients with chronic kidney disease[25] and is indicated even in this setting. MRI interpretation may be less intuitive to the surgeon in planning a complex case, and it can often be helpful to obtain an additional CT with 1 mm cuts if only MRI is available.

An angiographic venocavogram[26] can sometimes be helpful when venous occlusion or turbulence prevents proper delineation of tumor thrombus, which is critical to surgical planning.

Although all attempts should be made to characterize a thrombus preoperatively, the surgical team should always be prepared for a more extensive thrombus than anticipated with a plan for how this should be approached. At times the precise nature of a tumor thrombus may only be discovered on intraoperative transesophageal echocardiography[27] or intraoperative paracaval ultrasound.[28,29]

Venous Implications

Understanding the implications of an IVC thrombus on the remaining vasculature is important. Even when transesophageal echocardiography is planned, a preoperative transthoracic echocardiogram will assess ejection fraction, valvulopathy, septal defects, right heart strain, intraatrial thrombus extension, and friability of the cephalad extent of a level 4 thrombus and will rule out free-floating thrombus fragments. A CT pulmonary angiogram will assess for any preexisting emboli, for which patients with IVC thrombus are at risk. Finally, if indicated based on extent of IVC thrombus and/or physical signs/symptoms, duplex sonography of the lower extremities to assess for the presence of iliofemoral bland thrombus should be considered, as results will affect decision-making on IVC management following thrombectomy.

Anticoagulation

Therapeutic anticoagulation is not indicated for every RCC with IVC thrombus.[3,30–32] Indications for therapeutic anticoagulation generally include pulmonary emboli, iliofemoral deep vein thrombosis, suspected bland thrombus component of IVC thrombus, significant IVC obstruction, or a tumor thrombus where subtle progression could increase surgical complexity. Consequences of anticoagulation include bleeding and heparin-induced thrombocytopenia that will significantly complicate cardiopulmonary bypass.[33] For the patient receiving anticoagulation, it is unclear what regimen and dosing (ie, therapeutic vs prophylactic) is optimal and if bridging is necessary. Fluctuations in renal function are common in these patients and need to be considered when deciding on how long an anticoagulant is held preoperatively.[34] Patients at particularly high risk of bland thrombus progression or bleeding warrant preoperative admission with a heparin drip to limit their interval off anticoagulation.

Preoperative Risk Assessment

Preoperative cardiac risk assessment is indicated.[35] For patients who are likely to need sternotomy, this should include assessment of patency of the coronary arteries, as coronary revascularization at the time of IVC thrombectomy may be indicated. Our routine preoperative study for all patients undergoing sternotomy is a coronary CT angiogram, as it is the least invasive, but a standard coronary angiogram may be performed as well. Echocardiography and an assessment of

pulmonary embolism burden are also important in risk stratification. An asymptomatic preoperative pulmonary embolism (PE) should not contraindicate surgery[36]—but a significant and symptomatic PE is an indication to consider neoadjuvant systemic therapy and await stabilization. Communication with the blood bank is important—should a blood shortage be in effect,[37] special preparation may be needed if autoantibodies are present or for the massive transfusion sometimes required in these cases. Pulmonary function testing and carotid Doppler may also be indicated for those with pulmonary or vascular disease. Relevant comorbidities should be optimized with specialty consultation.

Multidisciplinary Involvement

Multidisciplinary communication based on the aforementioned data is essential for the successful outcome of any IVC thrombectomy case. There are 4 key aspects to this that may be relevant.

i. Oncologic review: the decision to pursue IVC thrombectomy is fundamentally a surgical decision. Institutions regularly performing IVC thrombectomy would benefit from having designated urologic oncologists that focus on this and are involved in decision-making for relevant cases. Particularly in the metastatic setting, the decision to operate may be influenced by the systemic therapy options available. Even in the nonmetastatic patient, systemic therapy and stereotactic body radiotherapy (SBRT) may be an appropriate alternative for the patient at high risk of perioperative mortality.[38] Discussion of these cases with focused medical and radiation oncologists can be helpful. Assuming tumor board review can be conducted expediently without delaying management, this can also be an option.

ii. Surgical review: the urologic oncologist should be mindful of their own skillset to judge which cases can be safely performed independently or may require expertise from other surgical disciplines. A consistent multidisciplinary team will be important in developing expertise and coordinating timely care. There is no specific team specialty makeup that works in every setting and composition varies significantly by institution. At MGH our multidisciplinary team is composed of surgeons from urologic oncology, cardiac surgery and vascular surgery, cardiac anesthesia, and genitourinary radiology. At other institutions, it may be transplant or hepatobiliary surgeons who are most comfortable with the relevant para- and retrohepatic anatomy that level 3 and 4 thrombi require. Ultimately, teams are best built with a focus on covering all necessary skillsets rather than a dogmatic view on what specialty roles are. A conference between involved parties before the operation is critical. We invoke a case review conference between relevant team members for all IVC thrombus cases reaching level 2 or higher. All parties understanding and participating in the surgical plan contributes to a better outcome than a disjointed approach.

iii. Anesthesia review: depending on institutional structure and anesthesia scheduling, this may coincide with the surgical review described earlier or happen subsequently once anesthesia assignments are made. Anesthetic management is highly complex given the numerous physiologic stressors that occur during these operations.[27,39–41] Excellent peripheral intravenous access, central venous catheterization, arterial catheterization, and transesophageal echocardiography are helpful in most cases. Close involvement of the anesthesiologist handling the case with the surgical plan is necessary along with discussions surrounding fluid resuscitation, vasopressor use, timing of vascular clamping, and the plan for management of intraoperative complications should they occur.

Preoperative Procedures

As described earlier, angiographic procedures such as a coronary angiography or venocavogram may be needed in selected cases. In the patient who will be rendered anephric, a tunneled dialysis catheter should be inserted.

A tissue diagnosis is not generally required if imaging features are typical of RCC. Biopsy should be performed if an alternative diagnosis is suspected. Biopsy is not required in patients with metastatic disease but it can be helpful in confirming metastases,[14] assessing prognosis,[15] and deciding on nonsurgical alternatives.

Some surgeons elect to embolize the renal artery preoperatively. Studies have not clearly demonstrated a benefit to this practice with respect to reducing bleeding or complication rates,[42] and we do not routinely perform preoperative embolization. The main potential benefit of preoperative embolization is that it may allow for division of a thrombus-containing vein before the renal artery if not performing an en bloc IVC thrombectomy; this is relevant to the case where early arterial ligation is felt to be prohibitively difficult (eg, very bulky left-sided thrombus with hilar adenopathy). If preoperative embolization is performed, coils need to be placed distally enough for the renal artery stump to be safely ligated. It

should also be performed very close to the operation, as a prolonged interval between embolization and surgery may result in the dissection planes becoming obscured and an angioinfarction syndrome.

Preoperative placement of a permanent IVC filter is rarely indicated unless decided on as part of the bland thrombus management following IVC thrombectomy.[4] If this is being considered, it may be best placed intraoperatively or postoperatively, as preoperative placement may interfere with caval clamping or repair during thrombectomy. Studies have been conducted on devices that temporarily filter the IVC to prevent embolization.[43–45] These are also not routinely used given the rarity of this event[46] but could have a role in thrombi at high risk of embolization or in the patient at high risk of morbidity from an embolization event (eg, pulmonary emboli already present or a patent foramen ovale). If either a temporary or a permanent filter is being considered, placement via the superior vena cava will avoid traversing thrombus. Enough distance is needed between the cephalad thrombus tip and the hepatic veins to both clamp the vena cava during IVC thrombectomy and deploy the device.

Vascular Bypass

Preoperative preparation for vascular bypass or autotransfusion is necessary given the expertise and equipment that will be required.

Intraoperative cell salvage (ICS) involves a special suction setup that allows for collection of blood loss from the operative field and processing for autotransfusion. Often the amount of blood available for autotransfusion is significantly less than actual blood lost. ICS use during oncologic surgery is controversial because of theoretic dissemination of tumor cells into the bloodstream by infused blood.[47] It is unclear how relevant ICS oncologic concerns are during IVC thrombectomy given the presence of gross intravenous tumor and the common use of other mechanistically similar bypass techniques for high-level thrombi. Transfusion is more likely if ICS is not used, which may also have oncologic implications[48] and be unavailable amid recurrent blood shortages.[37]

In venovenous bypass (VVB), blood is bypassed from the infrarenal IVC via a surgically or percutaneously placed catheter toward another catheter directed into the superior vena cava, usually a cordis catheter in the jugular vein if sternotomy is not performed. VVB is most commonly used in level 3 IVC thrombus cases that do not tolerate suprahepatic clamping.[49] VVB may also be initiated during the surgical dissection in cases where significant blood loss is anticipated from venous hypertension secondary to an obstructive IVC thrombus. In these cases,

VVB serves to decompress venous collaterals and varices by shunting blood around the obstruction. VVB can be performed with or without heparinization. Although VVB can be helpful in certain indications, alternatives to VVB exist if it is unavailable or unfamiliar to the multidisciplinary team.

Cardiopulmonary bypass (CPB)[50] involves removal of venous blood, external oxygenation, and reinfusion into the arterial system. Heparinization is required to prevent coagulation in the external circuit. Additional suction connected to the external circuit is also available for recirculation of any blood spilled in the operative field while on bypass. Unlike intraoperative cell salvage that depletes the reinfused blood of coagulation factors, CPB sucker blood retains all these plasma factors helping to decrease the risk of late coagulopathy. Conventionally, CPB is setup via sternotomy, and the venous cannula is placed in the superior vena cava; this is often sufficient without the need for an additional venous cannula inferior to the IVC thrombus. However, use of a venous cannula inferior to the IVC thrombus may provide the additional benefit of limiting blood loss in the operative field as well as helping to decompress hypertensive collaterals similar to the VVB approach. An arterial cannula is then placed in the aorta for blood return. Alternatives to this approach without median sternotomy and using the femoral veins and artery have been described.[51]

Generally, CPB is required to open the atrium for any appreciable time given the amount of blood loss that will occur. CPB does not eliminate blood in the operative field but does allow for recirculation and hemodynamic tolerance of this blood loss. When direct inspection of the atrium and

Table 1
Incisions for inferior vena cava thrombectomy

Incision	Description	Comment
Chevron (or anterior subcostal if incision is unilateral)	2 finger-breadths below rib cage, through all abdominal wall musculature, transperitoneal. Some surgeons may modify this as a triradiate incision with an extension toward xiphoid.	Excellent access to entire upper abdomen. Limited pelvic access. Divides abdominal wall vessels that may be important collaterals during caval obstruction.
Midline laparotomy	Through linea alba, transperitoneal	Excellent pelvic access for large tumors but can have more limited upper abdominal access and can make liver mobilization more difficult. Avoids muscle and abdominal wall collateral vessel division. Connects easiest to sternotomy.
Modified thoracoabdominal	8th or 9th intercostal thoracotomy that joins to a midline laparotomy just above umbilicus, diaphragm divided circumferentially or radially, supine, transperitoneal.	Best exposure: upper abdominal exposure. More morbid than abdominal incisions. Not often required except for the most exceptional tumors. Does not extend well into sternotomy should cardiopulmonary bypass be needed for IVC thrombectomy.
Modified Makuuchi	L or Reverse—L shape; midline from xiphoid to just above umbilicus, then transverse, transperitoneal.	Allows for better unilateral upper abdominal exposure than a standard midline laparotomy while preserving contralateral abdominal wall muscles and collaterals. Less extension options than a chevron incision.
Flank, dorsal lumbotomy	Should not generally be used due to limited vascular access.	

cava is desired, as is often the case with tumor thrombectomy, deep hypothermic circulatory arrest (DHCA) is needed.[50] In DHCA, the patient is cooled to a temperature of 16°C to 18°C and a large portion of the total blood volume drained from the patient before circulatory arrest. Tumor thrombectomy is then performed in 30 to 40 minutes (ideally <30 minutes) to avoid neurologic sequelae,[52] which are mitigated by the hypothermia. Caution is warranted when performing dissection under DHCA, as following reperfusion transected vessels will bleed. Furthermore, the hypothermia used in this technique leads to profound coagulopathy until the patient is rewarmed. An eye toward meticulous hemostasis during initial tumor dissection is paramount.

PRINCIPLES OF OPEN INFERIOR VENA CAVA THROMBECTOMY

The surgical approach to IVC thrombectomy can be divided into 4 parts—abdominal dissection, thoracic dissection, IVC thrombectomy, and IVC reconstruction.

Abdominal Dissection

Opening
The first decision to make is choice of surgical incision. Considerations surrounding surgical incision are detailed in **Table 1**. Once the abdomen is entered, dissection should be performed as atraumatically as possible to avoid dislodging friable thrombus, which may lead to intraoperative embolization. The natural tissue planes may not be preserved, as parasitic vessels cross these planes or a desmoplastic reaction may obscure them. A vessel sealing device may be helpful in this setting.

Mobilization of the bowel may be more difficult than normal due to enlargement of collateral vessels, high venous pressure, tumor-related neovascularization, and a desmoplastic reaction. Limiting mesenteric resection is ideal to ensure bowel viability. Generally, the required mobilization for these cases significantly exceeds what is required in the standard nephrectomy. Regardless of the laterality of the primary tumor, mobilization of the root of the mesentery along with the right colon toward the foramen of Winslow (Cattell-Braasch maneuver[53]) can be helpful in obtaining the necessary exposure to the vena cava and interaortocaval space. The inferior mesenteric vein can be divided if necessary for this mobilization. For a left-sided tumor, en bloc mobilization of the spleen, pancreas, and stomach off the left retroperitoneum will expose the left renal vein to its confluence with the vena cava.[54] If a large tumor prevents mobilization of the spleen and distal pancreas, splenectomy (and sometimes distal pancreatectomy) can be performed; the surgeon then exposes the left kidney by mobilizing the splenic flexure and reflecting the remaining pancreas through the lesser sac.[55]

Renal artery ligation
Renal artery ligation is generally the first consideration once the retroperitoneum is exposed. Ligation of the renal artery will allow for a reduction in tumor vascularity and bulk of a vascular thrombus. If the intention is to divide the thrombus-containing renal vein, this can also be done once the renal artery is ligated. En bloc stapling of the hilum is to be avoided except in extreme circumstances because the renal artery stump will likely be difficult to separate from the thrombus-containing vein after being stapled together.

It is optimal to approach the right renal artery in the interaortocaval space, as the conventional right renal hilar approach is more difficult in these cases. This space is generally exposed well with the Cattell-Braasch maneuver described in the preceding section.

Ligation of the renal artery for a left-sided nephrectomy is approached from underneath the left renal vein. Sometimes entry into the lesser sac[55] may facilitate identification of the superior mesenteric artery and left renal artery above the left renal vein, a maneuver that may be useful with bulky left renal vein thrombus or adenopathy. If the renal artery is otherwise inaccessible by any other method, the kidney can be fully mobilized and lifted (Mattox maneuver[56]) to provide view of the entire abdominal aorta. The surgeon may then be able to identify the artery from underneath the kidney posteriorly. This approach should only be used if necessary, as renal mobilization risks thrombus dislodgement and may still not provide the necessary exposure with a large tumor.

In cases where preoperative embolization has been performed, unless performed shortly before the procedure, an inflammatory reaction may obscure tissue planes. In addition, it is important to ensure that there is enough length of the renal artery stump free of embolization coils for ligation. If sufficient length of renal artery is not available for standard control, a 3-0 prolene pledgeted suture on the aorta at the renal artery os will be required.

Vena caval control
Vena caval control follows renal artery ligation. Gentle manipulation of the vena cava is essential to prevent embolization. Performing thrombectomy first is thought to have a lower risk of embolization than performing the renal dissection first.[57] Vena caval control is obtained as necessary for the

level of thrombus as detailed later. Ligating any veins feeding the segment to be isolated will ensure a bloodless field. Ligation of infrarenal lumbar vessels is ideally avoided to prevent disruption of important collaterals in the context of caval occlusion.[58]

En bloc versus disconnected thrombectomy

Nephrectomy and IVC thrombectomy are ideally performed en bloc; this may not be feasible in some cases. If required, the IVC can be disconnected from the tumor-bearing renal vein with a surgical stapler device. A tall staple load for thick tissue is needed to staple a bulky thrombus; tthese are not vascular loads and should not be left on any retained vascular structures. If a thrombus is not as bulky, vascular loads can be used. When thrombectomy is performed, the staple line must be excised en bloc with the tumor thrombus.

Disconnected thrombectomy is considered in cases where exposure of the vena cava is limited by mass or obesity and more space is needed; this is particularly helpful for left-sided cases where, following nephrectomy, retraction can then focus on the right side alone. Significant renal bleeding may also be a relative indication for completing the nephrectomy expediently. Disconnected thrombectomy is contraindicated if stapling the tumor thrombus is thought to be likely to dislodge the thrombus.

Inferior Vena Cava Thrombectomy

Level 0

These tumor thrombi can be approached with limited deviation from a conventional radical nephrectomy. Ultrasonography is used to map out thrombus extent intraoperatively. Care should be taken to ensure that all of the thrombus is included with the kidney when the renal vein is ligated; this is straightforward during open surgery, as the renal vein can be clamped as close to the IVC as necessary and ligated with a running 4-0 prolene suture line. Although careful use of vascular stapler device is likely a safe and more familiar alternative, it requires a reasonable length of uninvolved renal vein for application, and it is important to ensure that all of the thrombus is included with the specimen and not stapled or dislodged during a "milking" maneuver. An alternative technique to the stapler device is to apply sequential clips to progressively push the thrombus toward the kidney.

Level 1

Ultrasonography is used to delineate the extent of a level 1 thrombus and determine whether it can be encompassed by a Satinsky clamp that surrounds the tumor thrombus and partially occludes the IVC. If the thrombus is too large for this maneuver it will need to be approached as a level 2 thrombus. Once clamped, a venotomy is made at the renal vein-IVC junction, and the renal vein and en bloc tumor thrombus can then be excised. The IVC is repaired at the renal vein os with limited narrowing. Even in the setting of a level 1 IVC thrombus amenable to this approach, obtaining full control of the juxtarenal IVC is ideal. The juxtarenal IVC can be fully clamped if the partial clamp is dislodged, must be repositioned to excise more vein wall, or if there is insufficient vein wall above the clamp to repair the IVC.

Level 2

Level 2 IVC thrombectomy is performed by fully clamping the juxtarenal IVC. The infrarenal IVC, followed by the contralateral renal vein, then the suprarenal IVC above the level of the tumor thrombus are clamped sequentially. On occasion it may also be necessary to place a bulldog clamp on the right adrenal vein (for left-sided tumors) along with any large lumbar veins that must be preserved. While obtaining control of the infrarenal IVC and contralateral renal vein, care should be taken to avoid injury to any lumbar veins that may be obscured by fibrosis, dilated, and under high pressure. To ensure a bloodless field when the cava is opened, the surgeon should be able to run their hands behind and around the cava before opening it to verify that all necessary veins entering that segment have been divided. Alternatively, specialized vascular clamps such as Profunda clamps can be slid behind the cava to occlude posterior lumbar branches; however, extreme care must be taken to avoid avulsion or trauma. Finally, in difficult cases where posterior dissection or control is not feasible, backbleeding lumbar vein ostia can be plugged with balloon occlusion catheters from within the caval lumen.

Depending on the cephalad extent of a level 2 IVC thrombus, it may be necessary to gain control of the retrohepatic cava for clamping. If the tumor extends above the level of the hepatoduodenal ligament, the lesser sac should be entered by dividing the pars flaccida of the gastrohepatic ligament. Immediately deep to this is the caudate lobe, which sits on top of the retrohepatic portion of the cava. Some upward mobilization of this portion of the liver is often required. Along with peritoneal attachments, division of short hepatic veins will be necessary for caudate lobe mobilization. Short hepatic veins can be difficult to ligate due to their short length, and use of a vessel sealer device can be helpful.[59] If a short hepatic vein stump is not controlled and bleeds from the caudate lobe, a pledgeted 5-0 prolene suture on the caudate lobe can be effectively used. Meticulous dissection and control of venous branches is needed for this portion of the operation, as injuries to the retrohepatic cava can result in substantially increased operative mortality.

For a right-sided thrombus, identification and ligation of the right adrenal vein is also prudent to prevent injury during suprarenal control. Suprarenal IVC control should be obtained well above the level that is necessary. Obtaining insufficient cephalad control may lead to dislodgement of friable thrombus fragments when attempting to clamp the suprarenal IVC. For the level 2 thrombus that extends many centimeters beyond the inferior border of the caudate, particularly one that is friable and free-floating, it may be preferrable to avoid prolonged mobilization of the caudate lobe alone and approach cephalad control as a level 3 thrombus.

Most patients will tolerate caval clamping below the main hepatic veins without significant hemodynamic compromise if they are appropriately resuscitated.[60] It is wise to ensure that the patient remains stable following clamping before the blood loss that may result when the cava is opened. After administering heparin, a test clamp should be applied to the cava followed by an observation period of approximately 3 to 5 minutes. If hypotension does develop, the clamps should be released and standard assessment for hypotension conducted, including looking for evidence of embolization on transesophageal echocardiography. A repeat clamp trial can generally be made after further resuscitation.

When the juxtarenal IVC is successfully clamped, a venotomy should be made beginning at the inferior border of the involved renal vein os and extending cephalad enough to allow for thrombus extraction. In rare circumstances, it may be necessary to carry the venotomy behind the hepatoduodenal ligament and onto the retrohepatic cava. Following venotomy, it may also be helpful to ligate or compress the tumor-bearing vein if the thrombus is partially occlusive—blood drainage from the kidney can be significant if collaterals remain and will obscure visualization.

For left-sided tumors the right renal vein will need to be periodically vented, as it is usually not collateralized. Clamping of the right renal artery is ideally avoided to prevent ischemia. Following thrombectomy, an obliquely placed clamp that allows the right renal vein to decompress into the infrarenal IVC may be optimal to ensure right-renal drainage during IVC closure. If a lumbar vessel bleeds into the IVC lumen obscuring visualization during thrombectomy, it can be ligated

from inside the IVC with a figure-of-8 5-0 prolene suture or temporarily occluded with a balloon occlusion catheter.

A special note should be made of the imporance of anticipating the degree to which the tumor thrombus can be extracted from the cava; this is particularly important in level 2 cases where suprahepatic control has not been achieved. The surgical team must be ready for the possibility that the tumor may be completely adherent to the tumor wall requiring en bloc partial or complete caval resection. Consequently, adequate exposure to sew a patch or graft may be necessary before cavotomy. In addition, the patient may tolerate the 5- to 10-minute period of caval clamping necessary for simple thrombectomy and primary closure but may develop hemodynamic collapse during the additional time necessary for caval reconstruction. In such cases, preemptive use of VVB should be considered, even for level 2 tumors.

Level 3

Level 3 IVC thrombectomy requires control of the suprahepatic cava, infrahepatic suprarenal cava, contralateral renal vein, infrarenal cava, and porta hepatis within the hepatoduodenal ligament (Pringle maneuver). Isolation of the suprahepatic cava requires division of some of the triangular and coronary ligaments, and care should be taken to avoid injury to the phrenic and hepatic veins.

The surgeon will need to decide on the extent of liver mobilization that will be required. Full liver mobilization can be avoided with an incompletely occlusive thrombus that will be easy to extract. Avoiding liver mobilization in this setting may also limit embolization risk. If a bulky thrombus is likely to require a longer cavotomy and some caval wall resection, or total suprarenal cavectomy and ligation is anticipated, full liver mobilization is essential.

Liver mobilization is straightforward except in cases of hepatic congestion or obesity; this is analogous to the dissection necessary to perform a piggyback transplantation where the liver is released from the cava with the exception of the main hepatic veins.[61] To perform this, the surgeon's hand is used to retract the liver caudally and the falciform ligament is divided toward the suprahepatic IVC. The right liver is then pulled to the left to divide the right anterior coronary ligament and triangular ligament. At least some of the left coronary ligaments must be divided for suprahepatic IVC control. The diaphragm is released from the bare area, and the right posterior coronary ligament is divided to release the liver from the kidney. When the posterolateral retrohepatic vena cava is in close proximity it is necessary to use a surgical stapler or vessel sealing device to divide the Makuuchi ligament.[62] The caudate is now lifted, and a vessel sealing device can be helpful to divide the short hepatic veins that attach the caudate to the vena cava. Although included in a piggyback liver mobilization, the remaining left-sided ligaments may not require division if the liver is sufficiently mobilized at this point.

Once adequate exposure has been obtained, the infrarenal cava is clamped first, followed by the contralateral renal vein, porta hepatis (Pringle maneuver), then suprahepatic cava.[63] Time should be given for the liver to decompress following the Pringle maneuver before suprahepatic clamping. If the infrarenal cava or contralateral renal vein are occluded with thrombus it would be wise to alter the clamp order and only manipulate these after cephalad control to avoid fragmenting the thrombus.

Suprahepatic clamping is more likely to result in hemodynamic changes, and clamping should be tested for 5 to 10 minutes before cavotomy. If significant hypotension results, the clamps should be released and the patient resuscitated further before another clamp trial. The Pringle and suprahepatic clamp portion of the thrombectomy can often be limited to a very short duration (<1–2 minutes) and so limited hypotension will likely be tolerated. In cases of nonbulky, mobile tumor thrombus, we have been successful in developing an additional infra- or retrohepatic clamp site. Following the standard clamp placement described earlier, the tumor is milked down to the level of the retro- or infrahepatic cava and then a new clamp is placed at this level above the tumor. The suprahepatic clamp is released, as is the Pringle clamp, allowing for reperfusion of the liver and restoration of hemodynamics. Now the cavotomy and standard level 2 thrombectomy can be performed. This maneuver effectively "downstages" the tumor level from 3 to 2 but can only be done in cases where the tumor thrombus is not adherent to the wall and there is little-to-no concern for distal embolization. Alternatively, if suprahepatic clamping cannot be tolerated, either venovenous bypass[64,65] or infrarenal aortic clamping[66] (to increase cardiac afterload and blood pressure) can be usd.

Once the IVC is clamped, venotomy is performed at the renal vein os. Because the hepatic veins will be draining into the isolated segment, bleeding is likely once the venotomy is performed. Once the thrombus is extracted or lowered below the hepatic veins, an infrahepatic suprarenal clamp is applied, and the suprahepatic and porta hepatis clamps are released.[63] Caval reconstruction is now performed on the juxtarenal IVC segment in a bloodless setting.

Level 4

Level 4 IVC thrombectomy usually requires a combined abdominal and thoracic approach (**Fig. 3**). The case often starts with the abdominal approach, particularly in cases just above the diaphragm where the tumor thrombus can sometimes be found to be lower than expected and a sternotomy can be avoided.[67] Some access to the supradiaphragmatic cava is possible through an abdominal incision with diaphragmatic division.[10,67] Indications for performing the thoracic dissection first are discussed in the following section. For cases outside the atrium that are felt to be

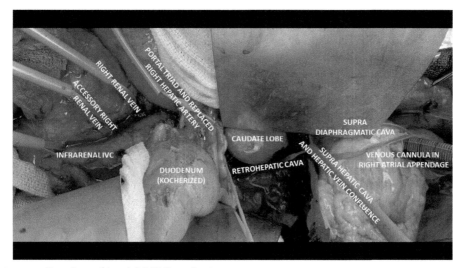

Fig. 3. Intraoperative view of level 4 IVC thrombectomy.

Table 2
Intraoperative findings during tumor thrombectomy

Category	Finding	Implication	Technique
0	No thrombus	The thrombus has embolized or imaging was inaccurate	Assess transesophageal echocardiography and patient stability. Standard radical nephrectomy.
1	Free-floating thrombus without wall contact, broad base	Extraction will be straightforward	Cava can be opened and closed, likely without reconstruction
2	Free-floating thrombus without wall contact, small freely mobile fragments visualized on inspection or ultrasonography	Extraction will be straightforward but higher risk for embolization or fragmentation	Care during dissection, careful inspection following cavotomy for all fragments, likely without need for reconstruction
3	Focal contact of IVC wall with flow seen around most of tumor thrombus	Thrombus extraction may not be straightforward due to focal adherence or IVC wall invasion	Focal dissection with Penfield dissector or focal cavectomy and closure. May be more likely to require patch cavoplasty
4	Significant contact with IVC wall by bulky thrombus with limited flow seen around tumor thrombus, significant collateralization, and atretic infrarenal cava	Thrombus will likely not extract intact—IVC is likely adherent/invaded and also significantly obstructed	Suprarenal cavectomy and ligation to be considered
5	Category 4, but with findings extending to hepatic veins and supradiaphragmatic IVC	Total clearance of unresectable portions of IVC will be difficult.	Technique focuses on clearance of gross disease. See text.

easily extractable and unlikely to be adherent, the procedure can be performed analogous to a level 3 thrombectomy with the cephalad clamp placed on the supradiaphragmatic infraatrial vena cava. Unless the thrombus is anticipated to be easy to extract, exposure of all of the retrohepatic IVC with liver mobilization is ideal so that the abdominal cavotomy can be extended upward as far as necessary, and this will facilitate suprarenal cavectomy and reconstruction or ligation.

If atriotomy is required, infraatrial clamping is not tolerated, or a bloodless field will aid in thrombectomy and inspection of the cava, CPB and DHCA are necessary. Although CPB and DHCA will provide unparalleled exposure of the IVC lumen, it does have several specific complications associated with it and requires heparinization.

PRINCIPLES OF THROMBECTOMY

Principles of thrombectomy based on intraoperative findings are detailed in **Table 2**.

Level 3 and 4 thrombi that are adherent to the hepatic veins or suprahepatic IVC pose a particular challenge. Unlike the infrahepatic IVC, it is generally not feasible to reconstruct or replace the hepatic veins or suprahepatic IVC in this situation. The segment of IVC from several centimeters below the hepatic veins up to the atrium is generally not opened. Significantly adherent thrombi often fragment during extraction and require prolonged debridement of all adherent fragments. CPB and DHA will greatly facilitate caval clearance in this setting. Options for optimizing outcomes include the following:

i. Use of a Penfield or laparotomy sponge for debridement of all gross visible fragments.
ii. Debridement of adherent fragments from the supradiaphragmatic cava from the atriotomy. The atriotomy may provide access to just above hepatic vein ostia.
iii. Passing a vascular tunneling clamp from the abdominal cavotomy up into the atrium,

which is then used to grab and pull a laparotomy sponge back through the atrium and retrohepatic cava and out of the cavotomy in order to clear the caval wall of residual debris.

iv. Gentle digital inspection of the caval lumen to ensure no residual fragments remain.

v. Instilling heparinized saline and visualizing the obscured cava with transesophageal echocardiography to assess for any residual fragments.

vi. Analogous to an arterial embolectomy, passing a Fogarty balloon or 20-Fr foley catheter through the obscured segment can also be helpful to ensure clearance.

vii. A flexible cystoscope may be useful to inspect the segment with umbilical tape or vessel loops occluding the segment to allow fluid distension.

Thoracic Dissection

The thoracic dissection is only necessary in patients with a level 4 thrombus. Median sternotomy is the conventional incision that most cardiac surgeons will be familiar with for cardiopulmonary bypass, although less invasive alternatives exist.[51] Some surgeons may also more routinely use a thoracoabdominal incision,[68] which can be particularly useful for right-sided tumors that will require extensive access to the retrohepatic cava. If major bleeding is anticipated and early bypass may be needed, embolization risk is high, or the thoracic dissection is anticipated to be complicated (eg, prior coronary artery bypass grafting), then consideration should be given to performing the thoracic dissection before the abdominal dissection. Planned concurrent coronary artery bypass grafting for patients with significant coronary artery lesions identified during preoperative assessment may also warrant starting thoracic dissection first to prepare for grafting to be performed during CPB. Sternotomy can also aid with exposure, as the ribcage will be much more mobile and diaphragm amenable to flattening for difficult abdominal dissections and for liver mobilization. Aortic and venous cannula placement can be avoided for infraatrial cases where one is hoping to avoid cardiopulmonary bypass although placement before cavotomy will make going on CPB much easier in the event of massive caval bleeding.

Working space is limited, and outside of the thrombectomy portion, it is usually not feasible for abdominal and cardiac teams to work synchronously in dissection or closure. Placing the abdominal retractor posts caudally can often be helpful during the thrombectomy to provide more space for the cardiac and abdominal surgeons to stand next to each other.

Inferior Vena Cava Reconstruction

Four options exist for IVC reconstruction following IVC thrombectomy (**Fig. 4**).

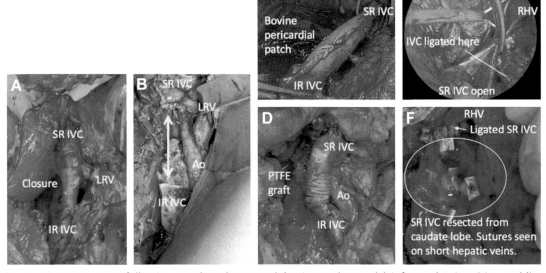

Fig. 4. IVC management following IVC thrombectomy. (*A*) Primary closure, (*B*) infrarenal IVC excision and ligation, (*C*) patch cavoplasty, (*D*) suprarenal cavectomy and tube graft, (*E* and *F*) suprarenal cavectomy and ligation. A final option is IVC filter placement for caudal bland thrombus (not depicted). AO, aorta; IR, infrarenal; LRV, left renal vein; RHV, right hepatic vein; SR, suprarenal.

i. Primary closure

It is often feasible to primarily close the IVC following thrombectomy with less than 50% luminal diameter narrowing; this is the preferred method of IVC closure if it is feasible. It should be avoided if primary repair will result in greater than 50% luminal narrowing or limit the oncologic completeness of the procedure. Conversely, the cava may be quite patulous following bulky tumor thrombectomy and primary repair patency may be increased by partially plicating the cava down to its pararenal diameter to accelerate blood flow through the area and theoretically avoid stasis and thrombus formation.

ii. Patch cavoplasty

Patch cavoplasty is indicated when the IVC luminal diameter will be narrowed greater than 50% with primary closure and ongoing IVC continuity is desired. The technique is also useful when R0 resection requires en bloc removal of a portion of the caval wall where the tumor is adherent or invasive. Bovine pericardium is often readily available in several sizes and is a common choice for patch material. Several other autologous and nonautologous options also exist for patch cavoplasty.

iii. Cavectomy and ligation

Suprarenal cavectomy is indicated for circumferential caval invasion. Suprarenal cavectomy is less complex for a right-sided primary tumor because the left renal vein will drain through collaterals. Suprarenal cavectomy can be done up to the level of the main hepatic veins and will require enough liver mobilization to achieve a circumferential retrohepatic clamp site. The infrarenal cavectomy margin is at the point where tumor thrombus extends to—and one should be especially careful of injury to the right common iliac artery that will cross the occluded IVC caudally and can be hidden amid the fibrosis resulting from chronic venous occlusion. Frozen section can be used to guide the infrarenal and left renal vein margins as necessary.

When performed for left-sided primaries, venous drainage of the right kidney needs to be considered. Sometimes the right kidney will have developed extensive collaterals if the right renal vein is obstructed. If this has not occurred, cavectomy can be performed obliquely, with the right renal vein continuing to drain into the retained IVC. Alternatively, the right renal vein can be anastomosed to another close vein such as the right gonadal vein. If the infrarenal IVC is obstructed, reimplantation of the right renal vein alone into a ringed polytetrafluoroethylene (PTFE) graft is possible but may lead to thrombotic complications due to a relatively small lumen.

Caval ligation is usually appropriate when suprarenal cavectomy is indicated because the infrarenal cava is often atretic and occluded by bland thrombus. Ligation can be performed with a vascular stapler device or 4-0 prolene suture.

iv. Caval replacement

Caval replacement is indicated when suprarenal cavectomy is performed but ligation is not desired due to residual infrarenal caval flow. A ringed PTFE graft can be used to anastomose the infrarenal to the suprarenal IVC, although other options exist. The renal vein can also be either reimplanted into this graft directly or bypassed with a separate PTFE side arm. This tube graft likely has the highest thromboembolism risk of all the options described earlier. For this reason, we prefer to use a graft that is 25% to 50% smaller in diameter than the infrahepatic cava in order to accelerate blood through the graft, thereby reducing stasis and thrombus formation.

Caval replacement is uncommon because either some portion of the IVC can be retained for patch cavoplasty or the IVC is completely occluded from circumferential invasion and ligation is likely to be hemodynamically insignificant and beneficial for prevention of embolus. Anastomosis of a tube graft to a low-flow chronically occluded infrarenal cava is not recommended, because this will have a high thromboembolism risk. An intraoperative doppler probe may be used to assess flow in the IVC after reconstruction is complete.

Bland thrombus management

Bland thrombus often coexists with tumor thrombus,[4] and a plan is needed for how any coexisting bland thrombus will be managed. Caval ligation will limit PE risk. If the cava is retained in continuity with either primary closure, patch cavoplasty, or replacement, infrarenal bland thrombus will require anticoagulation to be resumed as soon as feasible. An IVC filter can also be placed in the perioperative period.

POSTOPERATIVE MANAGEMENT

For high-level thrombectomies, intensive care unit admission is likely necessary for 1 or more days. Diet is advanced once postoperative ileus has resolved.

Anticoagulation postoperatively is dictated by thromboembolism risk. Pharmacologic deep vein

Table 3
Selected series detailing perioperative and oncologic outcomes

Study	Blute 2004[49]	Haddad 2014[91]	Vinzant 2022[41]
Study population	Mayo Clinic, 1970–2000, Level 0–4	Multiinstitutional, 2000–2013, level 3–4	Mayo Clinic, 2005–2017, level 3–4
Study size	540	166	65
Perioperative mortality (30-d)	Level 0: 1.8% Level 1: 1.5% Level 2: 3.9% Level 3: 14.2% Level 4: 15.0%	10.2%	4.6%
Cancer-specific survival (5-y)	Level 0: 49.1% Level 1: 31.7% Level 2: 26.3% Level 3: 39.4% Level 4: 37.0%	49.0% (pN0/Nx, M0 cohort n = 111)	n/a

thrombosis (DVT) prophylaxis for 28 days is indicated even for low-risk patients. For patients with known pulmonary emboli or deep vein thromboses, prophylactic dosing of heparin on the day of and day after surgery followed by a low-dose (500 u/h) heparin drip on day 2 is appropriate. This low-dose heparin can then be sequentially titrated to full dose should bleeding not develop and eventually transitioned to a more appropriate regimen for home. Patients with anything but an unnarrowed primary repair also likely benefit from antiplatelet therapy. Those having undergone patch cavoplasty receive long-term aspirin. Clopidogrel or low-dose oral anticoagulants can be used for those with a PTFE tube graft.

In patients undergoing cytoreductive nephrectomy and IVC thrombectomy, immunotherapy can be (re)started following hospital discharge. Complete wound healing is usually preferred before starting tyrosine kinase inhibitors. For nonmetastatic patients, adjuvant therapy is usually considered once fully recovered, and postoperative imaging demonstrates continued freedom from metastatic disease.

CLINICAL OUTCOMES

Perioperative and oncologic outcomes from selected series are detailed in **Table 3**. Numerous additional series describe analogous outcomes.[42,69] It is likely that outcomes are improving with time and will continue to improve with refinements in surgical technique, perioperative medicine, and nonsurgical alternatives for the poor surgical candidate.

PERIOPERATIVE COMPLICATIONS
Bleeding

Management of postoperative bleeding is similar to other major abdominal cases and is guided by the patient's clinical status. The cause of hemorrhage is often not clear and the stable patient not requiring immediate reexploration may benefit from a CT angiogram and correction of coagulopathy. Whenever possible, CT angiography should be performed with an additional prolonged delay or venous phase to assess for venous bleeding. Hemorrhage could result from the standard culprits following nephrectomy such as the renal arterial stump, IVC, or inadvertent injuries to the perirenal structures such as the spleen, liver, mesentery, omentum, or diaphragm. Abdominal wall collaterals originating from caval obstruction could be a unique source of hemorrhage following those cases performed through a muscle-dividing incision. The large renal masses that give rise to IVC thrombi are usually associated with significant neovascularization that may have been incompletely recognized or controlled. In cases where there has been both an abdominal and thoracic dissection, chest tube and abdominal drain output can be a signal as to the cavity from where hemorrhage originates.

Preoperative Pulmonary Embolism

Advances in systemic therapy provide flexibility in timing an operation in the patient with preexisting pulmonary emboli. Although the patient with a limited PE preoperatively will have limited perioperative risk,[36] those with pulmonary embolic burden that will result in excessive surgical mortality risk (eg, a main pulmonary embolism with a pulmonary infarct and oxygen requirement) could benefit from preoperative systemic therapy and anticoagulation to permit medical stabilization before IVC thrombectomy 3 to 6 months later.

It is unclear if a pulmonary embolus is tumor or bland. Although anticoagulation will presumably be less helpful in a tumor embolus, it may prevent additional bland thrombus forming on tumor emboli and prevent further bland emboli originating from the IVC thrombus. Fortunately, there is no clear risk of pulmonary seeding from tumor emboli.[36]

In patients who are clinically unstable, interventional measures can be considered, as several options exist for catheter-directed tumor thrombectomy,[70,71] and in some cases, mechanical cardiopulmonary support. Multidisciplinary discussions with cardiology, pulmonology, and interventional radiology will be helpful in these settings. All attempts should be made to continue anticoagulation despite hematuria that may originate from the primary renal tumor—and selective embolization or radiotherapy can be helpful in allowing for this.

When surgery is planned, patients with recent pulmonary emboli likely benefit from bridging anticoagulation, as progression could be challenging to manage in the perioperative period. The cava should be handled atraumatically to prevent further embolization. Hemostatic products and drain placement may be useful given the need for early postoperative anticoagulation. A transition toward full anticoagulation with a lower rate drip (eg, starting at 500 u/h on the second postoperative day before full dose on the following day) may be helpful.

Intraoperative Pulmonary Embolism

Mortality from an intraoperative embolism is high.[46] Specific signs of embolization include hypoxia accompanied by a drop in end-tidal CO_2 levels, which help distinguish it from hemodynamic instability from other causes. An embolus can be confirmed on transesophageal echocardiography or the loss of a known thrombus on intraoperative ultrasound or cavotomy.

Strong consideration should be given to a pulmonary artery embolectomy for intraoperative embolism. While awaiting the cardiac surgery and perfusion setup, the abdominal surgical team should expeditiously terminate the procedure. High doses of heparin (300–400 u/kg) will either have been administered or are imminent and attempts to prevent hemorrhage should be made

with packing and hemostatic products. If feasible, removing the kidney may control a significant potential source of bleeding. Temporary abdominal closure will facilitate a reoperation when the patient has stabilized. If an Abthera (Acelity) or analogous device is not immediately available, simply covering the bowel with laparotomy sponges and placing several sutures in the skin and/or fascia will facilitate termination. If preparation was not already made for sternotomy, the patient should be repositioned supine with arms tucked and sterile prep reapplied up to the neck. Following pulmonary artery embolectomy, return to the operating room once the patient has stabilized in 24 to 48 hours is important to ensure hemostasis, resect any additional areas of concern, assess for any inadvertent injury, and perform appropriate closure.

If pulmonary artery embolectomy is not feasible and the patient can be stabilized for transfer to the interventional radiology suite, several options exist for catheter-directed embolectomy.[70,71] Management with anticoagulation alone is likely appropriate for small emboli detected postoperatively in the hemodynamically stable patient.

Air Embolus

Air embolus may occur during cavotomy or after cavotomy closure and reperfusion, and clinical presentation is similar to that of pulmonary embolism. Specific care should be taken to prevent air embolism during the case by flushing extensively before caval closure and cephalad clamp release; this can be facilitated by letting the IVC bleed as the closure is completed (eg, by unclamping the contralateral renal vein).

Bland Thrombus

Bland thrombus can develop postoperatively in the retained IVC or any other large veins. Malignancy, altered venous dynamics, and venous clamping all predispose to the development of these deep vein thromboses. Therapeutic anticoagulation will generally allow for resolution of even significant thromboses. If the cava has not been ligated and there is significant iliofemoral DVT, consideration can be given to IVC filter placement.

Leg Edema

Leg edema either before or after IVC thrombectomy should prompt an assessment of iliofemoral venous drainage with duplex sonography. DVT generally indicates therapeutic anticoagulation, but edema is common enough even in the absence of DVT. Even with significant iliofemoral DVT, venous phlegmasia is unlikely but should be monitored for. In cases where phlegmasia develops, open venous thrombectomy or catheter-directed pharmacomechanical thrombectomy is effective, as prolonged catheter-directed thrombolysis will not be an option in the immediate postoperative period. Absent infrainguinal DVT should prompt pelvic or transabdominal imaging of the iliac veins and cava with either ultrasound or CT in cases of substantial edema. In most cases, however, leg edema is managed with conservative measures until its resolution. Even significant leg edema following IVC ligation will improve with conservative measures as collateralization occurs.

Hypotension from Inferior Vena Cava Syndrome

Postoperatively, patients with a ligated IVC or that develop bland caval and iliofemoral thrombosis can be at risk of hypotension and other sequelae of IVC syndrome[72]; this may be present at rest or only orthostatically and likely occurs due to inadequate venous return. It eventually improves but may require support with vasopressors and fluid resuscitation. It can be difficult to differentiate caval related hypotension from the myriad of other causes of hypotension in the early perioperative period and should be considered a diagnosis of exclusion. Midodrine can be helpful when this is persistent outside of the early perioperative period.

Chylous Ascites

Chylous ascites may rarely develop due to retroperitoneal lymphadenectomy and/or IVC resection. Chylous ascites will often resolve with conservative measures such as a low-fat diet and paracentesis. Options, should conservative measures fail, are well reviewed elsewhere.[73]

ON THE HORIZON
Shifting Case Mix

Cytoreductive nephrectomies comprise a significant proportion of most IVC thrombectomy series. As discussed previously, paradigms surrounding CN are shifting, and CN will be less frequently performed upfront. Meanwhile, deferred CN after response to systemic therapy may become routine.[74–76] Preoperative systemic therapy will reduce average thrombus level and bulk at the expense of a desmoplastic reaction that may be associated with systemic therapy.[77]

Systemic therapy and SBRT have a lower immediate morbidity and mortality risk in nonmetastatic patients.[38] Adoption of this SBRT will reduce upfront IVC thrombectomy rates at the expense of more complex salvage procedures.

Lymphadenectomy

Lymphadenectomy indication and template for advanced RCC has become controversial.[78] Indications and templates for concurrent lymphadenectomy will be solidified in the future.

Robotic Inferior Vena Cava Thrombectomy

Analogous to other procedures in urologic oncology, the robotic approach for highly selected renal vein and IVC thrombectomy cases is becoming more routine.[69] The perioperative benefits of minimally invasive renal surgery are appealing—including a lower blood loss during the renal dissection, reduced incisional pain and complications, and faster convalescence. Although these potential benefits are relevant to selected cases where major complication rates should be low, robotic IVC thrombectomy cannot mechanistically improve on the major perioperative complications that can occur during complex cases.

PREOPERATIVE CONSIDERATIONS

Mastery of open IVC thrombectomy along with advanced robotic retroperitoneal surgery are prerequisites to successful robotic IVC thrombectomy. The surgeon pursuing robotic IVC thrombectomy will also need to consider case selection, overcoming robotic limitations during intraoperative challenges, difficulty with left-sided tumors, how to position for open conversion, how to involve any necessary consulting surgeons that cannot perform robotic surgery, hemodynamic difficulties of pneumoperitoneum and a fixed position, inability to leave an open abdomen, and access difficulties for transesophageal echocardiography and emergent cardiopulmonary bypass.

Simpler IVC thrombectomy cases that may be initially considered for the robotic approach include absence of a bulky primary tumor, limited adenopathy, a thrombus that is not especially friable and does not significantly contact the IVC wall circumferentially, no anticipated vascular reconstruction, and a cephalad extent that will not require significant short hepatic division or liver mobilization. Although it may be appealing to perform minimally invasive surgery in the obese patient where a large incision for open surgery is likely to be necessary, robotic exposure can be similarly difficult and open conversion will also be more challenging.

The preoperative preparation before robotic IVC thrombectomy is analogous to the open approach. Transesophageal echocardiography may be facilitated by placing the probe before lateral positioning. Similarly, appropriate monitoring should be in place before positioning, as placing additional intravenous or arterial or central lines is challenging in the lateral position. A plan for massive transfusion is needed in the lateral approach, as this may be less familiar to both the surgical and anesthesia teams.

The AirSeal (Conmed) port should be placed in the nondependent position when major bleeding is expected because blood in the AirSeal (Conmed) tubing will stop the system and cause pneumoperitoneum to be lost. This issue can be common with an AirSeal (Conmed) assistant port placed in the midline and so consideration should be given to lateral placement.

Decisions on how the need for open conversion should be handled are important—a subcostal or extended flank incision conventionally considered for robotic nephrectomy conversions will have poor vascular access, particularly with a bulky renal mass or thrombus. Given the right lateral positioning, the optimal incision for exposure during emergent conversion for vascular catastrophe is likely a modified thoracoabdominal incision with an eighth or ninth rib thoracotomy connected to a midline or paramedian laparotomy with circumferential diaphragmatic division. Most of the juxtarenal and retrohepatic cava should be accessible with this approach but aortic access will be suboptimal. Repositioning to the supine position is likely best for nonemergent conversions. In the event of an on-table embolization requiring emergent cardiopulmonary bypass and embolectomy, plans should be discussed for how the case will be aborted and the patient positioned supine for sternotomy.

Operative Procedure

Technical aspects of robotic IVC thrombectomy are intuitive for those familiar with the open approach. Intraoperative ultrasound is helpful during robotic IVC thrombectomy to determine the location of the thrombus.

Options for vascular clamps are more limited robotically, and conventionally a doubly wrapped vessel loop with a sliding Weck Hem-O-Lok (Teleflex) clip is used instead of a Rummel tourniquet. Although a Foley catheter segment can be used to create a proper Rummel for robotic IVC thrombectomy, this is often unnecessary. Laparoscopic bulldog clamps are often not large enough for caval occlusion but may be helpful in occluding the ipsilateral or contralateral renal veins. A laparoscopic Satinsky should also be available but has limited utility, as it occupies an assistant port and cannot be manipulated by the console surgeon. "Tip-up" graspers have longer jaws that may facilitate the passing of vessel loops behind the cava and confirm the juxtarenal segment is isolated.

The surgical approach to a level 0 IVC thrombectomy involves clipping or stapling the renal vein distal to the thrombus. The level 0 thrombus with a friable tip or unclear distal extent should be approached as a level 1 thrombus to prevent embolization or a positive vascular margin.

Because options for salvage of a dislodged clamp are more limited, partial caval occlusion

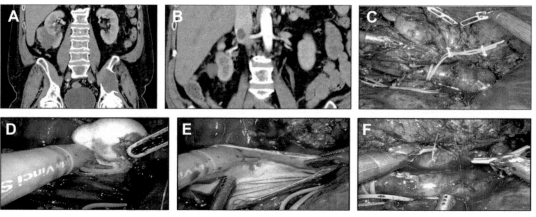

Fig. 5. Robotic level 2 IVC thrombectomy in a patient with oligometastatic RCC following systemic therapy response. (*A*) Coronal view of CT scan showing right renal mass and solitary left iliac bone lesion, which was subsequently treated with radiation. (*B*) Coronal view of CT scan showing level 2 IVC thrombus before surgery. (*C*) IVC (right of image is cephalad) with blue vessel loops placed around the infrarenal IVC, left renal vein, and suprarenal IVC (*left to right*). (*D*) IVC thrombus being resected with grossly negative IVC margin. (*E*) Intra-op image showing IVC lumen once tumor thrombus has been removed. (*F*) IVC has been repaired without visible narrowing.

and colporrhaphy for level 1 robotic thrombectomy should be approached with caution. Partial occlusion is likely only reasonable if there is also total control of the juxtarenal segment in the event of clamp dislodgement or failure.

Otherwise, level 1 to 2 thrombectomy are approached by clamping the infrarenal IVC, contralateral renal vein, and suprarenal IVC segments; performing cavotomy and thrombectomy; and completing caval repair (**Fig. 5**). The surgical approach to level 3 to 4 robotic IVC thrombectomy is beyond the scope of this review but has been well described elsewhere.[79]

Additional measures should be taken to prevent air embolism during the case that account for the effects of pneumoperitoneum. In addition to flushing the cava extensively before closure as described earlier, conducting a Valsalva maneuver with the cava surrounded by irrigant to create a water seal before final closure can be effective.

Neoadjuvant Systemic Therapy

Neoadjuvant therapy before IVC thrombectomy is not standard of care for the patient without metastatic disease. Its main indication in this setting is the rare patient where the tumor is felt to be unresectable due to a prohibitive mortality risk.

This paradigm may eventually change because of significant advances in systemic therapy for metastatic clear cell RCC. Objective response rates for first-line doublet therapy range from 42% to 73%.[80–82] Although there are case reports of complete resolution of significant tumor thrombi,[83] complete response in the primary tumor is exceedingly unlikely.[84]

Several studies have been conducted in the era of tyrosine kinase inhibitor monotherapy assessing neoadjuvant therapy before IVC thrombectomy.[85] Progression was uncommon and some patients were downstaged. These studies provide a proof of concept for neoadjuvant therapy before IVC thrombectomy. Prospective studies with doublet agents demonstrating perioperative and oncologic outcomes are improved with neoadjuvant therapy are required before adoption.

Postoperative Systemic Therapy

In nonmetastatic clear cell RCC with high-risk features, adjuvant immunotherapy with pembrolizumab (antiprogrammed cell death protein 1) for 1 year is known to reduce disease recurrence after nephrectomy by 37%.[86,87] Patients without distant metastases and an IVC thrombus generally meet one or more indications for adjuvant pembrolizumab treatment. Some may elect not to pursue adjuvant treatment because an overall survival benefit has not yet been demonstrated with pembrolizumab and other studies on adjuvant immunotherapy with atezolizumab and ipilimumab/nivolumab have been negative.[88,89] Ongoing clinical trials of adjuvant therapy will undoubtedly affect the adjuvant therapy options in the future.[90]

SUMMARY

Although surgical indications and operative approach may shift over time, the management of RCC with IVC thrombus is a perennial competency of the urologic oncologist. A multidisciplinary approach to the surgical techniques and perioperative management described herein has enabled these complex surgical cases to be performed safely for most of the patients.

CLINICS CARE POINTS

- Essential preoperative considerations before IVC thrombectomy includes: staging, IVC thrombus assessment, assessing venous implications, deciding on anticoagulation, preoperative risk assessment, and multidisciplinary assessment.
- IVC thrombectomy technique varies significantly by level, presence of preoperative bland thrombus, and intraoperative findings during tumor thrombectomy.
- A number of unique complications are attributable to IVC thrombectomy and familiarity with these is essential.
- Robotic surgery is being increasingly utilized for straight-forward IVC thrombectomy cases. Case selection and familiarity with the principles of open IVC thrombectomy are critical for a successful outcome.

DISCLOSURES

S. Dason—advisory board: Bristol Myers Squibb, Roche; education funding: Intuitive Surgical, United States. K. Salari—research support: Convergent Genomics.

REFERENCES

1. Siegel RL, Miller KD, Fuchs HE, et al. Cancer statistics, 2022. CA Cancer J Clin 2022;72(1):7–33. https://doi.org/10.3322/caac.21708.
2. Capitanio U, Bensalah K, Bex A, et al. Epidemiology of Renal Cell Carcinoma. Eur Urol 2019;75(1):74–84. https://doi.org/10.1016/j.eururo.2018.08.036.
3. Kaptein FHJ, van der HT, Braken SJE, et al. Prevalence, Treatment, and Prognosis of Tumor Thrombi

in Renal Cell Carcinoma. JACC CardioOncology 2022;4(4):522–31. https://doi.org/10.1016/j.jaccao.2022.07.011.

4. Blute ML, Boorjian SA, Leibovich BC, et al. Results of Inferior Vena Caval Interruption by Greenfield Filter, Ligation or Resection During Radical Nephrectomy and Tumor Thrombectomy. J Urol 2007;178(2):440–5. https://doi.org/10.1016/j.juro.2007.03.121.

5. Beveridge TS, Allman BL, Johnson M, et al. Considerations from a Cadaveric Study. J Urol 2016;196(6):1764–71. https://doi.org/10.1016/j.juro.2016.06.091.

6. Hostiuc S, Rusu MC, Negoi I. Dorobanţu B, Grigoriu M. Anatomical variants of renal veins: A meta-analysis of prevalence. Sci Rep 2019;9(1):10802. https://doi.org/10.1038/s41598-019-47280-8.

7. Cesmebasi A, Du Plessis M, Iannatuono M, et al. A review of the anatomy and clinical significance of adrenal veins. Clin Anat 2014;27(8):1253–63. https://doi.org/10.1002/ca.22374.

8. The minor hepatic veins. Anatomy and classification - Mehran - 2000-Clinical Anatomy - Wiley Online Library. Available at;. https://onlinelibrary.wiley.com/doi/epdf/10.1002/1098-2353%282000%2913%3A6%3C416%3A%3AAID-CA4%3E3.0.CO%3B2-H. Accessed December 1, 2022.

9. Loukas M, Louis RG, Hullett J, et al. An anatomical classification of the variations of the inferior phrenic vein. Surg Radiol Anat 2005;27(6):566–74. https://doi.org/10.1007/s00276-005-0029-0.

10. Shchukin D, Lesovoy V, Garagatiy I, et al. Surgical Approaches to Supradiaphragmatic Segment of IVC and Right Atrium through Abdominal Cavity during Intravenous Tumor Thrombus Removal. Adv Urol 2014;2014:e924269. https://doi.org/10.1155/2014/924269.

11. Singla N, Hutchinson RC, Ghandour RA, et al. Improved survival after cytoreductive nephrectomy for metastatic renal cell carcinoma in the contemporary immunotherapy era: An analysis of the National Cancer Database. Urol Oncol Semin Orig Investig 2020;38(6):604.e9. https://doi.org/10.1016/j.urolonc.2020.02.029.

12. Bakouny Z, El Zarif T, Dudani S, et al. Upfront Cytoreductive Nephrectomy for Metastatic Renal Cell Carcinoma Treated with Immune Checkpoint Inhibitors or Targeted Therapy: An Observational Study from the International Metastatic Renal Cell Carcinoma Database Consortium. Eur Urol 2022;S0302-2838(22):02713–20.

13. Méjean A, Ravaud A, Thezenas S, et al. Sunitinib Alone or after Nephrectomy in Metastatic Renal-Cell Carcinoma. N Engl J Med 2018;379(5):417–27. https://doi.org/10.1056/NEJMoa1803675.

14. Rathmell WK, Rumble RB, Van Veldhuizen PJ, et al. Management of Metastatic Clear Cell Renal Cell Carcinoma: ASCO Guideline. J Clin Oncol 2022;40(25):2957–95. https://doi.org/10.1200/JCO.22.00868.

15. Abel EJ, Spiess PE, Margulis V, et al. Cytoreductive Nephrectomy for Renal Cell Carcinoma with Venous Tumor Thrombus. J Urol 2017;198(2):281–8. https://doi.org/10.1016/j.juro.2017.03.011.

16. Renal mass and localized renal cancer: evaluation, management, and follow up. American Urological Association; 2021. Available at: https://www.auanet.org/guidelines-and-quality/guidelines/renal-mass-and-localized-renal-cancer-evaluation-management-and-follow-up. Accessed November 16, 2022.

17. Hallscheidt PJ, Fink C, Haferkamp A, et al. Preoperative Staging of Renal Cell Carcinoma With Inferior Vena Cava Thrombus Using Multidetector CT and MRI: Prospective Study With Histopathological Correlation. J Comput Assist Tomogr 2005;29(1):64–8.

18. Lawrentschuk N, Gani J, Riordan R, et al. Multidetector computed tomography vs magnetic resonance imaging for defining the upper limit of tumour thrombus in renal cell carcinoma: a study and review. BJU Int 2005;96(3):291–5. https://doi.org/10.1111/j.1464-410X.2005.05617.x.

19. Guzzo TJ, Pierorazio PM, Schaeffer EM, et al. The Accuracy of Multidetector Computerized Tomography for Evaluating Tumor Thrombus in Patients With Renal Cell Carcinoma. J Urol 2009;181(2):486–91. https://doi.org/10.1016/j.juro.2008.10.040.

20. Kallman DA, King BF, Hattery RR, et al. Renal vein and inferior vena cava tumor thrombus in renal cell carcinoma: CT, US, MRI and venacavography. J Comput Assist Tomogr 1992;16(2):240–7. https://doi.org/10.1097/00004728-199203000-00012.

21. Davenport MS, Perazella MA, Yee J, et al. Use of Intravenous Iodinated Contrast Media in Patients with Kidney Disease: Consensus Statements from the American College of Radiology and the National Kidney Foundation. Radiology 2020;294(3):660–8. https://doi.org/10.1148/radiol.2019192094.

22. Zhu. A hui, Hou X yan, Tian S, Zhang W fang. Diagnostic value of 18F-FDG PET/CT versus contrast-enhanced MRI for venous tumour thrombus and venous bland thrombus in renal cell carcinoma. Sci Rep 2022;12(1):587. https://doi.org/10.1038/s41598-021-04541-9.

23. Alayed A, Krishna S, Breau RH, et al. Diagnostic Accuracy of MRI for Detecting Inferior Vena Cava Wall Invasion in Renal Cell Carcinoma Tumor Thrombus Using Quantitative and Subjective Analysis. Am J Roentgenol 2019;212(3):562–9. https://doi.org/10.2214/AJR.18.20209.

24. Adams LC, Ralla B, Bender YNY, et al. Renal cell carcinoma with venous extension: prediction of inferior vena cava wall invasion by MRI. Cancer Imag

2018;18(1):17. https://doi.org/10.1186/s40644-018-0150-z.

25. Woolen SA, Shankar PR, Gagnier JJ, et al. Risk of Nephrogenic Systemic Fibrosis in Patients With Stage 4 or 5 Chronic Kidney Disease Receiving a Group II Gadolinium-Based Contrast Agent: A Systematic Review and Meta-analysis. JAMA Intern Med 2020;180(2):223–30. https://doi.org/10.1001/jamainternmed.2019.5284.

26. Shi T, Huang Q, Liu K, et al. Robot-assisted Cavectomy Versus Thrombectomy for Level II Inferior Vena Cava Thrombus: Decision-making Scheme and Multi-institutional Analysis. Eur Urol 2020;78(4):592–602. https://doi.org/10.1016/j.eururo.2020.03.020.

27. Calderone CE, Tuck BC, Gray SH, et al. The role of transesophageal echocardiography in the management of renal cell carcinoma with venous tumor thrombus. Echocardiography 2018;35(12):2047–55. https://doi.org/10.1111/echo.14187.

28. Li QY, Li N, Huang QB, et al. Contrast-enhanced ultrasound in detecting wall invasion and differentiating bland from tumor thrombus during robot-assisted inferior vena cava thrombectomy for renal cell carcinoma. Cancer Imag 2019;19(1):79. https://doi.org/10.1186/s40644-019-0265-x.

29. Li Q, Li N, Luo Y, et al. Role of intraoperative ultrasound in robotic-assisted radical nephrectomy with inferior vena cava thrombectomy in renal cell carcinoma. World J Urol 2020;38(12):3191–8. https://doi.org/10.1007/s00345-020-03141-y.

30. Agarwal S, Mullikin D, Scheurer ME, et al. Role of anticoagulation in the management of tumor thrombus: A 10-year single-center experience. Pediatr Blood Cancer 2021;68(9):e29173. https://doi.org/10.1002/pbc.29173.

31. Marcoux C, Al Ghamdi S, Manos D, et al. Natural History of Tumor Thrombus: A Single-Centre Retrospective Study. Blood 2019;134:2430. https://doi.org/10.1182/blood-2019-124476.

32. Hsu M. Balzer -Haas Naomi. When Clot Is Tumor. JACC CardioOncology 2022;4(4):532–4. https://doi.org/10.1016/j.jaccao.2022.10.005.

33. Pötzsch B, Klövekorn WP, Madlener K. Use of Heparin during Cardiopulmonary Bypass in Patients with a History of Heparin-Induced Thrombocytopenia. N Engl J Med 2000;343(7):515. https://doi.org/10.1056/NEJM200008173430718.

34. Douketis JD, Spyropoulos AC, Murad MH, et al. Perioperative Management of Antithrombotic Therapy: An American College of Chest Physicians Clinical Practice Guideline. Chest 2022;162(5):e207–43. https://doi.org/10.1016/j.chest.2022.07.025.

35. Smilowitz NR, Berger JS. Perioperative Cardiovascular Risk Assessment and Management for Noncardiac Surgery: A Review. JAMA 2020;324(3):279–90. https://doi.org/10.1001/jama.2020.7840.

36. Abel EJ, Wood CG, Eickstaedt N, et al. Preoperative Pulmonary Embolism Does Not Predict Poor Postoperative Outcomes in Patients with Renal Cell Carcinoma and Venous Thrombus. J Urol 2013;190(2):452–7. https://doi.org/10.1016/j.juro.2013.02.033.

37. Saillant NN, Kornblith LZ, Moore H, et al. The National Blood Shortage—An Impetus for Change. Ann Surg 2022;275(4):641–3. https://doi.org/10.1097/SLA.0000000000005393.

38. Freifeld Y, Pedrosa I, Mclaughlin M, et al. Stereotactic ablative radiation therapy for renal cell carcinoma with inferior vena cava tumor thrombus. Urol Oncol Semin Orig Investig 2022;40(4):166.e9.

39. Evans MA, Wolf FA. Anesthesia for Nephrectomy with Vena Cava Thrombectomy. In: Goudra BG, Duggan M, Chidambaran V, et al, editors. Anesthesiology: a practical approach. Springer International Publishing; 2018. p. 635–44.

40. Fukazawa K, Gologorsky E, Naguit K, et al. Invasive Renal Cell Carcinoma with Inferior Vena Cava Tumor Thrombus: Cardiac Anesthesia in Liver Transplant Settings. J Cardiothorac Vasc Anesth 2014;28(3):640–6. https://doi.org/10.1053/j.jvca.2013.04.002.

41. Vinzant NJ, Christensen JM, Smith MM, et al. Perioperative Outcomes for Radical Nephrectomy and Level III-IV Inferior Vena Cava Tumor Thrombectomy in Patients with Renal Cell Carcinoma. J Cardiothorac Vasc Anesth 2022;36(8, Part B):3093–100. https://doi.org/10.1053/j.jvca.2022.04.023.

42. Lardas M, Stewart F, Scrimgeour D, et al. Systematic Review of Surgical Management of Nonmetastatic Renal Cell Carcinoma with Vena Caval Thrombus. Eur Urol 2016;70(2):265–80. https://doi.org/10.1016/j.eururo.2015.11.034.

43. Yagisawa T, Kondo T, Yoshida K, et al. 1911 usefulness of temporary inferior vena cava filter in preventing intraoperative pulmonary embolism for patients with renal cell carcinoma extending into inferior vena cava thrombus. J Urol 2013;189(4S):e783–4. https://doi.org/10.1016/j.juro.2013.02.2330.

44. Zhang JP, Zhu Y, jun Liu Y, et al. Temporary Filters and Liver Mobilization Technique Improve the Safety and Prognosis of Radical Nephrectomy and Inferior Vena Cava Thrombectomy in Renal Cell Carcinoma with Subdiaphragmatic Thrombosis. Urol Int 2013;91(3):279–84. https://doi.org/10.1159/000350521.

45. Feng X, Bao J, Jing Z, et al. Tempofilter II for tumor emboli prevention during radical nephrectomy and inferior vena cava thrombus resection for renal cell carcinoma. J Surg Oncol 2009;100(2):159–62. https://doi.org/10.1002/jso.21303.

46. Shuch B, Larochelle JC, Onyia T, et al. Intraoperative Thrombus Embolization During Nephrectomy and Tumor Thrombectomy: Critical Analysis of the University of California-Los Angeles Experience. J Urol 2009;181(2):492–9. https://doi.org/10.1016/j.juro.2008.10.036.

47. Kinnear N, O'Callaghan M, Hennessey D, et al. Intra-operative cell salvage in urological surgery: a systematic review and meta-analysis of comparative studies. BJU Int 2019;123(2):210–9. https://doi.org/10.1111/bju.14373.

48. Iwata T, Kimura S, Foerster B, et al. Perioperative blood transfusion affects oncologic outcomes after nephrectomy for renal cell carcinoma: A systematic review and meta-analysis. Urol Oncol Semin Orig Investig 2019;37(4):273–81. https://doi.org/10.1016/j.urolonc.2019.01.018.

49. Blute ML, Leibovich BC, Lohse CM, et al. The Mayo Clinic experience with surgical management, complications and outcome for patients with renal cell carcinoma and venous tumour thrombus. BJU Int 2004;94(1):33–41. https://doi.org/10.1111/j.1464-410X.2004.04897.x.

50. Gaudino M, Lau C, Cammertoni F, et al. Surgical Treatment of Renal Cell Carcinoma With Cavoatrial Involvement: A Systematic Review of the Literature. Ann Thorac Surg 2016;101(3):1213–21. https://doi.org/10.1016/j.athoracsur.2015.10.003.

51. Faust WC, D'Agostino RS, Libertino J. Comparative Effectiveness of Median Sternotomy vs Minimal Access Cardiopulmonary Bypass and Circulatory Arrest for Resection of Renal Cell Carcinoma with Inferior Vena Caval Extension. J Cancer Ther 2016;7(10):752–61. https://doi.org/10.4236/jct.2016.710076.

52. Stecker MM, Cheung AT, Pochettino A, et al. Deep hypothermic circulatory arrest: I. Effects of cooling on electroencephalogram and evoked potentials. Ann Thorac Surg 2001;71(1):14–21. https://doi.org/10.1016/S0003-4975(00)01592-7.

53. Maclean W, Levy B, Rockall T. Trauma laparotomy and damage control surgery. Surg Oxf 2019;37(10):549–57. https://doi.org/10.1016/j.mpsur.2019.07.014.

54. Ciancio G, Vaidya A, Shirodkar S, et al. En Bloc Mobilization of the Pancreas and Spleen to Facilitate Resection of Large Tumors, Primarily Renal and Adrenal, in the Left Upper Quadrant of the Abdomen: Techniques Derived from Multivisceral Transplantation. Eur Urol 2009;55(5):1106–11. https://doi.org/10.1016/j.eururo.2008.12.038.

55. Application of Liver Transplant and Organ Procurement Techniques to Difficult Upper Abdominal Urological Cases. J Urol 1994;151(6):1652–6.

56. Mattox KL, Mccollum WB, Jordan GL, et al. Management of upper abdominal vascular trauma. Am J Surg 1974;128(6):823–8. https://doi.org/10.1016/0002-9610(74)90079-8.

57. "Thrombus-first" or "thrombus-last" approach for surgical management of renal cell carcinoma with inferior vena cava thrombus - Ishiyama - 2022-International Journal of Urology - Wiley Online Library. Available at: https://onlinelibrary.wiley.com/doi/abs/10.1111/iju.14846. Accessed December 2, 2022.

58. Xie L, Hong G, Nabavizadeh R, et al. Outcomes in Patients with Renal Cell Carcinoma Undergoing Inferior Vena Cava Ligation without Reconstruction versus Thrombectomy: A Retrospective, Case Controlled Study. J Urol 2021;205(2):383–91. https://doi.org/10.1097/JU.0000000000001354.

59. Olmez A, Karabulut K, Aydin C, et al. Comparison of Harmonic Scalpel Versus Conventional Knot Tying for Transection of Short Hepatic Veins at Liver Transplantation: Prospective Randomized Study. Transplant Proc 2012;44(6):1717–9. https://doi.org/10.1016/j.transproceed.2012.05.035.

60. Garg H, Kaushik D, Hui D, et al. Haemodynamic changes during radical nephrectomy with inferior vena cava thrombectomy: A pilot study. BJUI Compass 2022;3(5):327–30. https://doi.org/10.1002/bco2.154.

61. Tzakis A, Todo S, Starzl TE. Orthotopic liver transplantation with preservation of the inferior vena cava. Ann Surg 1989;210(5):649–52.

62. Close relation between the inferior vena cava ligament and the caudate lobe in the human liver - Kogure - 2007-Journal of Hepato-Biliary-Pancreatic Surgery - Wiley Online Library. Available at: https://onlinelibrary.wiley.com/doi/abs/10.1007/s00534-006-1148-7. Accessed December 3, 2022.

63. Dason S. V13-07 inferior vena cava management during left-sided level iii tumor thrombectomy. J Urol 2022;207(Supplement 5):e1033. https://doi.org/10.1097/JU.0000000000002646.07.

64. Simon RM, Kim T, Espiritu P, et al. Effect of utilization of veno-venous bypass vs. cardiopulmonary bypass on complications for high level inferior vena cava tumor thrombectomy and concomitant radical nephrectomy. Int Braz J Urol 2015;41(5):911–9.

65. The Mayo Clinic experience with surgical management, complications and outcome for patients with renal cell carcinoma and venous tumour thrombus - Blute - 2004-BJU International - Wiley Online Library. Available at: https://bjui-journals.onlinelibrary.wiley.com/doi/abs/10.1111/j.1464-410X.2004.04897.x. Accessed December 3, 2022.

66. Jibiki M, Iwai T, Inoue Y, et al. Surgical strategy for treating renal cell carcinoma with thrombus extending into the inferior vena cava. J Vasc Surg 2004;39(4):829–35. https://doi.org/10.1016/j.jvs.2003.12.004.

67. Dason S. V11-06 the open abdominal approach to level iii/iv vena caval tumor thrombi with caval obstruction. J Urol 2021;206(Supplement 3):e859. https://doi.org/10.1097/JU.0000000000002073.06.

68. Patil MB, Montez J, Loh-Doyle J, et al. Level III-IV Inferior Vena Caval Thrombectomy Without Cardiopulmonary Bypass: Long-Term Experience with

Intrapericardial Control. J Urol 2014;192(3):682–9. https://doi.org/10.1016/j.juro.2014.03.112.

69. Garg H, Psutka SP, Hakimi AA, et al. A Decade of Robotic-Assisted Radical Nephrectomy with Inferior Vena Cava Thrombectomy: A Systematic Review and Meta-Analysis of Perioperative Outcomes. J Urol 2022;208(3):542–60. https://doi.org/10.1097/JU.0000000000002829.

70. Enezate T, Alkhatib D, Raja J, et al. AngioVac for Minimally Invasive Removal of Intravascular and Intracardiac Masses: a Systematic Review. Curr Cardiol Rep 2022;24(4):377–82. https://doi.org/10.1007/s11886-022-01658-9.

71. Moriarty JM, Rueda V, Liao M, et al. Endovascular Removal of Thrombus and Right Heart Masses Using the AngioVac System: Results of 234 Patients from the Prospective, Multicenter Registry of AngioVac Procedures in Detail (RAPID). J Vasc Interv Radiol 2021;32(4):549–57. e3.

72. Inferior vena cava-syndrome | Vasa. Available at: https://econtent.hogrefe.com/doi/full/10.1024/0301-1526/a000919. Accessed December 3, 2022.

73. Rose KM, Huelster HL, Roberts EC, et al. Contemporary Management of Chylous Ascites after Retroperitoneal Surgery: Development of an Evidence-Based Treatment Algorithm. J Urol 2022;208(1):53–61. https://doi.org/10.1097/JU.0000000000002494.

74. Southwest Oncology Group. Phase III Trial of Immunotherapy-Based Combination Therapy With or Without Cytoreductive Nephrectomy for Metastatic Renal Cell Carcinoma (PROBE Trial). clinicaltrials.gov; 2022. Available at: https://clinicaltrials.gov/ct2/show/NCT04510597. Accessed November 14, 2022.

75. Fristrup N. Multicenter Randomized Trial of Deferred Cytoreductive Nephrectomy in Synchronous Metastatic Renal Cell Carcinoma Receiving Checkpoint Inhibitors: A DaRenCa and NoRenCa Trial Evaluating the Impact of Surgery or No Surgery. NORDIC-SUN-Trial. clinicaltrials.gov. 2022. Available at: https://clinicaltrials.gov/ct2/show/NCT03977571. Accessed November 14, 2022.

76. Runcie K, Singer EA, Ornstein MC, et al. Cyto-KIK: A phase II trial of cytoreductive surgery in kidney cancer plus immunotherapy (nivolumab) and targeted kinase inhibition (cabozantinib). J Clin Oncol 2021;39(15_suppl):TPS4598.

77. Pignot G, Thiery-Vuillemin A, Albigès L, et al. Oncological Outcomes of Delayed Nephrectomy After Optimal Response to Immune Checkpoint Inhibitors for Metastatic Renal Cell Carcinoma. Eur Urol Oncol 2022;5(5):577–84. https://doi.org/10.1016/j.euo.2022.07.002.

78. Unadkat P, Olumi AF, Gershman B. The Role of Lymphadenectomy in Patients with Advanced Renal Cell Carcinoma. Urol Clin North Am. 2020;47(3):371–7. https://doi.org/10.1016/j.ucl.2020.04.001.

79. Wang B, Huang Q, Liu K, et al. Robot-assisted Level III-IV Inferior Vena Cava Thrombectomy: Initial Series with Step-by-step Procedures and 1-yr Outcomes. Eur Urol 2020;78(1):77–86. https://doi.org/10.1016/j.eururo.2019.04.019.

80. Motzer RJ, Tannir NM, McDermott DF, et al. Nivolumab plus Ipilimumab versus Sunitinib in Advanced Renal-Cell Carcinoma. N Engl J Med 2018;378(14):1277–90. https://doi.org/10.1056/NEJMoa1712126.

81. Motzer R, Alekseev B, Rha SY, et al. Lenvatinib plus Pembrolizumab or Everolimus for Advanced Renal Cell Carcinoma. N Engl J Med 2021;384(14):1289–300. https://doi.org/10.1056/NEJMoa2035716.

82. Choueiri TK, Powles T, Burotto M, et al. Nivolumab plus Cabozantinib versus Sunitinib for Advanced Renal-Cell Carcinoma. N Engl J Med 2021;384(9):829–41. https://doi.org/10.1056/NEJMoa2026982.

83. Labbate C, Hatogai K, Werntz R, et al. Complete response of renal cell carcinoma vena cava tumor thrombus to neoadjuvant immunotherapy. J Immunother Cancer 2019;7(1):66. https://doi.org/10.1186/s40425-019-0546-8.

84. Albiges L, Tannir NM, Burotto M, et al. First-line Nivolumab plus Ipilimumab Versus Sunitinib in Patients Without Nephrectomy and With an Evaluable Primary Renal Tumor in the CheckMate 214 Trial. Eur Urol 2022;81(3):266–71. https://doi.org/10.1016/j.eururo.2021.10.001.

85. Stewart GD, Welsh SJ, Ursprung S, et al. A Phase II study of neoadjuvant axitinib for reducing the extent of venous tumour thrombus in clear cell renal cancer with venous invasion (NAXIVA). Br J Cancer 2022;127(6):1051–60. https://doi.org/10.1038/s41416-022-01883-7.

86. Choueiri TK, Tomczak P, Park SH, et al. Adjuvant Pembrolizumab after Nephrectomy in Renal-Cell Carcinoma. N Engl J Med 2021;385(8):683–94. https://doi.org/10.1056/NEJMoa2106391.

87. Powles T, Tomczak P, Park SH, et al. Pembrolizumab versus placebo as post-nephrectomy adjuvant therapy for clear cell renal cell carcinoma (KEYNOTE-564): 30-month follow-up analysis of a multicentre, randomised, double-blind, placebo-controlled, phase 3 trial. Lancet Oncol 2022;23(9):1133–44. https://doi.org/10.1016/S1470-2045(22)00487-9.

88. Pal SK, Uzzo R, Karam JA, et al. Adjuvant atezolizumab versus placebo for patients with renal cell carcinoma at increased risk of recurrence following resection (IMmotion010): a multicentre, randomised, double-blind, phase 3 trial. Lancet Lond Engl 2022;400(10358):1103–16. https://doi.org/10.1016/S0140-6736(22)01658-0.

89. Bristol Myers Squibb Provides Update on CheckMate -914 Trial Evaluating Opdivo (nivolumab) Plus Yervoy (ipilimumab) as Adjuvant Treatment of Localized Renal

Cell Carcinoma. Available at: https://news.bms.com/news/details/2022/Bristol-Myers-Squibb-Provides-Update-on-CheckMate–914-Trial-Evaluating-Opdivo-nivolumab-Plus-Yervoy-ipilimumab-as-Adjuvant-Treatment-of-Localized-Renal-Cell-Carcinoma/default.aspx. Accessed November 15, 2022.

90. Choueiri TK, Bedke J, Karam JA, et al. LITESPARK-022: A phase 3 study of pembrolizumab + belzutifan as adjuvant treatment of clear cell renal cell carcinoma (ccRCC). J Clin Oncol 2022;40(16_suppl):TPS4602.

91. Haddad AQ, Wood CG, Abel EJ, et al. Oncologic Outcomes Following Surgical Resection of Renal Cell Carcinoma with Inferior Vena Caval Thrombus Extending Above the Hepatic Veins: A Contemporary Multicenter Cohort. Journal of Urology 2014; 192(4):1050–6.

The Promise of Neoadjuvant and Adjuvant Therapies for Renal Cancer

Jeffrey J. Leow, MBBS, MPH, MRCS, FAMS(Urology)[a], Shagnik Ray, MD[b],
Shawn Dason, MD[b], Eric A. Singer, MD, MA, MS[b], Steven L. Chang, MD, MS[c],*

KEYWORDS

- Renal cancer • Kidney neoplasms • Radical nephrectomy • Systemic therapy
- Neoadjuvant therapy • Adjuvant therapy • Immunotherapy • Targeted therapy

KEY POINTS

- Metachronous metastatic disease will develop in 20% to 40% of patients with presumed localized RCC who undergo surgical resection.
- Neoadjuvant therapy could help select cases to improve resectability, avoid excessive morbidity, and prevent need for renal replacement therapy by enabling nephron-sparing surgery. However, there is no robust level 1 evidence to allow for guideline bodies to recommend this. Suitable patients should be recruited or referred to centers offering randomized controlled trials.
- Adjuvant therapy may improve disease-free survival in well-selected high-risk localized or locally advanced patients with RCC, particularly with pembrolizumab per KEYNOTE-564 trial; however, overall survival benefit is pending.

INTRODUCTION

Across a multitude of cancers, extirpative surgery is the cornerstone of treatment for patients with localized and locally advanced disease. However, a portion of these patients, especially those with locally advanced disease, will experience disease relapse at some point following surgery. In many cases, the recurrence of cancer is attributed to micrometastatic disease present at the time of surgery, which is not detectable on preoperative staging evaluation. To address this issue, it is common to manage patients with cancer using a multimodal treatment strategy to eliminate the primary tumor as well as the micrometastatic disease.

The idea of a sequential application of multiple cancer treatments to optimize the eradication of disease was initially proposed by Shapiro and Fugmann[1] in 1957 based on a mouse model of breast adenocarcinoma, which involved implantation of a larger and a smaller tumor into mice. The investigators reported improved effectiveness of chemotherapy after resection of the larger tumor leading to the hypothesis that postoperative chemotherapy as an adjunct to surgery "offers hope for cure of the microscopic metastases." However, it was another 2 decades before there was level I evidence for the use of postoperative adjuvant chemotherapy. In women with breast cancer and positive axillary nodes, Bonadonna and colleagues[2] demonstrated an improvement in initial disease-free recurrence rates as well as a trend for improved overall survival (OS) associated with adjuvant chemotherapy, thus setting the stage for a shift in the management of high-risk surgically resectable cancers from surgical alone to a multimodal approach.

a Department of Urology, Tan Tock Seng Hospital, 11 Jalan Tan Tock Seng, Annex 1-L04-Uro, Singapore 308433, Singapore; b Division of Urologic Oncology, The Ohio State University Comprehensive Cancer Center, 915 Olentangy River Road, Suite 3100, Columbus, OH 43212, USA; c Division of Urology, Brigham and Women's Hospital, 45 Francis Street, Suite ASBII-3, Boston, MA 02115, USA
* Corresponding author.
E-mail address: slchang@bwh.harvard.edu

Urol Clin N Am 50 (2023) 285–303
https://doi.org/10.1016/j.ucl.2023.01.011
0094-0143/23/© 2023 Elsevier Inc. All rights reserved.

Perioperative therapy can be applied before surgery (neoadjuvant therapy) and/or following surgery (adjuvant therapy). There is a multitude of strong arguments supporting and refuting these treatment strategies (**Table 1**). The term "neoadjuvant therapy" refers to treatments administered to decrease tumor burden and improve the eradication of disease with surgery. Historically, presurgical treatment was used in an effort to convert an inoperable cancer into a surgically resectable situation. Neoadjuvant therapy is now commonly used to treat potential micrometastatic disease before surgery to remove the primary tumor. In addition, neoadjuvant therapy may also decrease the burden of disease, thereby minimizing surgical morbidity and reducing the extent of surgery (ie, organ-sparing surgery). In contrast, "adjuvant therapy" is given after treatment of the primary tumor and in the absence of known disease with the intent of lowering the probability of recurrent disease in the future.

The role of neoadjuvant therapy and adjuvant therapy has been studied and recommended for many different cancers, including gastric, sarcoma, melanoma, pancreatic, breast, non–small cell lung, colon, bladder, and endometrial. In contrast, there is no widely accepted standard neoadjuvant or adjuvant therapy supported by high levels of evidence for patients with localized kidney cancer.

Current treatment guidelines recommend consideration for a clinical trial or simply pursuing active surveillance following extirpative surgery.[3,4]

In 2022, there were approximately 79,000 new cases of renal cell carcinoma (RCC) and 13,920 deaths attributed to RCC in the United States.[5] Localized RCC has numerous management options, but is definitively managed with surgical extirpation or ablation with excellent OS and disease-free survival (DFS) in these patients after definitive surgical management.[6] Unfortunately, 20% to 40% of all patients with RCC who undergo surgical resection will develop metachronous metastatic disease.[7,8] Thus, there remains significant room for improvement with regards to preventing progression to metastatic disease after surgical management in high-risk patients as well as in managing both synchronous and metachronous metastatic disease. This is where neoadjuvant and adjuvant systemic therapies may have a role in the clinical management of RCC patients.

NEOADJUVANT THERAPY TRIALS WITH ANTI–VASCULAR ENDOTHELIAL GROWTH FACTOR TYROSINE KINASE INHIBITOR AGENTS

Numerous prospective trials have investigated the use of targeted therapies with anti–vascular

Table 1
Advantages and disadvantages of neoadjuvant therapy before surgery and adjuvant therapy following primary cancer surgery

	Adjuvant Therapy Following Primary Surgery	Neoadjuvant Therapy Before Surgery
Advantages	Expeditious removal of tumor thus minimizing the population of potentially metastatic cancer cells and the possibility for evolving drug-resistant clones	Potentially convert a surgically unresectable disease to a surgically curable condition
	Provides a substantial amount of tissue for histopathologic evaluation, which then informs the selection of the ideal postoperative strategy	Decrease the morbidity of surgery by reducing the extent of surgery and increasing the preservation of the affected organ Early control of micrometastatic disease
Disadvantages	Recovery from surgery, especially if prolonged by complications, may delay adjuvant therapy, which is necessary to address micrometastatic disease	Persistence of a large burden of disease during neoadjuvant therapy may increase the possibility for developing drug-resistant clones
	Potentially increases the morbidity and mortality of surgery	Unnecessary treatment and potentially increased morbidity for patients who do not have micrometastatic disease and are curable with surgery alone The morbidity of neoadjuvant therapy may render surgery more challenging to tolerate

endothelial growth factor (VEGF) tyrosine kinase inhibitor (TKI) agents in the neoadjuvant setting, including axitinib, cabozantinib, pazopanib, sorafenib, and sunitinib (**Table 2**). Despite a substantial body of evidence gathered over the years, neoadjuvant targeted therapies have been barely mentioned, let alone recommended, in major guidelines bodies. This is due to the low quality of evidence. Most of these studies were generally small, with less than 50 patients each. Some included primary metastatic patients with multiple distant metastases and were therefore not carried out in a truly neoadjuvant setting for localized or locally advanced disease.

Some studies enrolled patients in whom nephrectomy was deemed not feasible. The median tumor size before neoadjuvant therapy ranged from 5.4 cm to 11.0 cm. Some studies included small renal masses as well (<4 cm). This may explain why there were only an average partial response of 24% (range, 5%–46%), given that larger tumors tend to respond better, show more downsizing, and achieve better partial response per RECIST criteria. The 3 best studies showing the highest proportion of partial response were from Rini 2015[9] (pazopanib, 36%), Hatiboglu[10] 2017 (sorafenib, 44%), and Karam[11] 2014 (axitinib, 46%). The lowest rates of partial response also came from Hellenthal 2010,[12] (sunitinib, 5%) and Cowey 2010[13] (sorafenib, 7%).

Although the translation of modest reductions in tumor size to overall clinical benefit is unclear in most patients, these findings have specific relevance to the patient deemed "unresectable." Notwithstanding that a locally advanced tumor that is "unresectable" should be rare in tertiary centers, neoadjuvant therapy may facilitate subsequent resection in these patients with reduced morbidity. In a retrospective review by Van der Veldt and colleagues,[14] 10 patients with metastatic RCC were deemed to have a surgically unresectable tumor of whom 3 were able to subsequently be surgically extirpated after neoadjuvant therapy following 4 weeks of neoadjuvant sunitinib. Rini and colleagues[15] performed a prospective phase II trial with neoadjuvant sunitinib in 28 patients with unresectable RCC (66% of patients had metastatic disease on presentation), with 13 (45%; 9 undergoing partial nephrectomy, 4 undergoing radical nephrectomy) of these patients able to undergo nephrectomy after neoadjuvant sunitinib therapy. Tumors deemed to be unresectable were classified based on the presence of large tumor size, bulky lymphadenopathy, high-level venous tumor thrombus, and/or proximity/invasion of adjacent structures. The investigators concluded that a modest decrease in

tumor size facilitated resection based on tumor characteristics and anatomic considerations, offering the example of allowing for partial nephrectomy versus radical in a tumor with hilar abutment, but may not allow for resection of a large primary tumor or bulky lymphadenopathy. Permitting partial nephrectomy instead of radical nephrectomy may be critical in very select situations, such as in a patient with a functionally solitary kidney who is declining post nephrectomy renal replacement therapy. Regardless, there are multiple case reports and case series in the literature reporting instances of tumors deemed to be unresectable that after a neoadjuvant course of modern systemic therapy were able to be successfully resected, such as with cabozantinib, pembrolizumab/ipilimumab, and sequential nivolumab/ipilimumab and pazopanib.[16–18]

Lebacle and colleagues[19] performed a phase II study of 18 patients with cT2 clear cell RCC not suitable for partial nephrectomy based on physician judgment receiving neoadjuvant axitinib with the goal of assessing whether a size reduction to less than 7 cm would allow for conversion from radical to partial nephrectomy. They found that 12 patients ultimately underwent partial nephrectomy for tumors less than 7 cm, notably with an additional 4 patients undergoing partial nephrectomy regardless. There was a median size reduction of 17%, with 16 tumors experiencing size reduction. At 6-year follow-up, unfortunately 6 patients had metastatic progression and 2 had recurrence. The investigators concluded that neoadjuvant axitinib for cT2 RCC can allow for tumor shrinkage to less than 7 cm and allow for partial nephrectomy to be performed when it may not have been technically feasible before, but note that these partial nephrectomies came with a significant complication burden, with 5 patients experiencing Clavien-Dindo grade 3 or higher complications. Ultimately, in patients with absolute indications for renal preservation (eg, solitary kidney) or in whom neoadjuvant therapy may facilitate the feasibility of partial nephrectomy, neoadjuvant therapy may be considered, but additional studies are required to determine the appropriateness of this practice and which patients are most likely to benefit from this.

In real-world settings, a locally advanced tumor deemed unresectable in the absence of metastatic disease is rare. It also depends on whether conventional staging (ie, cross-sectional computed tomography [CT] and/or MRI) or fluorodeoxyglucose [FDG] PET/CT scans were performed in search of occult metastasis that can change management. Although neoadjuvant therapy may decrease the primary tumor diameter or even

Table 2
Neoadjuvant vascular endothelial growth factor–targeting therapies for renal cell carcinoma

Author, Year (Trial Name, if Available) (Study Type)	Therapeutic Agent (in Alphabetical Order)	Dose and Duration	N	Period of Discontinuation Before Surgery	Median Tumor Size (Range) Before Neoadjuvant Therapy (cm)	Decrease in Tumor Diameter (Range)	Partial Response by RECIST Criteria	Downsize Primary Tumor(s) (Size or Tumor Volume)	Reduce RENAL Score; Facilitate NSS (Partial NSS Instead of Radical Nephrectomy)	Change of Tumor Status from Unresectable to Resectable
Karam, 2014 (prospective phase II)[11]	Axitinib	Dose: 5 mg BID Duration: 12 wk	24	36 h	10 (4.2–16.6)	28.3% (5.3–42.9)	46%	☑	☑	
Lebacle, 2019 (AXIPAN trial) (prospective phase II)[19]	Axitinib	Dose: 5 mg BID Duration: 8–32 wk	18	6 d	7.65 (7.0–9.8)	17% (4.8% to 29.4%)	22%	☑	☑	
de Velasco, 2022 (CABOPRE trial) (prospective phase II)[67]	Cabozantinib	Dose: 60 mg QD Duration: 12 wk	18	Not reported	Not reported	NA	27%	☑		☑
Rini, 2015 (prospective phase II)[9]	Pazopanib	Dose: 800 mg QD Duration: 8–16 wk	25	≥7 d	7.3 (2.3–10.7)	26% (−2% to 43%)	36%	☑	☑ Median RENAL nephrometry score of 11 was included. The RENAL nephrometry score decreased in 71% of tumor.	

Study	Agent	Dose/Duration						Comments
Cowey, 2010 (prospective phase II)[13]	Sorafenib	Dose: 400 mg BID Duration: median of 33 d (8–59 d)	30	3 d (range, 2–14 d)	8.7 (4.2–17)	9.6% (−16% to 40%)	7%	Six of 13 patients for whom PN was not possible at baseline were able to undergo PN after treatment
Zhang, 2015 (retrospective)[68]	Sorafenib	Dose: 400 mg BID Duration: 96 d (30–278 d)	18	12 d (range, 7–30 d)	7.8 (3.6–19.2)	NA	22%	
Hatiboglu, 2017 (prospective double-blinded randomized clinical trial)[10]	Sorafenib	Dose: 400 mg BID Duration: 4 wk	12	24 h	5.4 (4.3–7.3)	29% (4.9–61)	44%	
van der Veldt, 2008 (retrospective)[14]	Sunitinib	Dose: 50 mg QD Duration: 1.2–3.9 mo	17	Not reported	Not reported	0%–33%	24%	
Thomas, 2009 (retrospective)[69]	Sunitinib	Dose: 50 mg QD Duration: 4 cycles	19	≥28 d	Mean 10.5 (3–20)	24%	16%	

(continued on next page)

Table 2
(continued)

Author, Year (Trial Name, if Available) (Study Type)	Therapeutic Agent (in Alphabetical Order)	Dose and Duration	N	Period of Discontinuation Before Surgery	Median Tumor Size (Range) Before Neoadjuvant Therapy (cm)	Decrease in Tumor Diameter (Range)	Partial Response by RECIST Criteria	Downsize Primary Tumor(s) (Size or Tumor Volume)	Reduce RENAL Score; Facilitate NSS (Partial Nephrectomy Instead of Radical Nephrectomy)	Change of Tumor Status from Unresectable to Resectable
Bex, 2009 (retrospective)[70]	Sunitinib	Dose: 50 mg QD Duration: NA	10	Not reported	11.0 (8–15)	NA	20%	✓		✓
Silberstein, 2010 (retrospective)[71]	Sunitinib	Dose: 50 mg QD Duration: 12 wk	12	2 wk	7.1	21.1% (3.2–45)	16%	✓	✓	
Hellenthal, 2010 (prospective phase II)[12]	Sunitinib	Dose: 37.5 mg BID Duration: 3 mo	20	5 d (n = 5) 24 h (n = 15)	Mean 8.1 (4.7–11)	11.8% (–11% to 27%)	5%			✓
Rini, 2012 (prospective phase II trial)[15]	Sunitinib	Dose: 50 mg BID Duration: 6–120 wk (4 cycles)	28	≥7 d	7.2 (1.7–20.6)	22% (13% to 100%)	25%	✓	✓	
Kroon, 2013 (pooled data from selected retrospective and prospective studies)[72]	Sorafenib (n = 21) Sunitinib (n = 68)		89			Tumor size <5 cm: 32% (–46% to 11%) Tumor size 5–7 cm: 11% (–55%—16%)				

| Lane, 2015 (retrospective)[73] | Sunitinib | 72 | 7.2 (5.3–8.7) | 32% | Tumor size 7–10 cm: 18% (−39% to 2%) Tumor size >10 cm: 10% (−31% to 0%) |

Abbreviations: NSS, nephron-sparing surgery; PDGF, platelet-derived growth factor; RENAL, nephrometry score to assess kidney tumor complexity, denoted by Radius of tumor, Exophytic/endophytic, Nearness to collecting system, Anterior/posterior location, Location of tumor in relation to polar lines.[74]

Modified from "Westerman ME, Shapiro DD, Wood CG, Karam JA. Neoadjuvant Therapy for Locally Advanced Renal Cell Carcinoma. Urol Clin North Am . 2020 Aug;47(3):329-343. https://doi.org/10.1016/j.ucl.2020.04. PMID: 32600535".

reduce tumor volume, it is not likely to be the mainstay treatment of choice that dictates surgical planning in large, bulky disease.

Unfortunately, none of the trials listed in **Table 2** demonstrated an OS or progression-free survival (PFS) benefit for neoadjuvant therapies in RCC in a placebo-controlled double-blinded fashion. Interest to design and conduct such a neoadjuvant trial faded, in light of adjuvant trials coming to the forefront from 2017 onward with KEYNOTE-564, IMmotion010, Checkmate-914, and PROSPER trials having started their patient recruitment at that time. The proliferation of immunotherapeutic agents, efficacy demonstrated in the metastatic setting, and strong industry support created a "prime time" for neoadjuvant immunotherapy and combination therapies to be investigated in a prospective fashion.

NEOADJUVANT COMBINATION (IMMUNOTHERAPY + TYROSINE KINASE INHIBITOR) THERAPIES

Given that drugs targeting programmed cell death-1/programmed death ligand-1 (PD-1/PD-L1) combined with VEGF-inhibitors are considered first line for metastatic RCC, investigators aimed to evaluate if similar combinations used in the neoadjuvant setting can lead to downstaging and reduce recurrence risk. There is some scientific basis underlying such a combination, particularly in the locally advanced setting. Intratumoral immune components after pretreatment of human RCC suggest a potential synergism for TKI with anti–PD-L1 therapy. Given that axitinib is more effective than sunitinib in downsizing tumors during "pretreatment phases," it makes sense to combine axitinib with anti–PD-L1 therapy.[11,20] Two phase Ib dose-finding studies evaluating safety, pharmacokinetics, and pharmacodynamics of avelumab, an anti–PD-L1 monoclonal antibody, or pembrolizumab, an anti–PD-1 monoclonal antibody, in combination with axitinib were performed. These showed promising objective response rates of 67% to 70% and toxicity profiles as seen with VEGF receptor treatment. This helped pave the way for the NeoAvAx trial (NCT03341845) to begin recruitment in 2017. At the 2022 Genitourinary Cancers Symposium, the trial investigators reported partial response in 12 of 40 patients (30%). The primary tumor downsized by a median of 20% (range, +3.8% to 43.5%). Among the 12 patients with partial response, 11 were disease free at study cutoff (92%).[20] At a median follow-up period of 23.5 months, no patients suffered progression of disease. Longer-term follow-up is pending before further conclusions can be drawn,

but this may signal phase III multicenter intent in the future with comparison to standard of care for patients with intermediate- to high-risk nonmetastatic RCC.

Although not a neoadjuvant study, the neoadjuvant paradigm may be informed by the primary tumor response rates of patients receiving ipilimumab/nivolumab in Checkmate 214 that had a primary tumor in situ.[21] This is an inherently biased cohort because suitable patients likely received cytoreductive nephrectomy before study enrollment and thus did not have an evaluable primary tumor (82% of ipilimumab/nivolumab cohort had prior cytoreductive nephrectomy [CN]). Nonetheless, ≥30% primary tumor reduction was achieved in 35% of patients receiving ipilimumab/nivolumab versus 20% with sunitinib control in this study. An increase of primary tumor ≥20% occurred in 4.1% of patients with ipilimumab/nivolumab. This suggests that modern immuno-oncology/immuno-oncology (IO/IO) or IO/TKI regimens are likely more effective than TKI monotherapy. Although not strictly a neoadjuvant IO trial, the PROSPER RCC trial assessed 766 patients with clinical stage ≥T2 or TanyN + RCC planned for nephrectomy (partial or radical) as well as select oligometastatic disease if the patient could be rendered "no evidence of disease (NED)" within 12 weeks of surgery randomized to 1 dose of neoadjuvant and 9 doses of adjuvant nivolumab versus observation.[22] Notably, this did not show any difference between recurrence-free survival (RFS) between the experimental arm and placebo.

OTHER BENEFITS OF NEOADJUVANT THERAPY

A potential benefit of neoadjuvant therapy is in possibly mitigating surgical risk associated with inferior vena cava (IVC) tumor thrombus by decreasing tumor thrombus level. Field and colleagues[23] performed a multicenter retrospective review of 53 patients of whom 19 underwent neoadjuvant sunitinib, whereas 34 underwent surgery primarily. The IVC tumor thrombus decreased by a median of 1.3 cm, with tumor level decreasing in 8 of 19 (42.1%) patients, with it remaining stable in 10 of 19 (52.6%). Those undergoing neoadjuvant sunitinib had significantly less blood loss, but otherwise there were no differences in surgical outcomes between groups. Notably, although multivariate analysis showed that neoadjuvant sunitinib was associated with improved cancer-specific survival (CSS) (odds ratio = 3.28; $P = .021$), with a significantly longer median CSS for those undergoing neoadjuvant sunitinib (72 vs 38 months, $P = .023$), but on subgroup analysis of patients without metastatic disease this survival benefit did not persist. Keeping in mind the retrospective design of this study, although there was improvement in the size of the tumor thrombus, surgical approach and outcomes were largely similar between groups, without clear survival benefit. With regards to immune checkpoint inhibitor therapy, there are limited data published thus far, but there have been case reports detailing response to such therapy.[24]

FUTURE DIRECTIONS FOR NEOADJUVANT THERAPY

To address the dearth of prospective literature in this area, the NAXIVA phase II trial assessing 20 patients with clear cell RCC with tumor thrombus undergoing up to 8 weeks of neoadjuvant axitinib found that 7 of 20 patients (35%) had a reduction in thrombus level (6 of 16 with inferior vena cava tumor thrombus and 1 of 4 with renal vein without vena cava tumor thrombus).[25] In total,15 of 20 patients overall had a reduction in the length of the tumor thrombus, with 7 of 17 patients undergoing surgery that was less invasive than had been initially planned.

Although RCC has traditionally been viewed as radioresistant, this is increasingly being challenged. The use of neoadjuvant stereotactic ablative radiotherapy with subsequent nephrectomy and IVC thrombectomy is currently ongoing and may provide yet another potential method of neoadjuvant therapy in this specific clinical context.[26,27] Further studies are needed to better understand the safety and utility of different forms of neoadjuvant therapy for IVC tumor thrombus, with future investigation currently ongoing.[28]

ADJUVANT THERAPY IN HIGH-RISK RENAL CELL CARCINOMA

Historical stage-specific data reported the likelihood of recurrence in high-risk RCC patients postnephrectomy as 7% for T1 tumors, 26% for T2 tumors, and 39% for T3 tumors.[29] Up to 40% of patients with locoregional disease have a relapse with metastasis after nephrectomy.[7,30] Urologic oncologists are uniquely suited to counsel their patients about whether they may benefit from such therapies postoperatively and thus need to understand the current progress that has been made and continues to be made with regards to defining the role of such therapy in the modern systemic therapy era.

ADJUVANT THERAPY TRIALS IN THE CYTOKINE ERA

Before the advent of anti-VEGF TKI, the mainstay of systemic therapy was cytokine-based treatments. Observations that interleukin-2 (IL-2) and interferon-alpha (IFN-α) increased time to progression and improved OS in metastatic RCC[31,32] served as the rationale for using cytokine agents as adjuvant therapy for patients at high risk for RCC recurrence following potentially curative surgery.

Multiple randomized studies were then performed to investigate the potential benefits of adjuvant cytokine therapy following radical nephrectomy for high-risk localized disease or nephrectomy for locoregional disease (**Table 3**); however, none of these trials demonstrated statistically significant improvement of DFS or OS. Porzsolt,[33] Trump and colleagues,[34] Pizzocaro and colleagues,[35] and Messing and colleagues,[36] however, showed no improvements in DFS or OS for interferon-treated patients. The studies differ in the types of interferons used (L-IFN [lymphoblastoid], IFN-α2a, IFN-α2b), doses used, and duration of therapy (6–12 months).[37] An adjuvant clinical trial evaluating IL-2 compared with observation also failed to demonstrate benefit.[38] This study was designed and powered to show an improvement in predicted 2-year DFS from 40% for the observation group to 70% for the treatment group. Early closure occurred when an interim analysis determined that the improvement in 2-year DFS could not be achieved despite full accrual. Furthermore, the inclusion of chemotherapy (ie, 5-fluorouracil)[39] and hormone therapy[40,41] to adjuvant cytokine therapy did not achieve a meaningful improvement following surgery for high-risk RCC.

ADJUVANT THERAPY TRIALS WITH ANTI–VASCULAR ENDOTHELIAL GROWTH FACTOR TYROSINE KINASE INHIBITOR AGENTS

Beginning in 2005, the Food and Drug Administration (FDA) approved a multitude of novel drugs for the treatment of metastatic renal cell carcinoma (mRCC). These FDA-approved drugs belong to 2 broad categories: (1) VEGF inhibitors and (2) mammalian target of rapamycin inhibitors. More importantly, these agents were associated with unprecedented results, characterized by overall response rates of 20% to 40% and a median OS of greater than 24 months for patients with mRCC.[42] These agents were generally well tolerated and therefore immediately evaluated in phase III randomized double-blinded adjuvant clinical trials.

The first and largest adjuvant trial to date evaluating targeted therapeutic agents was the ASSURE (Adjuvant Sunitinib or Sorafenib for high-risk, non-metastatic renal-cell carcinoma)

Table 3
Adjuvant studies in the cytokine era for renal cell carcinoma

Trial	N	Patient Population	Comparison	Endpoint	Benefit?
Porzsolt, 1992[33]	270	pT3-4N0 or pTx N1-3	IFN-alpha vs observation	Time to treatment failure (TTF)/survival	No
Trump et al, 1996[34]	294	pT3-4aN0 or pTx N1-3	L-IFN-alpha vs observation	Recurrence	No
Pizzocaro et al, 2001[35]	247	pT3-4aN0 or pTx N1-3	IFN-alpha vs observation	5-y DFS	No
Messing et al, 2003[36,38]	283	pT3-4aN0 or pTx N1-3	IFN-alpha vs observation	5-y OS	No
Clark et al, 2003	138	pT3b-4Nx or pTx N1-3	IL-2 vs observation	2-y DFS	No
Atzpodien et al, 2005[37]	203	pT3b-4Nx or pTx N1-3	IL-2/IFN-alpha/5-FU vs observation	2-y DFS	No
Aitchison et al, 2014[39]	309	pT3b-4Nx or pTx Na-2 or + margin/vascular invasion	IL-2/IFN-alpha/5-FU vs observation	3-y DFS	No

trial, which investigated the efficacy of sunitinib or sorafenib versus placebo as adjuvant therapy in a cohort of 1943 patients after nephrectomy for high-risk RCC (**Table 4**). The trial did not achieve its primary endpoint, as there was no benefit in terms of median DFS in both treatment arms: for sunitinib versus placebo, respectively, 5.8 versus 6.6 years, hazard ratio (HR), 1.02 (97.5% confidence interval [CI], 0.85–1.23; $P = .8038$); for sorafenib versus placebo, respectively, 6.1 versus 6.6 years, for sorafenib versus placebo, respectively, HR, 0.97 (97.5% CI, 0.80–1.17; $P = .7184$). Furthermore, there was no significant difference in terms of OS between groups: for sunitinib versus placebo, HR, 1.17 (97.5% CI, 0.90–1.52; $P = .1762$); for sorafenib versus placebo, HR, 0.98 (97.5% CI, 0.75–1.28; $P = .8577$). Later, the follow-up at 5 years confirmed the lack of benefit in term of DFS and OS.[43]

After the negative results of the ASSURE trial, enthusiasm for adjuvant therapy returned with the phase III double-blinded S-TRAC (Sunitinib Treatment of Renal Adjuvant Cancer) clinical trial, which enrolled 615 patients diagnosed with high-risk resected RCC to compare adjuvant sunitinib versus placebo. The S-TRAC trial met its primary endpoint: at 5.4 years of follow-up, there was a modest improvement in terms of DFS associated with the sunitinib arm, compared with the placebo arm (6.8 vs 5.6 years; HR, 0.76 [95% CI, 0.59–0.98; $P = .03$]).[44] The magnitude of benefit was greater for patients at higher risk of relapse (defined as T3 N0/Nx, Fuhrman grade ≥ 2, and Eastern Cooperative Oncology Group Performance Status [ECOG PS] ≥ 1 or T4, local nodal involvement, or both), and DFS was 6.2 years compared with 4 years in the placebo arm (HR, 0.74 [95% CI, 0.55–0.99; $P = .04$]), leading the FDA to approve

sunitinib as adjuvant treatment following surgery for patients with locoregional disease.[45]

Despite the demonstrated benefit in terms of DFS in the S-TRAC trial, there was no evidence of an OS advantage for adjuvant sunitinib even with an updated analysis in 2017.[46] Because of this lack of OS benefit, the European Association of Urology did not recommend sunitinib as adjuvant treatment after nephrectomy for patients with RCC. Importantly, the investigators reported grade 3 to 4 adverse events (AEs) in about 65% of patients treated with sunitinib, potentially a result of the relatively high dose of sunitinib compared with other trials (see **Table 4**), in contrast to 23.3% in the placebo group. Ultimately, 28.1% of patients in the sunitinib arm discontinued treatment owing to AEs. The substantial number of AEs at the higher dose of sunitinib coupled with the results, which conflicted with the larger ASSURE trial, led to relatively limited use of adjuvant sunitinib following surgical resection of high-risk RCC despite FDA approval.

Disappointingly, none of the other phase III double-blinded adjuvant trials investigating anti-VEGF TKIs met their primary endpoints (see **Table 4**). One partial exception was the PROTECT (Pazopanib as an Adjuvant Treatment for Localized Renal Cell Carcinoma) trial, which enrolled 1538 patients and compared adjuvant pazopanib versus placebo. Because of drug-related hepatotoxicity, the original regimen on 800 mg daily was reduced to 600 mg daily, and the trial ultimately demonstrated no benefit in terms of DFS (HR, 0.94 [95% CI, 0.77–1.14; $P = .51$]). However, there was a subgroup of patients that continued with the original higher dose (800 mg daily), and among these subjects, there was a DFS advantage for the pazopanib arm versus placebo (HR, 0.66

Table 4
Adjuvant studies in the targeted therapy era for renal cell carcinoma

Trial	N	Comparison	Eligibility	Histology	Endpoint	Benefit?
ASSURE[43]	1943	Sunitinib vs Sorafenib vs Placebo	At least T1bNxM0	Any	DFS	No
SORCE[49]	1656	Sorafenib vs Placebo	Leibovich 3–11	Any	DFS	No
S-TRAC[44]	674	Sunitinib vs Placebo	UISS High-risk	Clear cell RCC	DFS	Yes
PROTECT[47]	1538	Pazopanib vs Placebo	pT2, pT3-4N0, or any N+	Clear cell RCC	DFS	No
ATLAS[48]	592	Axitinib vs Placebo	pT2, pT3-4N0, or any N+	Clear cell RCC	DFS	No
EVEREST[75]	1545	Everolimus vs Placebo	Intermediate-risk (pT2-3aN0) or high-risk (pT3a-4N0-1)	Any	DFS	No

[95% CI, 0.49–0.90; $P = .008$]). The updated final OS analysis however revealed no benefit associated with adjuvant pazopanib (HR, 1.0 [95% CI, 0.80–1.26; $P > .9$]) similar to the S-TRAC trial.[47] Furthermore, therapy with pazopanib was complicated by a higher rate of grade 3 or worse AEs in approximately 60% of patients in the 800-mg subgroup, whereas half (51%) of those in 600-mg group needed a further dose reduction owing to AEs.

In summary, although the advent of anti-VEGF TKI agents was a pivotal and meaningful improvement in the management of mRCC, it did not usher in a new era of adjuvant therapy for high-risk disease despite FDA approval of sunitinib based on the sole positive result from the S-TRAC trial. A plausible explanation for the negative results was the inability to achieve adequate dose intensity owing to poor tolerance of the anti-VEGF TKI therapies in the adjuvant setting evidenced by DFS benefit, albeit limited, seen only among the patients receiving the relatively high dose of sunitinib in the S-TRAC trial and those who remained in the original higher dose of pazopanib subgroup of the PROTECT trial. Another possible factor in the negative outcomes is the heterogeneity of RCC; only the S-TRACT,[44] PROTECT,[47] and ATLAS[48] (Adjuvant Axitinib Therapy of Renal Cell Cancer in High-risk Patients) trials limited enrollment to clear cell RCC. The nonclear cell variants can be highly dissimilar in pathophysiology and not often driven by aberrant activation of the angiogenic pathway, which is the target of the anti-VEGF TKI therapies. The inclusion of patients with nonclear cell variants may have negatively skewed the results of the ASSURE[43] and SORCE[49] (Sorafenib in Treating Patients at Risk of Relapse After Undergoing Surgery to Remove Kidney Cancer) trials, in which 21% and 16% of enrollees, respectively, had nonclear cell histologies.

ADJUVANT THERAPY TRIALS WITH IMMUNO-ONCOLOGY AGENTS

IO therapy, both as monotherapy or in combination, has dramatically altered the landscape of systemic therapy for mRCC.[50] Thus, it is not surprising that there have been multiple investigations centered on adjuvant therapy with IO agents.

KEYNOTE-564

The double-blind, randomized, phase III KEYNOTE-564 trial enrolled 994 patients with clear cell RCC at high risk of disease recurrence following nephrectomy between June 30, 2017 and September 20, 2019, to receive pembrolizumab (n = 496), a PD-1 inhibitor, versus placebo

(n = 498).[51] The updated efficacy and safety analysis with 30.1 months of follow-up showed that DFS was maintained for patients receiving pembrolizumab (HR, 0.63; 95% CI, 0.50–0.80) even though median DFS was not reached in either arm.[52] In addition, the DFS benefit for pembrolizumab was consistent among 3 distinct subgroups following surgery: intermediate-high-risk (HR, 0.68; 95% CI, 0.52–0.89), high-risk (HR, 0.60; 95% CI, 0.33–1.10), and M1 NED (HR, 0.28; 95% CI, 0.12–0.66). This most recent analysis also demonstrated a trend for an OS advantage associated with pembrolizumab, although this difference did not reach statistical significance. Because only 66 of the anticipated 200 events accrued at the most recent analysis, substantially longer follow-up is needed to determine if adjuvant pembrolizumab is associated with an OS benefit.[52]

All-cause grade 3 AEs or higher were observed in 157 (32%) of 488 patients in the pembrolizumab arm versus 88 (18%) of those in the placebo arm. Treatment toxicity resulting in dose interruptions and discontinuation of pembrolizumab occurred in 127 (26%) and 103 (21%) patients, respectively. The most common grade 3 or higher AEs associated with pembrolizumab were hypertension and increased alanine aminotransferase. As a point of comparison, the rate of treatment-related AEs was 18.6% in the KEYNOTE-564 trial compared with 57.2% in the S-TRAC trial; thus, this was a well-tolerated regimen overall.

Despite the immature OS analysis, the robust DFS advantage seen in the KEYNOTE-564 trial coupled with its tolerability has established pembrolizumab as a legitimate adjuvant strategy for patients with high-risk clear cell RCC following surgery. FDA approval was announced on November 17, 2021, followed soon thereafter by the European Commission approval on January 27, 2022.

IMmotion010, CheckMate 914, and PROSPER

Despite the positive results of the KEYNOTE-564 trial, the results of 3 phase III clinical trials evaluating adjuvant immunotherapy were presented at 2022 ESMO Congress, all of which disappointingly showed no benefit of adjuvant systemic therapy for surgically resected high-risk RCC (**Table 5**).

The phase III IMmotion010 trial compared adjuvant monotherapy atezolizumab (n = 390), a PD-L1 inhibitor, versus placebo (n = 388) for patients with high-risk clear cell RCC.[53] After a median follow-up of 44.7 months, there was no DFS benefit associated with atezolizumab, although it was found to be well tolerated by patients. This study highlights the possibility that PD-L1

Table 5
Adjuvant studies in the immunotherapy era for renal cell carcinoma

Trial	N	Comparison	Stage/Grade	Histology	Endpoint	Benefit for Adjuvant Therapy?
KEYNOTE-564[52]	994	Pembrolizumab vs placebo	pT2 (G4), pT3a (G3-4), pT3b-T4 (Gx), pTxN1, pTxNxM1 (resected to NED within 1 y)	Clear cell RCC	DFS	Yes
IMmotion010[53]	778	Atezolizumab vs placebo	pT2 (G4), pT3a (G3-4), pT3b-T4 (Gx), pTxN1, pTxNxM1 (resected to NED)	Clear cell RCC	DFS	No
CheckMate-914[54]	1600	Nivolumab + ipilimumab vs nivolumab + placebo vs placebo	pT2aN0 (G3-4), pT2b-T4N0 (Gx), pTxN1 (Gx)	Clear cell RCC	DFS	No (part A/combination), part B pending
PROSPER	766	Nivolumab vs active monitoring	T2Nx, TxN1, TxNxM1 (resected to NED)	Any RCC	DFS	No
RAMPART	1750	Durvalumab + tremelimumab vs durvalumab vs active monitoring	Leibovich score 3-11	Any RCC	DFS, OS	Accruing
LITESPARK-022	1600	Belzutifan + pembrolizumab vs pembrolizumab	pT2 (G4/sarcomatoid), pT3, pT4, pTxN1, pTxNxM1 (resected to NED)	Clear cell RCC	DFS	Accruing

inhibitors may simply have limited efficacy in the management of RCC. Multiple studies investigating PD-L1 agents, such as atezolizumab and avelumab, have consistently underperformed compared with PD-1 inhibitors, such as nivolumab and pembrolizumab, and thus have failed to achieve regulatory approval in RCC.[54] In addition, the negative results may have also been influenced by the unique definition for the M1 NED category: although patients with synchronous metastatic disease were included, those with metachronous metastatic disease were only included if the disease recurrence was beyond 1 year from the time of the surgery. This potentially excluded the higher-risk M1 patients, who may be the patients to benefit most from adjuvant therapy, based on the KEYNOTE-564 trial.

The CheckMate 914 trial evaluated adjuvant nivolumab and ipilimumab compared with placebo (part A), as well as adjuvant nivolumab as monotherapy compared with placebo (part B) for patients with resected clear cell RCC and a high risk of rephase. This study was a natural extension of the prior CheckMate 214 trial,[55] which demonstrated significant benefit in OS for the combination of nivolumab and ipilimumab as first-line treatment in the management of metastatic clear cell RCC. Surprisingly, in the primary analysis for part A, including 816 patients receiving nivolumab and ipilimumab (n = 405) or placebo (n = 411), the primary efficacy objective of DFS was not met at a median follow-up of 37 months (HR, 0.92; 95% CI, 0.71–1.19), as DFS probabilities were essentially identical at 24 months at 76.4% for the treatment arm and 74% for the control arm. The negative results for CheckMate 914 may be attributed to the shorter 6-month regimen, compared with 12-month regimen of adjuvant pembrolizumab in the KEYNOTE-564 trial. Another factor may have been the relatively toxic regimen of nivolumab and ipilimumab, which was associated with any treatment-related AEs in 88% of patients and treatment discontinuation in 43% of patients in the treatment arm. In addition, CheckMate 914 did not include M1 NED patients, which is arguably the patient population most likely to benefit from adjuvant therapy following surgery based on KEYNOTE-564 trial. Part B, evaluating nivolumab alone as adjuvant therapy compared with placebo, is ongoing, although there is a low degree of confidence that it will meet the primary endpoint of DFS given the negative results of part A.

Single-agent nivolumab was also studied as adjuvant therapy in the RandOmized Study Comparing PErioperative Nivolumab versus Observation in Patients with RCC Undergoing Nephrectomy (PROSPER, ECOG-ACRIN EA8143), which was an unblinded phase III randomized study as perioperative therapy for patients with high-risk RCC. Unlike other studies, this trial examined the effect of priming the immune system with neoadjuvant nivolumab before nephrectomy followed by adjuvant nivolumab. Eligible patients had high-risk RCC of clinical stage T2 or greater, or any T stage with clinical regional lymph node involvement of any histology. Patients randomized to the treatment arm received a single dose of nivolumab 7 to 28 days before nephrectomy followed by 9 adjuvant doses, whereas patients in the control arm proceeded directly to surgery without a placebo. In total, 819 patients were randomized to perioperative nivolumab (n = 404) or surgery alone (n = 415). At a median follow-up of 16 months, the primary endpoint, RFS, was not met (HR, 0.97; 95% CI, 0.74–1.28), and the trial was stopped early owing to futility. This trial was characterized by a high degree of attrition with only approximately 75% (314 of 404) actually receiving adjuvant nivolumab. Furthermore, this trial may have been handicapped by enrichment of patients unlikely to respond to immunotherapy, including 34% who had pT1/T2 disease, 22% who had nonclear cell RCC, and 5% who had benign renal masses.

ONGOING ADJUVANT TRIALS WITH IMMUNOTHERAPY

Investigators may look to ongoing trials to clarify the role of adjuvant systemic therapy.

The RAMPART (Renal Adjuvant Multiple Arm Randomized Trial; NCT03288532) is a United Kingdom–led multiarm and multistage clinical trial, which is designed to accommodate additional arms in the future to address new research questions over time. Eligible patients include patients with histologically proven, resected, locally advanced RCC (both clear and nonclear cell types), and be at high or intermediate risk of relapse based on a Leibovich score between 3 and 11. Currently, there are 3 arms: patients in arm A will be actively monitored for 1 year; patients in arm B will receive the durvalumab every 4 weeks for 1 year; and patients in arm C will receive the combination of durvalumab every 4 weeks for 1 year plus 2 doses of tremelimumab on day 1 of the first 2 cycles of durvalumab. The primary endpoints of this study are DFS and OS. This study opened in 2018 and is actively accruing with a target enrollment of 1750 participants.

In addition, LITESPARK-022 (NCT05239728) is a phase III study investigating the efficacy and safety of pembrolizumab plus belzutifan compared with pembrolizumab plus placebo as adjuvant therapy for patients with clear cell RCC after nephrectomy. This study builds on the positive results of KEYNOTE-564 and studies demonstrating that belzutifan, an HIF-2α inhibitor, has efficacy and tolerability in patients with metastatic clear cell RCC as well as with von Hippel-Lindau disease–associated RCC. Combining belzutifan with pembrolizumab may therefore be a therapeutic option as adjuvant treatment of clear cell RCC. This study opened in 2022 and is actively accruing with a target enrollment of 1600 participants.

FUTURE DIRECTIONS FOR ADJUVANT THERAPY
Better Selection with Prognostication Tools

Optimizing selection of patients for adjuvant systemic therapy has been the subject of research long before any of the above-mentioned trials even started. There exist combination prognostic tools incorporating clinical information that help predict the risk of relapse and hence may be used to better select patients for adjuvant therapy. For example, the UCLA Integrated Staging System (UISS),[56,57] the Leibovich system,[58] and the Stage, Size, Grade and Necrosis score[59] are recommended for use in guidelines.

Another way to select patients for adjuvant systemic therapy could be simply to follow the same inclusion criteria of existing clinical trials. These criteria had been determined by these clinical trials' investigators in order to maximize recruitment in a select group of patients in whom they believe will best benefit from the trial drug and therefore demonstrate efficacy for regulatory authorities. The inclusion/exclusion criteria of adjuvant immunotherapy trials (PROSPER, CheckMate 914, KEYNOTE-564, IMmotion010, RAMPART) had been scrutinized against existing retrospective cohorts, such as the SEER database (2001–2015, n = 116,750)[60] and a multicenter European database called RECUR (2006–2011, n = 3024) capturing patient and tumor characteristics, recurrence patterns, and survival of those curatively treated for nonmetastatic RCC without any adjuvant therapy.[61] This may have helped clinicians to refer appropriate patients to trial enrollment. Palumbo and colleagues,[60] based on the SEER database analysis, concluded that "participation in adjuvant immunotherapy trials should be predominantly encouraged for patients with high-grade stage T3, T4, and N1 and patients with any stage with sarcomatoid pathologic features."

Some may want to only use the inclusion criteria from a positive trial or trials demonstrating

survival benefit, to guide their recommendation to patients for adjuvant therapy. Being the only randomized trial for RCC showing survival benefit in the adjuvant setting (see **Table 5**), scrutinizing the categorization of KEYNOTE-564 participants is important.[51] They were categorized as follows:

1. M0 intermediate-high risk of disease recurrence (pathologic tumor stage 2 [pT2] with nuclear grade 4 or sarcomatoid differentiation, no nodal involvement [N0], and no metastasis [M0]; or pT3, any grade, N0, M0);
2. M0 high risk of disease recurrence (pT4, any grade, N0, M0; or any pT, any grade, N+, M0); or
3. M1 stage with NED after complete resection of oligometastases synchronously or within 1 year of nephrectomy (M1 with NED).

Although subgroup analyses can only be hypothesis-generating, it was interesting to note that only the M0 intermediate-high-risk group (HR, 0.68; 95% CI, 0.52–0.89) and the M1 NED group (HR, 0.28; 95% CI, 0.12–0.66) had DFS benefit. The M0 high-risk group seemed to have no DFS benefit (HR, 0.60) with wide 95% CI of 0.33 to 1.10.

Beyond these clinical parameters using TNM staging and histologic information, there are also tools that incorporate molecular or genetic features. The expression of 34 genes, ClearCode34, has been proposed to categorize patients with clear cell nonmetastatic RCC in 2 subgroups (ccA vs ccB) with different prognosis.[62] This had been externally validated in another cohort of patients.[63] Another tool based on 16 genes, the Recurrence Score, aimed to detect patients who can benefit from adjuvant treatment, and has been validated in the S-TRAC population to select for who can benefit from adjuvant sunitinib.[64,65] Unfortunately, these 2 genetic tools are not widely used in routine clinical practice yet, possibly owing to access and cost issues.

Of late, there is increasing enthusiasm for circulating tumor DNA (ctDNA) with 19 studies investigating its use for RCC.[66] However, although cell-free methylated DNA immunoprecipitation and high-throughput sequencing may be a very sensitive method for ctDNA detection in RCC, ctDNA levels are still found to be low.[66] RCC tends not to be a cell-shedding cancer; hence, so far, there appears to be limited clinical utility and thus ctDNA has not been routinely incorporated yet in to combined scoring/prognostication tools. This is a space to watch for in the future.

Combination Adjuvant Therapy, and Disease Progression Among Those Who Received Adjuvant Therapy

In the metastatic RCC space, combination therapy is recommended as a standard of care in the first-line treatment of clear cell metastatic RCC (eg, pembrolizumab/axitinib in KEYNOTE-426).[21] Although these treatments may be of interest for future adjuvant trials in RCC, there may be a higher toxicity profile compared with a single systemic agent, making them less suitable for use in the adjuvant setting.

In addition, it is currently unclear as to what systemic therapy options are best for patients who already received adjuvant therapy and subsequently progress. It will likely be up to the clinician's discretion based on existing burden of disease, ECOG status, medical comorbidities, and tolerability to further lines of treatment. Future trials will be needed to determine the preferred sequencing of therapy for such patients.

SUMMARY

Surgery remains the cornerstone of treatment of locoregional renal cancers. The story of neoadjuvant and adjuvant therapies for renal cancer is one of ups and downs. Neoadjuvant systemic therapy for RCC may have a role particularly for locally advanced disease, which would otherwise be inoperable and treated with metastatic intent. However, its promise to improve survival has not been fulfilled yet—with disappointing performance overall with the anti-VEGF TKI agents. There is still hope in the ongoing evaluation of immunotherapeutic agents because efficacy had been demonstrated in the metastatic setting. With strong industry support, neoadjuvant immunotherapy and combination therapies can be investigated in a prospective fashion and can be a promising option to keep a lookout for.

As for adjuvant therapies, the history from the cytokine era to the anti-VEGF TKI agents and to the current paradigm of immunotherapy has hailed numerous lessons for medical and urologic oncologists as well as for clinical trialists. Adjuvant pembrolizumab will likely feature strongly as an option in the standard care of high-risk patients with RCC. Better selection of candidates for adjuvant pembrolizumab via clinical nomograms and biomarkers like ctDNA and integrating these into routine clinical care will be promising in the future, to help patients receive optimal care. The future of multimodal therapies for high-risk RCC will be dictated by close coordination between extirpative surgery and the rapidly changing landscape of systemic therapies and nonsurgical treatment options for RCC.

CLINICS CARE POINTS

- Despite notable advancements in systemic treatments for advanced renal cell carcinoma, numerous recent clinical studies have failed to demonstrate a clear clinical benefit associated with neoadjuvant and adjuvant therapies for localized renal cell carcinoma.

- While limited data report that neoadjuvant systemic therapy may facilitate extirpative surgery and adjuvant therapies (pembrolizumab and high-dose sunitinib) can improvement disease-free survival, multimodal therapies have yet to demonstrate improvement in overall survival survival for this patient population.

- There remains optimism for a benefit associated with neoadjuvant and adjuvant therapies with the continued progress for systemic therapies and promising advancements in biomarkers for renal cell carcinoma.

DISCLOSURE

J.J. Leow, S. Ray, S.L. Chang: no disclosures. S. Dason: Bristol Myers Squibb, Roche, Advisory Board; Intuitive Surgical Education, funding. E.A. Singer: Astellas/Medivation, research support for clinical trial; Merck, advisory board; Johnson & Johnson, advisory board; Vyriad, advisory board; Aura Biosciences, data safety monitoring board.

REFERENCES

1. Shapiro DM, Fugmann RA. A role for chemotherapy as an adjunct to surgery. Cancer Res 1957;17(11): 1098–101.
2. Bonadonna G, Rossi A, Valagussa P, et al. The CMF program for operable breast cancer with positive axillary nodes. Updated analysis on the disease-free interval, site of relapse and drug tolerance. Cancer 1977;39(6 Suppl):2904–15.
3. Ljungberg B, Albiges L, Abu-Ghanem Y, et al. European Association of Urology Guidelines on Renal Cell Carcinoma: The 2022 Update. Eur Urol 2022; 82(4):399–410.
4. Campbell SC, Clark PE, Chang SS, et al. Renal Mass and Localized Renal Cancer: Evaluation, Management, and Follow-Up: AUA Guideline: Part I. J Urol 2021;206(2):199–208.

5. Siegel RL, Miller KD, Fuchs HE, et al. Cancer statistics, 2022. CA Cancer J Clin 2022;72(1):7–33.

6. Van Poppel H, Da Pozzo L, Albrecht W, et al. A prospective, randomised EORTC intergroup phase 3 study comparing the oncologic outcome of elective nephron-sparing surgery and radical nephrectomy for low-stage renal cell carcinoma. Eur Urol 2011;59(4):543–52.

7. Janzen NK, Kim HL, Figlin RA, et al. Surveillance after radical or partial nephrectomy for localized renal cell carcinoma and management of recurrent disease. Urol Clin North Am 2003;30(4): 843–52.

8. Lam JS, Leppert JT, Belldegrun AS, et al. Novel approaches in the therapy of metastatic renal cell carcinoma. World J Urol 2005;23(3):202–12.

9. Rini BI, Plimack ER, Takagi T, et al. A Phase II Study of Pazopanib in Patients with Localized Renal Cell Carcinoma to Optimize Preservation of Renal Parenchyma. J Urol 2015;194(2):297–303.

10. Hatiboglu G, Hohenfellner M, Arslan A, et al. Effective downsizing but enhanced intratumoral heterogeneity following neoadjuvant sorafenib in patients with non-metastatic renal cell carcinoma. Langenbeck's Arch Surg 2017;402(4):637–44.

11. Karam JA, Devine CE, Urbauer DL, et al. Phase 2 trial of neoadjuvant axitinib in patients with locally advanced nonmetastatic clear cell renal cell carcinoma. Eur Urol 2014;66(5):874–80.

12. Hellenthal NJ, Underwood W, Penetrante R, et al. Prospective clinical trial of preoperative sunitinib in patients with renal cell carcinoma. J Urol 2010; 184(3):859–64.

13. Cowey CL, Amin C, Pruthi RS, et al. Neoadjuvant clinical trial with sorafenib for patients with stage II or higher renal cell carcinoma. J Clin Oncol 2010; 28(9):1502–7.

14. van der Veldt AAM, Meijerink MR, van den Eertwegh AJM, et al. Sunitinib for Treatment of Advanced Renal Cell Cancer: Primary Tumor Response. Clin Cancer Res 2008;14(8):2431–6.

15. Rini BI, Garcia J, Elson P, et al. The effect of sunitinib on primary renal cell carcinoma and facilitation of subsequent surgery. J Urol 2012;187(5):1548–54.

16. Nishimura K, Miura N, Sugihara N, et al. Sequential immune-targeted surgical therapy resulted in disease-free survival in a case with advanced renal cell carcinoma. BMC Urol 2021;21(1):124.

17. Hess KJ, Bascoy S, Vadher U, et al. Neoadjuvant Immunotherapy in the Treatment of Renal Cell Carcinoma: A Case Series. Cureus 2022;14(7): e27019.

18. Roy AM, Briggler A, Tippit D, et al. Neoadjuvant Cabozantinib in Renal-Cell Carcinoma: A Brief Review. Clin Genitourin Cancer 2020;18(6):e688–91.

19. Lebacle C, Bensalah K, Bernhard J-C, et al. Evaluation of axitinib to downstage cT2a renal tumours and allow partial nephrectomy: a phase II study. BJU Int 2019;123(5):804–10.

20. Bex A, Abu-Ghanem Y, Thienen JVV, et al. Efficacy, safety, and biomarker analysis of neoadjuvant avelumab/axitinib in patients (pts) with localized renal cell carcinoma (RCC) who are at high risk of relapse after nephrectomy (NeoAvAx). J Clin Oncol 2022; 40(6_suppl):289.

21. Rini BI, Plimack ER, Stus V, et al. Pembrolizumab plus Axitinib versus Sunitinib for Advanced Renal-Cell Carcinoma. N Engl J Med 2019;380(12): 1116–27.

22. Phase III randomized study comparing perioperative nivolumab (nivo) versus observation in patients (Pts) with renal cell carcinoma (RCC) undergoing | OncologyPRO. Available at: https:// oncologypro.esmo.org/meeting-resources/esmo-congress/phase-iii-randomized-study-comparing-perioperative-nivolumab-nivo-versus-observation-in-patients-pts-with-renal-cell-carcinoma-rcc-undergoing. Accessed September 30, 2022.

23. Field CA, Cotta BH, Jimenez J, et al. Neoadjuvant Sunitinib Decreases Inferior Vena Caval Thrombus Size and Is Associated With Improved Oncologic Outcomes: A Multicenter Comparative Analysis. Clin Genitourin Cancer 2019;17(3): e505–12.

24. Labbate C, Hatogai K, Werntz R, et al. Complete response of renal cell carcinoma vena cava tumor thrombus to neoadjuvant immunotherapy. Journal for ImmunoTherapy of Cancer 2019; 7(1):66.

25. Stewart GD, Welsh SJ, Ursprung S, et al. A Phase II study of neoadjuvant axitinib for reducing the extent of venous tumour thrombus in clear cell renal cell cancer with venous invasion (NAXIVA). Br J Cancer 2022;127(6):1051–60.

26. Freifeld Y, Pedrosa I, McLaughlin M, et al. Stereotactic ablative radiation therapy for renal cell carcinoma with inferior vena cava tumor thrombus. Urol Oncol 2022;40(4):166. e169-e113.

27. Margulis V, Freifeld Y, Pop LM, et al. Neoadjuvant SABR for Renal Cell Carcinoma Inferior Vena Cava Tumor Thrombus-Safety Lead-in Results of a Phase 2 Trial. Int J Radiat Oncol Biol Phys 2021;110(4): 1135–42.

28. Margulis V. Safety and Efficacy of Neoadjuvant Lenvatinib and Pembrolizumab in Patients With Renal Cell Carcinoma and IVC Tumor Thrombus 2022/06/ 28 2022. NCT05319015.

29. Levy DA, Slaton JW, Swanson DA, et al. Stage specific guidelines for surveillance after radical nephrectomy for local renal cell carcinoma. J Urol 1998;159(4):1163–7.

30. Janowitz T, Welsh SJ, Zaki K, et al. Adjuvant Therapy in Renal Cell Carcinoma—Past, Present, and Future. Semin Oncol 2013;40(4):482–91.

31. Amin A, White RL. Interleukin-2 in Renal Cell Carcinoma: A Has-Been or a Still-Viable Option? J Kidney Cancer VHL 2014;1(7):74–83.

32. Fisher RI, Rosenberg SA, Fyfe G. Long-term survival update for high-dose recombinant interleukin-2 in patients with renal cell carcinoma. Cancer J Sci Am 2000;6(Suppl 1):S55–7.

33. Porzsolt F on behalf of the Delta-P Study Group. Adjuvant therapy of renal cell cancer (RCC) with interferon alfa-2A. Proc Am Soc Clin Oncol 1992; 11:202 (abstract).

34. Trump D, Elson P, Propert K, et al. Randomized controlled trial of adjuvant therapy with lymphoblastoid interferon (L-IFN) in resected, high-risk renal cell carcinoma (HR-RCC. Proc Am Soc Clin Oncol 1996; 15:253 (abstract).

35. Pizzocaro G, Piva L, Colavita M, et al. Interferon adjuvant to radical nephrectomy in Robson stages II and III renal cell carcinoma: a multicentric randomized study. J Clin Oncol 2001;19(2):425–31.

36. Messing EM, Manola J, Wilding G, et al. Phase III study of interferon alfa-NL as adjuvant treatment for resectable renal cell carcinoma: an Eastern Cooperative Oncology Group/Intergroup trial. J Clin Oncol 2003;21(7):1214–22.

37. Atzpodien J, Schmitt E, Gertenbach U, et al. Adjuvant treatment with interleukin-2- and interferon-alpha2a-based chemoimmunotherapy in renal cell carcinoma post tumour nephrectomy: results of a prospectively randomised trial of the German Cooperative Renal Carcinoma Chemoimmunotherapy Group (DGCIN). Br J Cancer 2005;92(5):843–6.

38. Clark JI, Atkins MB, Urba WJ, et al. Adjuvant high-dose bolus interleukin-2 for patients with high-risk renal cell carcinoma: a cytokine working group randomized trial. J Clin Oncol 2003;21(16):3133–40.

39. Aitchison M, Bray CA, Van Poppel H, et al. Adjuvant 5-flurouracil, alpha-interferon and interleukin-2 versus observation in patients at high risk of recurrence after nephrectomy for renal cell carcinoma: results of a phase III randomised European Organisation for Research and Treatment of Cancer (Genito-Urinary Cancers Group)/National Cancer Research Institute trial. Eur J Cancer 2014;50(1): 70–7.

40. Pizzocaro G, Piva L, Di Fronzo G, et al. Adjuvant medroxyprogesterone acetate to radical nephrectomy in renal cancer: 5-year results of a prospective randomized study. J Urol 1987;138(6):1379–81.

41. Karr JP, Pontes JE, Schneider S, et al. Clinical aspects of steroid hormone receptors in human renal cell carcinoma. J Surg Oncol 1983;23(2):117–24.

42. Daste A, Grellety T, Gross-Goupil M, et al. Protein kinase inhibitors in renal cell carcinoma. Expert Opin Pharmacother 2014;15(3):337–51.

43. Haas NB, Manola J, Dutcher JP, et al. Adjuvant Treatment for High-Risk Clear Cell Renal Cancer: Updated Results of a High-Risk Subset of the ASSURE Randomized Trial. JAMA Oncol 2017;3(9): 1249–52.

44. Ravaud A, Motzer RJ, Pandha HS, et al. Adjuvant Sunitinib in High-Risk Renal-Cell Carcinoma after Nephrectomy. N Engl J Med 2016;375(23):2246–54.

45. Food and Drug Administration. FDA approves sunitinib malate for adjuvant treatment of renal cell carcinoma 2018. Available at: https://www.fda.gov/drugs/resources-information-approved-drugs/fda-approves-sunitinib-malate-adjuvant-treatment-renal-cell-carcinoma.

46. Motzer RJ, Ravaud A, Patard JJ, et al. Adjuvant Sunitinib for High-risk Renal Cell Carcinoma After Nephrectomy: Subgroup Analyses and Updated Overall Survival Results. Eur Urol 2018;73(1):62–8.

47. Motzer RJ, Russo P, Haas N, et al. Adjuvant Pazopanib Versus Placebo After Nephrectomy in Patients With Localized or Locally Advanced Renal Cell Carcinoma: Final Overall Survival Analysis of the Phase 3 PROTECT Trial. Eur Urol 2021;79(3):334–8.

48. Gross-Goupil M, Kwon TG, Eto M, et al. Axitinib versus placebo as an adjuvant treatment of renal cell carcinoma: results from the phase III, randomized ATLAS trial. Ann Oncol 2018;29(12):2371–8.

49. Eisen T, Frangou E, Oza B, et al. Adjuvant Sorafenib for Renal Cell Carcinoma at Intermediate or High Risk of Relapse: Results From the SORCE Randomized Phase III Intergroup Trial. J Clin Oncol 2020;38(34): 4064–75.

50. Choueiri TK, Motzer RJ. Systemic Therapy for Metastatic Renal-Cell Carcinoma. N Engl J Med 2017; 376(4):354–66.

51. Choueiri TK, Tomczak P, Park SH, et al. Adjuvant Pembrolizumab after Nephrectomy in Renal-Cell Carcinoma. N Engl J Med 2021;385(8):683–94.

52. Powles T, Tomczak P, Park SH, et al. Pembrolizumab versus placebo as post-nephrectomy adjuvant therapy for clear cell renal cell carcinoma (KEY-NOTE-564): 30-month follow-up analysis of a multicentre, randomised, double-blind, placebo-controlled, phase 3 trial. Lancet Oncol 2022;23(9): 1133–44.

53. Pal SK, Uzzo R, Karam JA, et al. Adjuvant atezolizumab versus placebo for patients with renal cell carcinoma at increased risk of recurrence following resection (IMmotion010): a multicentre, randomised, double-blind, phase 3 trial. Lancet 2022; 400(10358):1103–16.

54. Bedke J, Albiges L, Capitanio U, et al. The 2022 Updated European Association of Urology Guidelines on the Use of Adjuvant Immune Checkpoint Inhibitor Therapy for Renal Cell Carcinoma. Eur Urol 2023; 83(1):10–4.

55. Motzer RJ, McDermott DF, Escudier B, et al. Conditional survival and long-term efficacy with nivolumab plus ipilimumab versus sunitinib in patients with

advanced renal cell carcinoma. Cancer 2022; 128(11):2085–97.

56. Zisman A, Pantuck AJ, Dorey F, et al. Improved prognostication of renal cell carcinoma using an integrated staging system. J Clin Oncol 2001;19(6): 1649–57.

57. Patard JJ, Kim HL, Lam JS, et al. Use of the University of California Los Angeles integrated staging system to predict survival in renal cell carcinoma: an international multicenter study. J Clin Oncol 2004; 22(16):3316–22.

58. Leibovich BC, Blute ML, Cheville JC, et al. Prediction of progression after radical nephrectomy for patients with clear cell renal cell carcinoma: a stratification tool for prospective clinical trials. Cancer 2003; 97(7):1663–71.

59. Frank I, Blute ML, Cheville JC, et al. An outcome prediction model for patients with clear cell renal cell carcinoma treated with radical nephrectomy based on tumor stage, size, grade and necrosis: the SSIGN score. J Urol 2002;168(6):2395–400.

60. Palumbo C, Mazzone E, Mistretta FA, et al. A Plea for Optimizing Selection in Current Adjuvant Immunotherapy Trials for High-risk Nonmetastatic Renal Cell Carcinoma According to Expected Cancer-specific Mortality. Clin Genitourin Cancer 2020;18(4): 314–321 e311.

61. Marconi L, Sun M, Beisland C, et al. Prevalence, Disease-free, and Overall Survival of Contemporary Patients With Renal Cell Carcinoma Eligible for Adjuvant Checkpoint Inhibitor Trials. Clin Genitourin Cancer 2021;19(2):e92–9.

62. Brooks SA, Brannon AR, Parker JS, et al. ClearCode34: A prognostic risk predictor for localized clear cell renal cell carcinoma. Eur Urol 2014; 66(1):77–84.

63. Haake SM, Brooks SA, Welsh E, et al. Patients with ClearCode34-identified molecular subtypes of clear cell renal cell carcinoma represent unique populations with distinct comorbidities. Urol Oncol 2016; 34(3):122 e121–e127.

64. Rini B, Goddard A, Knezevic D, et al. A 16-gene assay to predict recurrence after surgery in localised renal cell carcinoma: development and validation studies. Lancet Oncol 2015;16(6):676–85.

65. Rini BI, Escudier B, Martini JF, et al. Validation of the 16-Gene Recurrence Score in Patients with Locoregional, High-Risk Renal Cell Carcinoma from a Phase III Trial of Adjuvant Sunitinib. Clin Cancer Res 2018;24(18):4407–15.

66. Geertsen L, Koldby KM, Thomassen M, et al. Circulating Tumor DNA in Patients with Renal Cell Carcinoma. A Systematic Review of the Literature. Eur Urol Open Sci 2022;37:27–35.

67. de Velasco G, Carril-Ajuria L, Guerrero-Ramos F, et al. A case series of advanced renal cell carcinoma patients treated with neoadjuvant cabozantinib prior to cytoreductive nephrectomy within the phase 2 CABOPRE trial. Oncotarget 2020;11(47): 4457–62.

68. Zhang Y, Li Y, Deng J, et al. Sorafenib neoadjuvant therapy in the treatment of high risk renal cell carcinoma. PLoS One 2015;10(2):e0115896.

69. Thomas AA, Rini BI, Lane BR, et al. Response of the primary tumor to neoadjuvant sunitinib in patients with advanced renal cell carcinoma. J Urol 2009; 181(2):518–23. ; discussion 523.

70. Bex A, van der Veldt AA, Blank C, et al. Neoadjuvant sunitinib for surgically complex advanced renal cell cancer of doubtful resectability: initial experience with downsizing to reconsider cytoreductive surgery. World J Urol 2009;27(4):533–9.

71. Silberstein JL, Millard F, Mehrazin R, et al. Feasibility and efficacy of neoadjuvant sunitinib before nephron-sparing surgery. BJU Int 2010;106(9): 1270–6.

72. Kroon BK, de Bruijn R, Prevoo W, et al. Probability of downsizing primary tumors of renal cell carcinoma by targeted therapies is related to size at presentation. Urology 2013;81(1):111–5.

73. Lane BR, Derweesh IH, Kim HL, et al. Presurgical sunitinib reduces tumor size and may facilitate partial nephrectomy in patients with renal cell carcinoma. Urol Oncol 2015;33(3):112 e115–e121.

74. Kutikov A, Uzzo RG, The RENAL. Nephrometry score: a comprehensive standardized system for quantitating renal tumor size, location and depth. J Urol 2009;182(3):844–53.

75. Ryan CW, Tangen C, Heath EI, et al. EVEREST: Everolimus for renal cancer ensuing surgical therapy—A phase III study (SWOG S0931, NCT01120249). J Clin Oncol 2022;40(17_suppl):LBA4500.

The Great Masquerader's New Wardrobe in the Modern Era
The Paraneoplastic Manifestations of Renal Cancer

Kevin R. Loughlin, MD, MBA

KEYWORDS

- Renal cancer • Great masquerader symptoms • Paraneoplastic manifestations

KEY POINTS

- The classic triad of palpable mass, hematuria, and flank pain occurs in less than 15% of patients with renal cell carcinoma.
- The paraneoplastic manifestations of renal cancer may occur in 10% to 40% of patients.
- The common paraneoplastic manifestations include fever, anemia, polycythemia, hepatic dysfunction, hypercalcemia, and hypertension.
- Less common paraneoplastic manifestations include neuromyopathies, endocrinopathies, and cutaneous abnormalities.
- In the absence of metastatic disease, some of these paraneoplastic abnormalities resolve with resection of the primary tumor and in that circumstance can be used as biomarkers to follow the disease.

INTRODUCTION

It is estimated that in 2022, approximately 79,000 new cases of kidney cancer will be diagnosed, 50,290 in men and 28,710 in women, and about 13,920 people, 8960 men and 4960 women, will die from this disease.[1] Risk factors for developing cancer of the kidney include smoking, obesity, hypertension, family history, workplace exposures, gender, race (more common in African-Americans) and certain medications such as acetaminophens.[1]

Paraneoplastic syndromes (PNS) can occur in 8% to 20% of individuals with malignancies.[2] They can occur in a variety of cancers that include breast, gastric, leukemia, lung, ovarian, pancreatic, prostate, testicular, as well as kidney.[2] The classic presentation of the triad of mass, hematuria, and flank pain occurs in less than 15% of patients with renal cancer.[3] However, 10% to 40% of individuals with kidney cancer will develop paraneoplastic syndrome of some type.

Because of the protean presentations of renal cell cancer, it has been referred to as the internist's tumor or the great masquerader.[4] In the modern era, there has been an increased understanding of some of the underlying mechanisms that mediate the paraneoplastic presentations of renal cancers. This article will provide a review of the causes of these symptoms.

CONSTITUTIONAL AND HEMATOLOGIC PRESENTATIONS

In as many as one-third of cases, the symptoms of fever, weight loss, and fatigue are the first symptoms of renal cancer.[5] Fever is detected in 20% to 30% of patients with renal cell carcinoma (RCC) and is the

Karp Family Research Laboratories, Boston Children's Hospital, Longwood Avenue, Boston, MA 02115, USA
E-mail address: KLOUGHLIN@PARTNERS.ORG

Urol Clin N Am 50 (2023) 305–310
https://doi.org/10.1016/j.ucl.2023.01.005

only presenting complaint in about 2% of patients.[6] Other constitutional symptoms can include malaise, anorexia, night sweats, and chills.[7] It has been suggested by some investigators that constitutional symptoms do not auger well for a good prognosis.[7] However, other studies have not confirmed this.[3]

In the modern era, there has been increasing evidence that at least some of the paraneoplastic manifestations of RCC are mediated by cytokines. Some patients with RCC have been found to have elevated serum levels of tumor necrosis factor-alpha, a cytokine known to alter adipocyte metabolism and affect appetite control.[3] In addition, interleukin-6 (IL-6) has been identified as a possible pyrogen in RCC. In one report, 18 of 71 patients with RCC were found to have increased levels of IL-6 and 78% of those with elevated IL-6 had fever.[8] There has also been evidence that IL-1 and some interferons and prostaglandins may also mediate some of the constitutional symptoms associated with RCC. It should also be recognized that fevers in some apparently organ-confined renal cancers may subside after radical nephrectomy, and a return of the fever may be a harbinger of disease recurrence.[9]

A variety of hematological findings has also been identified as presenting signs of RCC. These may include anemia, polycythemia, dysfibrinogenemia, thrombocytosis, and leukocytosis. An association of anemia and renal carcinoma has been reported ranging from 20% to 52% of patients.[7,10,11]

The anemia of renal cancer that is out of proportion to the amount of gross hematuria observed has been thought to be associated, in most cases, to low serum iron.[12,13] Loughlin and colleagues[12] reported the utility of serum iron as a tumor marker following nephrectomy, and this was confirmed by Yu and colleagues.[13] Further investigation by Loughlin and colleagues[14] identified lactoferrin as the mediator of the low serum iron and anemia in selected cases. Lactoferrin is a glycoprotein contained in neutrophils, which binds free iron and shunts the iron-laden lactoferrin into the reticuloendothelial system. The normal physiologic role of lactoferrin seems to be antibacterial.[15]

Unlike the low serum iron observed in some patients with RCC, the elevation of serum ferritin has been observed in some patients with renal cancer. This observation was made by Essen and colleagues[16] and confirmed by Partin and colleagues.[17] The study by Partin and colleagues[17] reported that ferritin levels were not correlated with increasing stage but did correlate with tumor volume. Additional studies have confirmed this association between ferritin and some renal cancers.[18,19]

Erythrocytosis has been reported in 1% to 8% of renal carcinoma patients.[20,21] Sufrin and colleagues measured increased levels of erythropoietin in 63% of their 57 patients with renal carcinoma.[22] However, Gross and colleagues reported doubts about the clinical utility of serum erythropoietin in patients with RCC and did not identify immunoreactive erythropoietin in monolayer cultures of 14 RCC cell lines.[23]

Abnormalities of platelet and while blood cell counts have also been observed as part of the PNS associated with RCC. Men and colleagues[24] published a metanalysis of 8735 patients with renal cancer and identified thrombocytosis in 1059 patients (12.1%). Those patients who exhibited thrombocytosis had a 1.61-fold higher risk of death at 5 years compared with those patients with normal platelet counts. The cancer-specific mortality at 5 years was 2.56-fold higher compared with normal controls.

Mandel and colleagues[25] reported a patient with RCC who exhibited leukocytosis. This paraneoplastic syndrome has been seen with other malignancies and is thought to be due to increased production of granulocyte-stimulating factor, granulocyte-macrophage colony-stimulating factor, IL-6, and other cytokines produced by the tumor cells.

Dawson and colleagues[26] published a case report of a patient with RCC who exhibited dysfibrinogenemia characterized by prolongation of the thrombin and reptilase times and increased sialic acid context of the purified fibrinogen. The thrombin and reptilase times returned toward normal values after nephrectomy but became abnormal with the development of nonhepatic metastases. They concluded that the acquired dysfibrinogenemia can be part of a paraneoplastic syndrome and is a sensitive plasma marker for tumor progression.

STAUFFER SYNDROME

Stauffer syndrome, a paraneoplastic disorder associated with RCC, is characterized by hepatic dysfunction in the absence of metastases and elevated alkaline phosphatase, amino transferases, and prolonged prothrombin time. It was first described by Herbert Maurice Stauffer in 1961.[27] It has been further characterized by a reversible anicteric elevation of liver enzymes, erythrocyte sedimentation rate, thrombocytosis, prolongation of prothrombin time and hepatosplenomegaly by the absence of direct hepatobiliary obstruction.[28] Recent reports have also described cholestatic jaundice as a paraneoplastic manifestation of renal cell carcinoma.[28,29] The size of the primary lesion does not seem to be predictive of the clinical manifestations,[30] and the typical paraneoplastic hepatology consists of unexplained elevation in liver enzymes without evidence of anatomic obstruction, infection, or neoplastic involvement of the liver or bile ducts.[28]

Although Stauffer syndrome is most commonly associated with RCC, it has also been associated with prostate cancer, soft tissue sarcomas,[31] pancreatic cancer, bladder cancer,[32] malignant lymphoproliferative diseases,[33] bronchogenic carcinoma,[34] gastrointestinal carcinoma,[35] and thrombocytopenia variant.[36]

In the absence of metastatic disease, a curative radical nephrectomy seems to achieve resolution of the symptoms.[30] IL-6 has been considered to mediate the major manifestations of the syndrome.[30]

ROLE OF INTERLEUKIN 6 AND CYTOKINES

Tsukamoto and colleagues studied the relationship between IL-6 and RCC. They identified IL-6 production in 3 of 4 renal cancer cell lines and in 25% of the 71 patients that they assayed, although the IL-6 level did not directly correlate with the tumor volume or grade of the carcinoma.[36] When the IL-6 was elevated, the patients had a significantly higher frequency of unexplained fever.

Blay and colleagues investigated this association further in a series of 119 patients with metastases.[37] Those patients with detectable serum IL-6 (n = 90, 76%) had significantly higher serum C-reactive protein (CRP), haptoglobin, serum alkaline phosphatase, and gamma glutamyl transferase levels. In addition, platelets, polymorphonuclear neutrophil, and monotype counts were also significantly higher in patients with detectable serum IL-6 and hemoglobin levels were lower.

Interestingly, in 3 patients who were entered into an anti-IL-6 treatment protocol, it was observed that reductions were observed in CRP, haptoglobin, and serum alkaline phosphatase during the anti-IL-6 administration. These studies demonstrate the role of IL-6 in several of the paraneoplastic manifestations of RCC.

HYPERCALCEMIA

Hypercalcemia has been reported in up to 30% of patients who have a malignancy.[38] Hypercalcemia of malignancy is classified into 4 types: malignant humoral hypercalcemia (80%), local osteolytic hypercalcemia (20%), secretion of 1,25-dihydroxy vitamin D (<0.1%), and ectopic hyperparathyroidism (<0.1%)[39,40]

Albright was the first to describe the association of hypercalcemia with RCC in 1941.[41] Hypercalcemia is one of the most common PNS associated with renal cancer, affecting 13% to 20% of patients.[42–44] Of the patients with RCC who have

hypercalcemia, about 75% will have higher stage lesions but neither the presence nor the degree of hypercalcemia is correlated with grade or survival.[45,46] Approximately 50% of all patients with hypercalcemia and RCC have bone metastases.[47] Osseous metastatic RCC lesions seem to elaborate substances that activate osteoclasts, which release calcium from bone.[3]

Humoral factors associated with increased remodeling and resultant hypercalcemia include IL-1, IL-3, IL-6, tumor necrosis factor alpha, transforming growth factor alpha and beta, lymphotoxins, and E series prostaglandins.[48–50]

However, nonmetastatic hypercalcemia in patients with RCC can occur and seems to be mediated by the elaboration of hormonal peptides by renal tumor cells. It has been demonstrated that some renal cancer cells can produce parathormone or parathyroid hormone-related peptide.[3]

NEUROLOGICAL MANIFESTATIONS

A variety of neurological symptoms can present as part of PNS associated with RCC. These include limbic encephalitis,[51–54] opsoclonus myoclonus,[55–57] myasthenia gravis,[58] amyotrophic lateral sclerosis,[59] and bilateral diaphragmatic paralysis.[60] The presentation and management of the neurological PNS are largely limited to case reports and must be managed on a case-by-case basis, although there have been reports of regression of the neurological symptoms after treating the primary lesion.[55,61]

CUTANEOUS MANIFESTATIONS

Cutaneous manifestations of the constellation of PNS associated with RCC are rare, but do occur. Corven and colleagues reported a case of an elderly man who presented with a blister, which revealed a subepidermal bulla with neutrophils. Further investigation revealed a vasculitis with fibrinoid necrosis. Radiologic examination revealed a 6 × 7-cm tumor of the right kidney and the patient underwent a right radical nephrectomy. After 12 months of reported follow-up, there was no evidence of recurrent bullous dermatosis.[62]

Acanthosis nigricans (AN) is characterized by eruption of multiple, symmetric, velvety hyperkeratotic lesions with brownish hyperpigmentation. The occurrence of AN in adults is usually associated with cancers[63] and often is an indicator of a bad prognosis.[64]

GLUCOSE MANIFESTATIONS

Abnormalities of glucose metabolism can also be part of the paraneoplastic manifestation of renal cancer. Palgon and colleagues reported a patient who had complete resolution of hyperglycemia after surgical removal of clear cell type of renal cell carcinoma.[54] A similar case was presented by Jobe and colleagues.[65] The mechanism of the hyperglycemia was unknown in both cases.

In contrast, hypoglycemia has also been reported in association with RCC.[66] It has been proposed that this may be due to tumor production of the proprotein of insulin-like growth factor-II, which mimics the effects of insulin due to its structure.[67,68]

MISCELLANEOUS MANIFESTATIONS

Renal cell carcinoma is indeed the great masquerader because it can have protean presentations where the underlying cause may be subtle. Myositis,[69,70] thyroiditis,[71] hypertension,[72] Cushing syndrome,[73] and amyloid[74] have all been associated with renal cancer. Often, the key to making the underlying diagnosis of RCC is having an index of suspicion that the presenting symptoms bear further investigation.

PARANEOPLASTIC SYNDROMES AS BIOMARKERS

Throughout the literature, there have been repeated observations of the utility of paraneoplastic manifestations as biomarkers. When the disease is organ-confined to the kidney, the symptoms typically resolve after treatment of the primary lesion, when disease recurs, the symptoms typically reappear. These observations can be very useful when following this subset of patients with RCC.

SUMMARY

Renal cell carcinoma can present in a variety of ways. The astute clinician will be familiar with the many manifestations of the great masquerader and consider the diagnosis as part of the differential when the clinical presentation is elusive.

CLINICS CARE POINTS

- Renal cellcarcinoma should always be part of the differential in patients with fever of unknown origin.
- Renal cell carcinoma should be considered in unexplained anemia in the abscence of hematuria.
- In some cases, the paraneoplastic manifestations of renal cancer cah serve as tumor markers.

REFERENCES

1. American Cancer Society. Available at: Cancer.org/cancer/kidney-cancer/about/key-statistics.html#. Accessed September 12, 2022.
2. Paraneoplastic Syndromes, Available at: my.clevelandclinic.org/health/diseases/17938-paraneoplastic-syndrome. Accessed September 12, 2022.
3. Palapattu GS, Kristo B, Rajfer J. Paraneoplastic syndrome in urologic malignancy: the many faces of renal cell carcinoma. Rev Urol 2002;4(4):163–70.
4. McCullough DL, Harris RD. Renal cell carcinoma (hypernephroma): the great masquerader. J Med Assoc State Ala 1976;45(12):33–7.
5. McDougal WS, Garrick MB, et al. Clinical signs and symptoms of renal carcinoma. In: Vogelzang NJ, Shipley WU, Scardino PT, et al, editors. Comprehensive textbook of genitourinary oncology. Baltimore (MA): Williams and Wilkins; 1995. p. 154–9.
6. Lasla ME, Vugin D. Paraneoplastic syndromes in hypernephroma. Semin Nephrol 1987;7:12–30.
7. Kim HL, Belldegrun AS, Freitas DG, et al. Paraneoplastic signs and symptoms of renal cell carcinoma-implications for prognosis. J Urol 2003;170:1742–6.
8. Tsukamoto T, Kumamoto Y, Miyao, et al. Interleukin-6 in renal cell carcinoma. J Urol 1992;148:1778–82.
9. Barrington JL, Kradjian RM. Renal carcinoma. Philadelphia: Saunders; 1967. Presenting signs and symptoms.
10. Gold PJ, Fefer A, Thompson JA. Paraneoplastic manifestations of renal cell carcinoma. Semin Urol 1996;14(4):216–22.
11. Marshall FF, Walsh PC. Extrarenal manifestations of renal cell carcinoma. J Urol 1977;117:439–40.
12. Loughlin KR, Gittes RF. Serum iron: a tumor marker in renal carcinoma. Br J Urol 1986;58(6):617–20.
13. Yu CC, Chan KK, Chen MT. Serum iron as tumor marker in renal cell carcinoma. Eur Urol 1991;19(1):54–8.
14. Loughlin KR, Gittes RF, Partridge D, et al. The relationship of lactoferrin to the anemia of renal cell carcinoma. Cancer 1987;59:566–71.
15. Klugar M, Rotheberg B. Fever and reduced iron. Their interaction as a host defense response to bacterial infection. Science 1979;203:374–6.
16. Essen A, Ozein H, Ayhan A, et al. Serum ferritin: a tumor marker for renal cell carcinoma. J Urol 1991;45(6):1134–7.
17. Partin A.W., Criley S.R., Steiner M.S., et al., Serum ferritin as a clinical marker for renal cell carcinoma : influence of tumor volume, Urology, 45 (2), 1995, 211–217.
18. Kirkali Z, Guzelsay M, Mungan M, et al. Serum ferritin as a clinical marker for renal cell carcinoma: influence of tumor size and volume. Urol Int 1999;62:21–5.
19. Ozen H, Uygur C, Sahin A, et al. Clinical significance of serum ferritin in patients with renal cell carcinoma. Urology 1995;46(4):494–8.

20. Karzal LA, Erslev AJ. Erythropoietin production in renal tumors. Ann Clin Lab Sci 1975;5:98–109.

21. Ljungberg B, Rasmuson T, Grankuist K. Erythropoietin in renal cell carcinoma : elevation of its usefulness as a tumor marker. Eur Urol 1992;21:160–3.

22. Sufrin G, Mirand EA, Moore RH, et al. Hormones in renal cancer. J Urol 1977;117:433–8.

23. Gross AJ, Wolff M, Fandrey WD. Prevalence of paraneoplastic erythropoietin production by renal cell carcinoma. Clin Investig 1994;72:337–40.

24. Men H, Liang C, Yu M. Thrombocytosis as a prognostic factor in patients with renal cell carcinoma: a meta-analysis of literature. J Cancer Res 2015; 11(1):67–72.

25. Mandal SK, Ganguly J, Silk, et al. Renal cell carcinoma with paraneoplastic leucocytosis. J. Cancer Res Ther 2015;11(3):660.

26. Dawson NA, Barr CF, Alving BM. Acquired dysfibrinogenemia: paraneoplastic syndrome in renal cell carcinoma. Am J Med 1985;78(4):682–6.

27. Stauffer HM. Nephrogenic hepatosplenomegaly. Gastroenterology 1961;40:694–6.

28. Sharma N, Darr U, Darr A, et al. Stauffer syndrome: a comprehensive review of the icteric variant of the syndrome. Cureus 2019;11(10):e6032. Available at: ncbi.nlh.gov/pmc/articles/PMC6886655. Accessed September 13, 2022.

29. Dourakis SP, Sinani C, Deutsch M, et al. Cholestatic jaundice as a paraneoplastic manifestation of renal cell carcinoma. Eur J Gastroenterol Hepatol 1997; 9(3):311–4.

30. Chavarriago J, Fakih N, Cantano J, et al. Stauffer syndrome, clinical implications and knowledge gaps, does size matter? Case report. BMC Urol 2020;20:105–9.

31. Fontes-Sausa M, Magalhaes H, da Silva F, et al. Stauffer's syndrome: a comprehensive review and proposed updated diagnostic criteria. Urol Oncol 2018;36:321–6.

32. Harris D, Saif M. Stauffer's syndrome in pancrear﹨tic cancer: first case report. Cureus 2017;9:5–6.

33. Karakolio A, Kasapisa C, Kallinekidisa, et al. Cholestatic jaundice as a paraneoplastic manifestations of prostate adenocarcinoma. Cline Gastroenterol Hepatol 2003;6:480–3.

34. Marla D, Alazemi S, Lichstein D. Stauffer's syndrome variant with cholestatic jaundice : a case report. J Gen Intern Med 2006;21:11–3.

35. Mehta D, Chugh P, Chawla L, et al. Paraneoplastic hepatology associated with gastrointestinal carcinoma. ACG Case Rep J 2017;4:117–8.

36. Tsukamato T, Kumamoto Y, Miyan N, et al. Interleukin-6 in renal cell carcinoma. J Urol 1992;148:1178–781.

37. Blay JY, Rossi JF, Wijdenes J, et al. Role of interleukin-6 in the paraneoplastic inflammatory syndrome associated with renal cell carcinoma. Int J Cancer 1997;75:424–30.

38. Goldrier W. Cancer-related hypercalcemia. J Oncol Pract 2016;12(5):426–32.

39. Gomes L, Kulak C, Costa T, et al. Association of primary hyperthyroidism and humoral hypercalcemia of malignancy in a patient with clear cell renal carcinoma. Arch Endocrinol Metab 2015;59(1):84–8.

40. Stewart AF. Hypercalcemia associated with cancer. N Engl J Med 2005;352:372–9.

41. Albright F. Case records of the Massachusetts General Hospital -Case 39061. N Engl J Med 1941;225: 789–96.

42. Muggia FM. Overview of cancer-related hypercalcemia: epidemiology and etiology. Semin Oncol 1990; 17:3–9.

43. Warren WD, Utz DC, Kelalis PP. Concurrence of hypernephroma and hypercalcemia. Ann Surg 1971; 174:863–5.

44. Murdy GR, Ibbotson KJ, D'Suza SM, et al. The hypercalcemia of cancer. N Engl J Med 1984;310:1718–27.

45. Buckner RM, McMillian M, Mallinson C. Ectopic secretion of parathyroid hormone by a renal adenocarcinoma in a patirnt with hypercalcemia. Br Med J 1970;4:724–6.

46. Plimpton CH, Gellhorn A. Hypercalcemia in malignant disease without evidence of bone destruction. Am J Med 1956;21:750–9.

47. Chason SA, Pothel RL, Huben RP. Management and prognostic significant of hypercalcemia in renal cell carcinoma. Urology 1989;33:167–71.

48. Mirralehimou AE. Hypercalcemia of malignancy. An update on pathogens and management N. Am J Med Sci 2015;7:483–93.

49. Climes GA, Guise TA. Hypercalcemia of malignancy and basic research on mechanisms responsible for osteolytic and osteoblastic metastasis to bone. Endocr Relat Cancer 2005;12:549–85.

50. Seyberth HW, Segre GV, Morgan JL, et al. Prostaglandins as mediators of hypercalcemia associated with certain types of cancer. N Engl J Med 1975;293: 1278–83.

51. Newman NJ, Bell IR, McKee AC. Paraneoplastic limbic encephalitis: neuropsychiatric presentation bio. Psychology 1990;27:529–42.

52. Bell B, Tognomi PG, Bihrle R. Limbic encephalitis as a paraneoplastic manifestation of renal cell carcinoma. J Urol 1998;160:828.

53. Kararizou E, Markov I, Zalonis I, et al. Paraneoplastic limbic encephalitis presenting as acute viral encephalitis. J Neurooncol 2005;75:229–32.

54. Palgon N, Greenstein F, Noretsky AD, et al. Hyperglycemia associated with renal cell carcinoma. Urology 1986;28:516–7.

55. Vigliani MC, Palmucci L, Polo P, et al. Paraneoplastic opsoclonus-myoclones associated with renal cell carcinoma and responsive to tumor ablation carcinoma and responsive to tumor ablation. J Neurol Neurosurg Psychiatry 2001;70:814–5.

56. Koukoulis A, Cimas I, Gomaras S. Paraneoplastic opsoclonus associated with papillary renal cell carcinoma. J Neurol Neurosurg Psychiatry 1998;64(1): 137–8.

57. DeLuca S, Terrane C, Crivellaro S, et al. Opsoclonous-mypclonus syndrome as a paraneoplastic manifestation of renal cell carcinoma. Urol Int 2002;68:206208.

58. Torgerson EL, Khalil R, Dobkin BH, et al. Myasthemia gravis as a paraneoplastic syndrome associated with renal cell carcinoma. J Urol 1999;162:154.

59. Evans BK, Fagan C, Arnold, et al. Paraneoplastic moter neuron disease and renal cell carcinoma. Neurologgy 1990;40:960–2.

60. Thomas NE, Passamonte PM, Sunder Rajan EV, et al. Bilateral diaphragmatic paralysis as a possible paraneoplastic syndrome from renal cell carcinoma. Am Rev Respir Dis 1984;129(3):507–9.

61. Zhu L, Deng X, Tan W. Paraneoplastic limbic encephalitis cured with nephron-sparing surgery in a patient with clear cell carcinoma: a case report. J Int Med Res 2019;47(10):5318–22.

62. Corven CB, Khala FA, Courville P, et al. Renal chromophobe cell carcinoma and paraneoplastic IgA bullous dermatosis. J Urol 2003;169:270.

63. Sacco E, Pinto F, Sasso F, et al. Paraneoplastic syndromes in patients with urological malignancies. Urol Int 2009;83:1–11.

64. Moscardi L|JL, Macedo NA, Espasandin JA, et al. Malignant acanthosis migraines associated with a renal tumor. Int J Dermatol 1993;32:893–4.

65. Jobe BA, Bierman MH, Mezzacappa FJ, et al. Hyperglycemia as a paraneoplastic endocrinopathy in renal cell carcinoma. Nebr Med J 1993;349–51.

66. Dilenno N, Han E, Maritland C, et al. Hypoglycemia in renal cell carcinoma: a rare paraneoplastic syndrome. Urology 2019;124:10–3.

67. Philips LS, Roberston DG. Insulin-like growth factors and non-islet cell tumor hypoglycemia. Metabolism 1993;42:1093–101.

68. Maki RG. Small is beautiful: Insulin-like growth factors and their role in growth development and cancer. J Clin Oncol 2010;28:4985–95.

69. Wurzer H, Brandstatter G, Harnoncourt K, et al. Paraneoplastic polymyositis associated with a renal carcinoma. J Intern Med 1993;234:521–4.

70. Solon AA, Gilbert CS, Meyer C. Myopath as a paraneoplastic manifestation of renal cell carcinoma. Am J Med 1994;97:491–2.

71. Algune E, Alici S, Topal C, et al. Coexistence of subacute thyroiditis and renal cell carcinoma: a paraneoplastic syndrome. CMAJ 2003;168(8):985–6.

72. Ram MD, Chisolm GD. Hypertension due to hypernephroma. Br Med J 1969;4:87–9.

73. Riggs BL, Sprange RG. Association of Cushing's syndrome and neoplastic disease. Arch Intern Med 1961;108:841–9.

74. Fischer K, Thail G, Hoda R, et al. Serum amyloid: a biomarker for renal cancer. Anticancer Res 2012; 32:1801–4.

Integrating Surgery in the Multidisciplinary Care of Advanced Renal Cell Carcinoma

Shagnik Ray, MD, Shawn Dason, MD, Eric A. Singer, MD, MA, MS*

KEYWORDS

- Renal cell carcinoma • Neoadjuvant • Adjuvant • Lymphadenectomy • Cytoreductive nephrectomy
- Metastasectomy

KEY POINTS

- Distant metastatic disease will be present in 20% to 30% of patients with renal cell carcinoma (RCC) at diagnosis. Metachronous metastatic disease will develop in 20% to 40% of patients with presumed localized RCC who undergo surgical resection.
- No prospective trial has shown a survival benefit to regional lymphadenectomy in patients with locally advanced RCC. Nonetheless, some retrospective studies have shown an overall survival benefit as well as the possible utility of optimally staging select patients given mounting evidence that patients with stage 3 disease with lymph node involvement may have disease characteristics more akin to stage 4 disease.
- The role and timing of cytoreductive nephrectomy (CN) in the modern era of systemic therapy remains unclear. Multiple randomized controlled trials are underway to define the role of CN in the context of contemporary systemic therapy.
- Metastasectomy may be considered in properly selected patients after careful consideration of the site-specific complication profile, and additional prospective trials are needed to clarify exactly which patients will benefit from metastasectomy in the modern systemic therapy era.

INTRODUCTION

Approximately 79,000 cases of renal cell carcinoma (RCC) will be diagnosed in the United States in 2022, with 13,920 deaths attributed to RCC.[1] Localized RCC has numerous management options but is definitively managed with surgical extirpation or ablation, with ~50% and ~11% of these patients presenting with cT1 or cT2 disease, respectively, with excellent overall survival (OS) and disease-free survival (DFS) in these patients after definitive surgical management.[2] Unfortunately, 20% to 40% of all patients with RCC who undergo surgical resection will develop metachronous metastatic disease.[3] Furthermore, 20% to 30% of patients who are diagnosed with RCC are found to have synchronous distant metastatic disease.[4] Thus,

there remains significant scope for improvement with regards to preventing progression to metastatic disease after surgical management in high-risk patients as well as in managing both synchronous and metachronous metastatic disease.

Therapeutic advances in advanced RCC during the past 2 decades have leveraged our molecular insight into the carcinogenesis of clear cell RCC. Our understanding of clear cell RCC is centered on the Von Hippel Lindau (VHL) pathway, which is altered in 91% of patients with clear cell RCC.[5] VHL is a tumor suppressor gene, which functions as a component of a larger complex that is responsible for targeting hypoxia inducible factor (HIF)-1 alpha to mark it for proteosomal degradation.[6] With VHL loss, constitutional activation of HIF-1 alpha results in the transcription of downstream

Division of Urologic Oncology, The Ohio State University Comprehensive Cancer Center, 915 Olentangy River Road, 3rd Floor, Urology Suite 3100, Columbus, OH 43212, USA
* Corresponding author.
E-mail address: singere@georgetown.edu

Urol Clin N Am 50 (2023) 311–323
https://doi.org/10.1016/j.ucl.2023.01.013
0094-0143/23/© 2023 Elsevier Inc. All rights reserved.

targets (including vascular endothelial growth factor (VEGF), glucose transporter 1 (GLUT-1), platelet derived growth factor (PDGF)) that propagate growth, angiogenesis, and avoidance of cell death.[5] Understanding this pathway was instrumental in the transition from the cytokine era of systemic therapies (interferon alfa, interleukin 2) to the targeted VEGF tyrosine kinase inhibitor (TKI) era of advanced RCC management in the mid-2000s. In 2005, the United States Food and Drug Administration approved sorafenib as the first anti-VEGF TKI, with subsequent multiple anti-VEGF TKIs and mammalian target of rapamycin (mTOR) pathway inhibitors being approved in the years to come.[7,8] Newer generations of TKIs have focused on increasing tolerability (axitinib, pazopanib) and overall targeting efficacy (cabozantinib, lenvatinib). A subsequent leap forward was made with the development of immune checkpoint inhibitors (ICIs), which interface with targets such as PD-1, its ligand PD-L1, and CTLA-4. These antigens are central to tumor-related immune evasion, which can be countered with ICIs. The FDA first approved nivolumab, a monoclonal antibody that blocks the PD-1 receptor, in the second-line setting in 2015.[9(p5)] ICI (a subset of the broader immuno-oncology [IO] therapies) and TKI therapy have subsequently been used synergistically.[10] By 2022, combination therapy has become standard with survival benefits seen for a number of IO/IO or IO/TKI combinations over sunitinib monotherapy, with preferred regimens for clear cell RCC including ipilimumab/nivolumab, axitinib/pembrolizumab, lenvantinib/pembrolizumab, and cabozantinib/nivolumab.[11]

Although significant advances have been made with systemic therapies for RCC, in all facets of RCC-related care for localized, locally advanced, and metastatic disease, surgery likely has some role in well-selected patients. Notably, the complete response (CR) rate for targeted therapy remains low for cytokine, VEGF, and ICI-related therapies.[12–16] In the metastatic setting, cytoreductive nephrectomy (CN) refers to the surgical extirpation of the primary renal tumor, whereas metastasectomy refers to the resection of distant metastatic sites, with both interlinked interventions likely having some role in select patients. We present the findings of a narrative review on how surgery can be integrated into our contemporary treatment paradigm of advanced RCC.

RETROPERITONEAL LYMPHADENECTOMY FOR NODE-POSITIVE DISEASE

For multiple other urological malignancies, lymph node dissection (LND) has shown utility from both a disease staging and therapeutic standpoint. However, the role of LND for RCC at the time of radical nephrectom (RN) or partial nephrectomy (PN) is less clear despite the presence of lymph node metastases in both locally advanced and metastatic disease being associated with a poorer prognosis.[17–20] Notably, Capitanio and colleagues[19] found in a retrospective multi-institution review that of patients with cT1, cT2, and cT3 disease, 1.1%, 4.5%, and 12.3% of patients had pathological nodal metastases, respectively. The accuracy of clinical lymph node staging has been assessed in numerous studies across varying modalities.[21] Computed tomography (CT) remains the most commonly used imaging modalities for the clinical staging of RCC, demonstrating sensitivity ranging from 60% to 100% and specificity ranging from 75% to 82% across various studies.[22–28] In a retrospective analysis of the National Cancer Database (NCDB), Radadia and colleagues[29] found that the sensitivity and specificity to detect pathological lymph node (LN) involvement of preoperative clinical LN staging clinical were 95% and 67%, respectively, with associated positive predictive value of 74% and negative predictive value of 94%. Despite this, the AUA guidelines recommend on the basis of expert opinion surgical resection of clinically positive LNs. Capitanio and colleagues[30] performed a systematic review noting that cT3-T4 disease, high-grade tumor, Sarcomatoid features, and tumor necrosis were associated with an increased incidence of nodal disease, with patients with 2 or more of these factors having a greater than 40% increased risk of this. Such factors together along with radiographic evidence of nodal metastases will likely play a role in determining which patients would possibly benefit from LND but at present, there exists no such framework. Furthermore, the optimal template of nodal dissection remains unclear, in part due the unpredictable lymphatic drainage of the kidneys, where despite knowledge that the right kidney drains to the paracaval, precaval, retrocaval, and interaortocaval nodes, and the left kidney drains into the para-aortic, preaortic, and retroaortic nodes, there exists connections between the different elements of the retroperitoneal lymphatic system as well as posterior efferent lymphatic vessels that can drain into the thoracic duct and contribute to distant metastases without evidence of regional nodal disease.[31–33]

EORTC 30881, the only phase 3 prospective randomized trial assessing the impact of LND during nephrectomy for RCC, did not demonstrate any differences in terms of progression-free and OS between the LND with nephrectomy versus nephrectomy alone group. Notably, the patients in this trial represented a lower risk group of patients undergoing nephrectomy for RCC with resectable masses at clinical stage N0M0.[34] There have been multiple retrospective trials assessing the impact of LND as well as nodal yield on higher risk cohorts with suggestion of survival benefit.[35–37] However, a study using the NCDB by Faber and colleagues[38] found no difference in OS for those undergoing LND at the time of nephrectomy for RCC, and found that of those undergoing LND, 5% and 23% occurred with cT1 and cT2, respectively, suggesting that LND may be being overutilized in a subset of lower risk patients. Supplementing this, Gershman and colleagues[39] performed a retrospective cohort analysis of 1797 patients treated for M0 RCC from 1990 to 2010, with 606 (34%) of patients having undergone LND, and did not identify any oncologic benefit to LND in the overall cohort or among those at an increased risk of nodal disease (including those with preoperative radiographic lymphadenopathy). The same group retrospectively assessed the utility of LND in patients undergoing CN for metastatic RCC and similarly did not identify an oncologic benefit overall or even among higher risk subgroups (including those with preoperative lymphadenopathy).[40] Ultimately, prospective data analyzing the impact of LND on a higher risk cohort is necessary to determine whether LND will have any OS benefit for such patients in the future. Furthermore, recent data has called into the question of grouping patients with nodal metastases into the stage 3 RCC category. Yu and colleagues,[18] retrospectively, reviewed patients with $pT_{1-3} N_1 M_0$ disease, $pT_3 N_0 M_0$ disease, and $pT_{1-3} N_{0/x} M_1$, and found that those with $pT_{1-3} N_1 M_0$ disease had significantly worse OS than those with $pT_3 N_0 M_0$ disease, and that overall and cancer-specific survival (CSS) were similar for those with $pT_{123} N_1 M0$ disease and those with $pT_{1-3} N_{0/x} M_1$ disease (stage IV). These findings were further supported by a review of the NCDB by Srivastava and colleagues,[41] where patients with lymph node-negative stage III disease had improved OS (61.9% 5-year survival) compared with those with lymph node-positive stage III disease (22.7% 5-year survival), that those patients with stage III nodal disease had similar OS to those with stage IV RCC (15.6% 5-year survival), with 5-year OS rates of 61.9% (95% confidence interval [95% CI], 60.3%–63.4%), 22.7% (95% CI, 20.6%–24.9%), and 15.6% (95% CI, 11.1%–23.8%), respectively. This difference in natural history of disease with nodal involvement may lend evidence suggesting possible utility in LND for staging purposes and for the selection patients for adjuvant systemic therapy given their high risk for recurrence.

CYTOREDUCTIVE NEPHRECTOMY

CN for the removal of the primary renal tumor in the setting of metastatic RCC has had an evolving role over time as progresses have been made in systemic therapy. Cytoreductive surgery is used in metastatic RCC as well as a variety of other malignancies such as ovarian and breast cancer with the goal of debulking and ideally removing a primary lesion with the goal of addressing local symptoms, treating paraneoplastic syndromes, and improving progression-free survival (PFS) and OS by possibly enhancing the response to a patient's own immune system as well as systemic therapies.[42–45] Notably, there are rare case reports of complete regression of metastatic RCC after CN, suggesting that the primary tumor may have a key role in the interactions between one's immune system and metastatic disease.[46,47] The benefits of CN must be taken in the context of the notable risks of CN.[48] A review of the Registry for Metastatic RCC found a 10.9% intraoperative complication rate with 29.5% of patients experiencing any grade complication with 6.1% of patients experiencing high-grade complications.[49] Importantly, CN caseload correlated with lower high-grade morbidity, possibly suggesting that if CN is to be pursued, it should be done at a center that performs this complex procedure at a high volume.

Two landmark studies gave evidence in favor of CN in select patients with metastatic RCC during the earlier cytokine era. The SWOG-8949 RCT assessed patients with metastatic RCC who either underwent radical nephrectomy with subsequent interferon alfa-2b compared with interferon alfa-2b alone.[50] This trial found a significant improvement with CN compared with interferon alfa-2b therapy alone, with a median OS of 11.1 months (95% CI: 5.4–9.5 months) versus 8.1 months (95% CI: 9.2–16.5 months), respectively. The EORTC 30947 RCT similarly compared patients with metastatic RCC who either underwent radical nephrectomy with subsequent interferon immunotherapy and those undergoing interferon immunotherapy alone.[51] This study found a significantly improved median duration of survival (17 vs 7 months, HR: 0.54, 95% CI: 0.31–0.94) and time to progression (5 vs 3 months, HR: 0.60, 95% CI: 0.36–0.97) in the group receiving CN versus interferon therapy alone. A metanalysis combining the results from these similar trials further corroborated these results, finding a median survival of 13.6 months for nephrectomy plus interferon versus 7.8 months for interferon alone.[52] Although these results are not directly applicable in the modern era of VEGFR and IC-centered therapies, they do suggest that there is a certain subset of patients who may benefit from CN.

Numerous retrospective studies have suggested that there is a survival benefit to CN in the setting of targeted therapies toward VEGFR and mTOR in select patients with clear cell and nonclear cell histologies.[53–56] A large retrospective review by Heng and colleagues[57] of 1658 patients with metastatic RCC who underwent targeted therapy from the International Metastatic Renal Cell Carcinoma Database Consortium of whom 982 patients underwent CN while the remaining 676 did not and found that those undergoing CN had better IMDC prognostic profiles compared with those without (favorable, intermediate, or poor in 9%, 63%, and 28% vs 1%, 45%, and 54%, respectively). When controlling for IMDC criteria, the HR of death was 0.60 (95% CI, 0.52–0.69; $P < .0001$) for those undergoing CN. Notably, they concluded that those with an estimated survival of less than 12 months may only receive marginal benefit from CN, and those with 4 or more IMDC criteria did not benefit from CN. These studies when assessed via systematic review with metanalysis suggest that properly selected patients with limited metastatic burden, good performance status, and good/intermediate IMDC/MSKCC may receive the most benefit from CN and targeted therapy compared with targeted therapy alone.[58,59]

To further assess the role of CN in the era of targeted therapies, 2 prospective phase III RCTs were performed, the CARMENA and the SURTIME trials.[60,61] The CARMENA trial was designed as a noninferiority trial comparing sunitinib alone versus sunitinib with CN and found that there was noninferior OS in the sunitinib alone arm (18.4 months) versus the sunitinib with CN arm (13.9 months; HR: 0.89, 95% CI: 0.71–1.10). The implications of the CARMENA trial continue to be debated to this day. The trial was criticized for only including intermediate and poor risk (57%) patients with relatively high tumor burden, as prior retrospective studies had suggested that CN was most likely to benefit those with more favorable risk profiles.[62] This study was notably underpowered with slow accrual, accruing 450 out of planned 576 patients during 8 years across 79 centers. Results are further complicated by notable crossover, with 15% of patients undergoing CN not receiving sunitinib, and 17% of patients in the sunitinib alone arm receiving CN. These limitations ultimately limit the generalizability of these results. The SURTIME trial approached the question of the utility of CN in the ERA of VEGR and mTOR targeted therapies differently, instead assessing the timing of CN with regards to

systemic therapy for metastatic RCC. Trial participants were randomized to sunitinib therapy followed by CN in the absence of progression versus immediate CN followed by sunitinib with a primary endpoint of PFS. For this, a sample size of 458 was needed but secondary to poor accrual, the intention-to-treat 28-week PFS was reported instead (42% in the immediate CN arm [n = 50] and 43% in the deferred CN arm [n = 49] [P = .61]), with 99 patients accrued total. When assessing for OS, the OS hazard ratio (HR) for deferred compared with immediate CN was 0.57 (95% CI, 0.34–0.95; $P = .03$), with median OS 32.4 months (95% CI, 14.5–65.3 months) and 15.0 months (95% CI, 9.3–29.5 months) in the deferred and immediate CN arms, respectively. Authors concluded that pretreatment with sunitinib may identify those patients with resistance to systemic therapy that may not benefit from planned CN. A post hoc analysis of the trial found that those undergoing immediate CN had decreased rates of sunitinib administration (80% [95% CI 66.9–88.7%, n = 40] compared with 97.7% [95% CI 89.3–99.6%; n = 48]), increased time to sunitinib administration (39.5 vs 4.5 days), and decreased duration of sunitinib administration (172.5 vs 248 days), which may have contributed to the difference in survival noted between the 2 groups.[63] Considered together, these 2 studies emphasize the importance of appropriate patient selection for CN.

With the advent of novel ICIs and data that has led to combination therapy with such ICIs becoming the first-line treatment of metastatic RCC, the role of CN in this era is actively being assessed. Singla and colleagues queried the NCDB and analyzed 391 patients from 2015 to 2016 who were surgical candidates with metastatic clear cell RCC treated with ICIs with or without CN (without other systemic therapies). A total of 221 of these patients received CN in conjunction with immune checkpoint inhibition, whereas 170 received immune checkpoint inhibition only. During a median follow-up of 14.7 months, those undergoing CN had significantly improved survival (median NR vs 11.6 mos.; HR 0.23, $P < .001$). Further analysis revealed that those undergoing immune checkpoint therapy before CN had lower pT stage, grade, tumor size, and lymphovascular invasion rates compared with upfront CN. Notably, 2 out of 20 patients undergoing delayed CN after ICI therapy achieved complete pathologic response pT0 in the primary tumor. Importantly, those undergoing delayed CN had no positive surgical margins, 30-day readmissions, or prolonged length-of-stay, suggesting that in properly selected patients delayed CN can be a safe intervention. Of course, such a retrospective design carries with it significant bias, with those receiving CN possibly having had more favorable patient or tumor characteristics.

Further supplementing these results, a multi-center retrospective analysis of 367 patients treated from 2000 to 2020 at the Seattle Cancer Care Alliance and The Ohio State University with metastatic RCC (232 treated with CN and IO [of whom 30 patients underwent deferred CN] and 135 treated with IO alone) found a longer median OS (56.3 months IQR 50.2–79.8) compared with the IO only group (19.1 months IQR 12.8–23.8).[64] The authors' multivariable analysis revealed a 67% reduction in risk of all-cause mortality (P <.0001) in patients CN and IO compared with IO alone. Notably, although there was variability to what line of therapy IO was (first-line in 28.1%, second-line in 17.4%, and third or subsequent line (3L+) in 54.5% of patients), similar results were noted on subgroup analysis of those receiving first-line IO. Additionally, upfront and deferred CN did not demonstrate significant differences in OS, keeping in mind the relatively small number of patients undergoing deferred CN. These retrospective results suggest that CN in conjunction with IO can be appropriate for select patients with metastatic RCC. A recent analysis of the International Metastatic RCC Database Consortium found 4639 patients with metastatic RCC, of whom 4202 patients treated with targeted therapy and 437 patients treated with IO. 2326 (55%) and 234 (54%) patients received upfront CN, with multivariable analysis showing that CN was associated with significantly improved OS in both the IO treated (HR: 0.61; 95% CI, 0.41–0.90, P =.013) and the targeted therapy treatment (HR: 0.72; 95% CI, 0.67–0.78, P <.001) groups, without a OS survival difference between groups (P =.6).[65] These retrospective results ultimately highlight the importance of prospective clinical trials in elucidating which patients in which contexts may benefit from CN.

To date, no phase 3 trials have assessed the impact of CN for patients with metastatic RCC treated with ICI-combination therapy but multiple randomized controlled trials are actively underway to assess this (**Table 1**). The NORDIC-SUN study will assess patients standard of care nivolumab plus ipilimumab.[66] These patients will then be assessed by a multidisciplinary tumor board, and those with less than or equal to 3 IMDC risk factors and who are eligible for CN will be randomized to CN plus maintenance nivolumab versus maintenance nivolumab alone. Notably, those with more than 3 IMDC risk factors or who are not eligible for CN will undergo 3 months of additional nivolumab therapy, and if there is favorable response (ie,

those patients then have less than or equal to 3 IMDC risk factors and are CN eligible) then will be randomized as above, but if still not eligible or if greater than 3 IMDC risk factors, then will undergo maintenance nivolumab. The PROBE study will assess ICI regimens after 12 weeks, and if there is stable disease or PR with surgical candidacy after urologist evaluation, they will be randomized to CN and subsequent continued systemic therapy versus continued systemic therapy alone.[67] The Cyto-KIK trial takes an alternate approach to this question, with investigators assessing the CR rate in patients receiving neoadjuvant nivolumab and cabozantinib followed by nephrectomy and subsequent systemic therapy, with patients notably having renal mass biopsies performed before beginning treatment.[68]

ROLE OF METASTASECTOMY

To date, there have been no randomized controlled trials analyzing the benefit of metastasectomy in patients with metastatic RCC, and much of the current understanding in the field is predicated on multiple retrospective studies with active investigation underway (**Table 2**). Broadly speaking, these studies typically categorize patients as having received (complete) metastasectomy, incomplete metastasectomy, and no metastasectomy.

Alt and colleagues[69] retrospectively reviewed 887 patients from 1976 to 2006 who underwent nephrectomy for RCC with subsequent development of multiple metastases, of whom 125 underwent complete surgical resection of all metastases. Complete metastasectomy was associated with significant improvement in CSS (4.8 years vs 1.3 years; P < .001). Multivariate analysis found that complete resection, Eastern Cooperatie Oncology Group (ECOG) performance status, lung only metastases, and asynchronous metastases were significantly prognostic. Dragomir and colleagues[70] performed a retrospective review of the Canadian Kidney Cancer Information System to compare patients (n = 229) who underwent complete metastasectomy each with up to 4 propensity-matched patients who did not undergo metastasectomy (n = 803), finding a 5-year OS of 63.2% and 51.4%, respectively, with multivariate analysis showing that patients who underwent metastasectomy had a significantly lower risk of mortality than those who did not (HR: 0.41, 95% CI 0.27–0.63). Of course, such retrospective reviews even with propensity matching are plagued by significant selection bias, with patients possibly being selected for metastasectomy based on feasibility of resection of metastatic sites as well as overall health and surgical candidacy, possibly

Table 1
Select ongoing trials assessing the role of cytoreductive nephrectomy in the modern immuno-oncology therapy era for metastatic renal cell carcinoma

Trial Name	Clinical Trial Number	Intervention	Primary Endpoint	Status
NORDIC-SUN (Deferred Cytoreductive Nephrectomy in Synchronous Metastatic Renal Cell Carcinoma)	NCT03977571	Nivolumab, ipilimumab, CN	OS	Recruiting
PROBE (Comparing the Outcome of Immunotherapy-Based Drug Combination Therapy with or Without Surgery to Remove the Kidney in Metastatic Kidney Cancer)	NCT04510597	CN, active comparator	OS	Recruiting
CYTO-KIK (CYTO-reductive Surgery in Kidney Cancer Plus Immunotherapy and Targeted Kinase Inhibition)	NCT04322955	Cabozantinib, nivolumab, CN	CR rate	Recruiting
Nivolumab With or Without Bevacizumab or Ipilimumab Before Surgery in Treating Patients with Metastatic Kidney Cancer That Can Be Removed by Surgery	NCT02210117	Bevacizumab, ipilimumab, nivolumab, metastasectomy, therapeutic conventional surgery, laboratory biomarker analysis, biopsy	Adverse events	Active, not recruiting
Pembrolizumab With or Without Axitinib for Treatment of Locally Advanced or Metastatic Clear Cell Kidney Cancer in Patients Undergoing Surgery	NCT04370509	Axitinib, pembrolizumab, metastatectomy, CN	Proportion of participants with >2-fold increase in tumor-infiltrating immune cells	Recruiting

Data from Lichtbroun BJ, Srivastava A, Doppalapudi SK, Chua K, Singer EA. New Paradigms for Cytoreductive Nephrectomy. Cancers (Basel). 2022 May 27;14(11):2660. https://doi.org/10.3390/cancers14112660. PMID: 35681638; PMCID: PMC9179532.

alluding to a more limited extent of disease. In order to better predict which patients may benefit from metastasectomy, Wu and colleagues[71] developed a nomogram that has yet to be validated based on a retrospective review of 2911 patients who had undergone CN from the SEER database, finding that those undergoing metastasectomy had improved OS (HR = 0.875, 95% CI 0.773–0.991; P = .015). They stratified these patients into low, medium, and high-risk groups based on T stage, N stage, presence of different types of metastases (bone, brain, liver, lung),

Table 2
Selected ongoing clinical trials including patients undergoing metastatectomy for metastatic RCC

Trial Name	Clinical Trial Number	Intervention	Primary Endpoint	Status
Follow-up After Metastasectomy in Patients with Kidney Cancer	NCT00918775	Follow-up and evaluation during and after metastasectomy every 6 mo up to 5 y (metastasectomy alone)	Progression-free/relapse-free survival	Active, not recruiting
Pembrolizumab With or Without Axitinib for Treatment of Locally Advanced or Metastatic Clear Cell Kidney Cancer in Patients Undergoing Surgery	NCT04370509	Pembrolizumab alone vs pembrolizumab + axitinib, followed by CN or metastasectomy (neoadjuvant therapy + nephrectomy or metastasectomy)	Proportion with ≥2-fold increase in the number of tumor-infiltrating immune cells	Recruiting
Nivolumab With or Without Bevacizumab or Ipilimumab Before Surgery in Treating Patients with Metastatic Kidney Cancer That Can Be Removed by Surgery	NCT02210117	Nivolumab alone vs Nivolumab with bevacizumab or ipilimumab, Followed by nephrectomy, metastasectomy or biopsy (neoadjuvant therapy + nephrectomy, metastasectomy or biopsy)	Safety and tolerability	Active, not recruiting
Daratumumab in Treating Patients with Muscle Invasive Bladder Cancer or Metastatic Kidney Cancer	NCT03473730	Daratumumab followed by biopsy, nephrectomy, or metastasectomy. Restart daratumumab postprocedure (neoadjuvant therapy + nephrectomy, metastasectomy or biopsy + adjuvant therapy)	Incidence of adverse events	Active, not recruiting
PROSPER RCC (Nivolumab in Treating Patients with Localized Kidney Cancer Undergoing Nephrectomy)	NCT03055013	Neoadjuvant and adjuvant nivolumab and nephrectomy ± metastasectomy versus surgery alone (neoadjuvant therapy + nephrectomy, metastasectomy or biopsy + adjuvant therapy)	Event-free survival	Active, not recruiting

(continued on next page)

Table 2
(continued)

Trial Name	Clinical Trial Number	Intervention	Primary Endpoint	Status
RESORT (Evaluate the Efficacy of Sorafenib in Renal Cell Carcinoma Patients After a Radical Resection of the Metastases)	NCT01444807	Adjuvant sorafenib vs supportive care (Metastasectomy ± Adjuvant Therapy)	Recurrence-free survival	Active, not recruiting
SMAT (Resection of Pulmonary Metastasis in Clear Cell Renal Cell Carcinoma ± Adjuvant Sunitinib Therapy)	NCT01216371	Adjuvant sunitinib vs placebo (metastasectomy ± adjuvant therapy)	2-year recurrence-free survival	recruiting
Pazopanib Hydrochloride in Treating Patients with Metastatic Kidney Cancer Who Have No Evidence of Disease After Surgery	NCT01575548	Adjuvant pazopanib vs placebo (metastasectomy ± adjuvant therapy)	Disease-free survival	Active, not recruiting
KEYNOTE-564 (Safety and Efficacy Study of Pembrolizumab (MK-3475) as Monotherapy in the Adjuvant Treatment of Renal Cell Carcinoma Post Nephrectomy)	NCT03142334	Nephrectomy ± metastasectomy with adjuvant pembrolizumab vs placebo (metastasectomy ± adjuvant therapy)	Disease-free survival	Active, not recruiting

Data from Mikhail M, Chua KJ, Khizir L, Tabakin A, Singer EA. Role of metastasectomy in the management of renal cell carcinoma. Front Surg. 2022 Jul 29;9:943604. https://doi.org/10.3389/fsurg.2022.943604. PMID: 35965871; PMCID: PMC9372304.

tumor grade, and found that those in the low-risk group who underwent complete metastasectomy had a 12.8% reduction of 3-year cancer-specific mortality, whereas such a survival benefit was not noted in the medium and high-risk groups. The exact risk factors and optimal risk stratification tool to determine which patients may benefit from metastasectomy remains to be seen.

Unsurprisingly, the survival benefit and complication profile of metastasectomy differ based on number of sites of metastasis and location of metastases, with multiple studies revealing that metastasectomy is more feasible with improved survival with fewer sites of disease, although without any set definition in the literature for what constitutes oligometastatic versus polymetastatic disease.[69,72,73] The potential benefits of metastasectomy must be carefully weighed against the site-dependent complication profile. For example, the most common metastatic site in metastasectomy is the lung, with a large retrospective review by Sun and colleagues[74] of 6994 patients with mRCC from the NCDB, of whom 1976 underwent metastasectomy for lung metastases, finding those undergoing lung metastasectomy had improved survival compared with those who did not (HR: 0.83, 95% CI: 0.77–0.90, P <.001). Although there is potential benefit in well-selected patients, reported complications include pneumonia, chylothorax, bronchial stump fistula, nerve injury, and arrhythmia.[75] There exists robust data describing this for bone, liver, adrenal, brain, and pancreatic metastases in the literature.[76] How to manage patients postmetastasectomy also remains unclear. On a subgroup analysis of patients with M1 disease with no evidence of disease (NED) after surgical extirpation in the Keynote 564 trial assessing the utility of adjuvant pembrolizumab for high-risk RCC, there was DFS benefit of adjuvant pembrolizumab (HR: 0.28, 95% CI: 0.12–0.66).[77] Contrasting this, the E2810 phase III RCT assessed the role of pazopanib in patients with NED after metastasectomy.[78] This study evaluated 129 patients randomized to either 52 weeks of pazopanib versus placebo with a median follow-up time after randomization of 30 months (range 0.4–66.5 months), and found no improvement in DFS with pazopanib, even finding that the HR for OS was 2.65 (95% CI: 1.02–6.9, P = .05) in favor of placebo. Additional investigation is needed into which patients may benefit from systemic therapy after metastasectomy. Ultimately, metastasectomy may be considered in properly selected patients after careful consideration of the specific complication profile, and additional prospective trials are needed to clarify exactly which patients will benefit from metastasectomy in the modern systemic therapy era.

SUMMARY

Surgery remains a cornerstone of advanced RCC management. Rapid advances in systemic therapies have outpaced our knowledge of how to best integrate surgical therapy into advanced RCC management. Although this provides significant opportunities for further study, it complexifies decision-making today. Given the current paucity of evidence in this space, shared decision-making on how best to integrate surgical and medical treatments is essential. Prospective clinical trials are needed to define the optimal roles of regional lymphadenectomy, CN, and metastasectomy. As our understanding of the molecular and immunological basis of RCC continues to develop along with the advent of novel systemic therapies and regimens, well-designed randomized controlled trials will be needed to determine the ideal combinations of surgery and systemic therapy needed for each individualized patient. The future of RCC care will likely be predicated on a multidisciplinary model involving the urologic oncologist, medical oncologist, other relevant medical providers, and those involved in the complex care coordination for these patients.

CLINICS CARE POINTS

- While regional lymphadenectomy is not routinely indicated at the time of nephrectomy nor is a set template defined, it can be considered in patients with abnormal lymph nodes either detected preoperatively on imaging or intraoperatively as well as in those with high risk features such as tumor stage/size & histology if available.

- Cytoreductive nephrectomy can be considered in patient's with limited metastatic disease burden with the potential for subsequent active surveillance or metastasis directed therapy following nephrectomy, with 1 IMDC risk factor with the majority of their tumor burden deriving from the kidney, and/or notable local symptoms. Contrasting this, upfront systemic therapy may be preferred in patients with high volume extra renal disease, significant morbidity associated with surgery, 2 or more IMDC risk factors, or poor performance status.

- Metastasectomy can be considered in favorable surgical candidates who are likely to become disease free upon metastasectomy (after or in conjunction with nephrectomy), or in those requiring palliation from metastases.

FUNDING

This study is supported by a grant from the National Cancer Institute (2P30CA016058), United States.

DECLARATION OF INTERESTS

E.A. Singer: Astellas/Medivation, research support for clinical trial; Merck, United States, advisory board; Johnson & Johnson, United States, advisory board; Vyriad, advisory board; and Aura Biosciences, data safety monitoring board.

REFERENCES

1. Siegel RL, Miller KD, Fuchs HE, et al. Cancer statistics, 2022. CA Cancer J Clin 2022;72(1):7–33.
2. Van Poppel H, Da Pozzo L, Albrecht W, et al. A prospective, randomised EORTC intergroup phase 3 study comparing the oncologic outcome of elective nephron-sparing surgery and radical nephrectomy for low-stage renal cell carcinoma. Eur Urol 2011;59(4):543–52.
3. Janzen NK, Kim HL, Figlin RA, et al. Surveillance after radical or partial nephrectomy for localized renal cell carcinoma and management of recurrent disease. Urol Clin North Am 2003;30(4):843–52.
4. Lam JS, Leppert JT, Belldegrun AS, et al. Novel approaches in the therapy of metastatic renal cell carcinoma. World J Urol 2005;23(3):202–12.
5. Haase VH. The VHL Tumor Suppressor: Master Regulator of HIF. Curr Pharm Des 2009;15(33): 3895–903.
6. Stebbins CE, Kaelin WG, Pavletich NP. Structure of the VHL-ElonginC-ElonginB complex: implications for VHL tumor suppressor function. Science 1999; 284(5413):455–61.
7. Dutcher JP, Flippot R, Fallah J, et al. On the shoulders of giants: the evolution of renal cell carcinoma treatment—cytokines, targeted therapy, and immunotherapy. Am Soc Clin Oncol Educ Book 2020;(40):418–35. https://doi.org/10.1200/EDBK_280817.
8. Srivastava A, Doppalapudi SK, Patel HV, et al. The roaring 2020s: a new decade of systemic therapy for renal cell carcinoma. Curr Opin Oncol 2022; 34(3):234–42.
9. Tsimafeyeu I. Nivolumab: 5 years since FDA approval of the first checkpoint inhibitor for renal cell carcinoma. Kidney Cancer 2021;5(2):63–71.
10. Rini BI, Plimack ER, Stus V, et al. Pembrolizumab plus axitinib versus sunitinib for advanced renal-cell carcinoma. N Engl J Med 2019;380(12): 1116–27.
11. Tran J, Ornstein MC. Clinical review on the management of metastatic renal cell carcinoma. JCO Oncol Pract 2022;18(3):187–96.
12. Fishman M, Dutcher JP, Clark JI, et al. Overall survival by clinical risk category for high dose interleukin-2 (HD IL-2) treated patients with metastatic renal cell cancer (mRCC): data from the PROCLAIMSM registry. J Immunother Cancer 2019;7(1):84.
13. Iacovelli R, Alesini D, Palazzo A, et al. Targeted therapies and complete responses in first line treatment of metastatic renal cell carcinoma. A meta-analysis of published trials. Cancer Treat Rev 2014;40(2): 271–5.
14. Choueiri TK, Powles T, Burotto M, et al. Nivolumab plus Cabozantinib versus Sunitinib for Advanced Renal-Cell Carcinoma. N Engl J Med 2021;384(9): 829–41.
15. Zambrana F, Carril-Ajuria L, Gómez de Liaño A, et al. Complete response and renal cell carcinoma in the immunotherapy era: The paradox of good news. Cancer Treat Rev 2021;99:102239.
16. Powles T, Plimack ER, Soulières D, et al. Pembrolizumab plus axitinib versus sunitinib monotherapy as first-line treatment of advanced renal cell carcinoma (KEYNOTE-426): extended follow-up from a randomised, open-label, phase 3 trial. Lancet Oncol 2020;21(12):1563–73.
17. Kroeger N, Pantuck AJ, Wells JC, et al. Characterizing the impact of lymph node metastases on the survival outcome for metastatic renal cell carcinoma patients treated with targeted therapies. Eur Urol 2015;68(3):506–15.
18. Yu KJ, Keskin SK, Meissner MA, et al. Renal cell carcinoma and pathologic nodal disease: Implications for American Joint Committee on Cancer staging. Cancer 2018;124(20):4023–31.
19. Capitanio U, Jeldres C, Patard JJ, et al. Stage-specific effect of nodal metastases on survival in patients with non-metastatic renal cell carcinoma. BJU Int 2009;103(1):33–7.
20. Rodríguez-Covarrubias F, Castillejos-Molina R, Sotomayor M, et al. Impact of lymph node invasion and sarcomatoid differentiation on the survival of patients with locally advanced renal cell carcinoma. Urol Int 2010;85(1):23–9.
21. Vig SV, Zan E, Kang SK. Imaging for Metastatic Renal Cell Carcinoma. Urol Clin North Am 2020; 47(3):281–91.
22. Tadayoni A, Paschall AK, Malayeri AA. Assessing lymph node status in patients with kidney cancer. Transl Androl Urol 2018;7(5):766–73.
23. Türkvatan A, Akdur PO, Altinel M, et al. Preoperative staging of renal cell carcinoma with multidetector CT. Diagn Interv Radiol Ank Turk 2009;15(1):22–30.
24. Kang DE, White RL, Zuger JH, et al. Clinical use of fluorodeoxyglucose F 18 positron emission tomography for detection of renal cell carcinoma. J Urol 2004;171(5):1806–9.
25. Spahn M, Portillo FJ, Michel MS, et al. Color Duplex sonography vs. computed tomography: accuracy in

the preoperative evaluation of renal cell carcinoma. Eur Urol 2001;40(3):337–42.

26. Studer UE, Scherz S, Scheidegger J, et al. Enlargement of regional lymph nodes in renal cell carcinoma is often not due to metastases. J Urol 1990; 144(2 Pt 1):243–5.

27. Johnson CD, Dunnick NR, Cohan RH, et al. Renal adenocarcinoma: CT staging of 100 tumors. AJR Am J Roentgenol 1987;148(1):59–63.

28. Nazim SM, Ather MH, Hafeez K, et al. Accuracy of multidetector CT scans in staging of renal carcinoma. Int J Surg Lond Engl 2011;9(1):86–90.

29. Radadia KD, Rivera-Núñez Z, Kim S, et al. Accuracy of clinical nodal staging and factors associated with receipt of lymph node dissection at the time of surgery for nonmetastatic renal cell carcinoma. Urol Oncol 2019;37(9):577.e17–25.

30. Capitanio U, Becker F, Blute ML, et al. Lymph node dissection in renal cell carcinoma. Eur Urol 2011; 60(6):1212–20.

31. Karmali RJ, Suami H, Wood CG, et al. Lymphatic drainage in renal cell carcinoma: back to the basics. BJU Int 2014;114(6):806–17.

32. Parker AE. Studies on the main posterior lymph channels of the abdomen and their connections with the lymphatics of the genito-urinary system. Am J Anat 1935;56(3):409–43.

33. Brouwer OR, Noe A, Olmos RAV, et al. Lymphatic Drainage from Renal Cell Carcinoma along the Thoracic Duct Visualized with SPECT/CT. Lymphat Res Biol 2013;11(4):233–8.

34. Blom JHM, van Poppel H, Maréchal JM, et al. Radical Nephrectomy with and without Lymph-Node Dissection: Final Results of European Organization for Research and Treatment of Cancer (EORTC) Randomized Phase 3 Trial 30881. Eur Urol 2009;55(1):28–34.

35. Whitson JM, Harris CR, Reese AC, et al. Lymphadenectomy Improves Survival of Patients With Renal Cell Carcinoma and Nodal Metastases. J Urol 2011;185(5):1615–20.

36. Crispen PL, Breau RH, Allmer C, et al. Lymph Node Dissection at the Time of Radical Nephrectomy for High-Risk Clear Cell Renal Cell Carcinoma: Indications and Recommendations for Surgical Templates. Eur Urol 2011;59(1):18–23.

37. Capitanio U, Suardi N, Matloob R, et al. Extent of lymph node dissection at nephrectomy affects cancer-specific survival and metastatic progression in specific sub-categories of patients with renal cell carcinoma (RCC). BJU Int 2014;114(2): 210–5.

38. Farber NJ, Rivera-Núñez Z, Kim S, et al. Trends and outcomes of lymphadenectomy for nonmetastatic renal cell carcinoma: A propensity score-weighted analysis of the National Cancer Database. Urol Oncol Semin Orig Investig 2019;37(1):26–32.

39. Gershman B, Thompson RH, Moreira DM, et al. Radical Nephrectomy With or Without Lymph Node Dissection for Nonmetastatic Renal Cell Carcinoma: A Propensity Score-based Analysis. Eur Urol 2017; 71(4):560–7.

40. Gershman B, Thompson RH, Moreira DM, et al. Lymph Node Dissection is Not Associated with Improved Survival among Patients Undergoing Cytoreductive Nephrectomy for Metastatic Renal Cell Carcinoma: A Propensity Score Based Analysis. J Urol 2017;197(3, Part 1):574–9.

41. Srivastava A, Rivera-Núñez Z, Kim S, et al. Impact of pathologic lymph node-positive renal cell carcinoma on survival in patients without metastasis: Evidence in support of expanding the definition of stage IV kidney cancer. Cancer 2020;126(13):2991–3001.

42. Dehal A, Smith JJ, Nash GM. Cytoreductive surgery and intraperitoneal chemotherapy: an evidence-based review—past, present and future. J Gastrointest Oncol 2016;7(1). https://doi.org/10.3978/j.issn.2078-6891.2015.112.

43. Makar AP, Tropé CG, Tummers P, et al. Advanced Ovarian Cancer: Primary or Interval Debulking? Five Categories of Patients in View of the Results of Randomized Trials and Tumor Biology: Primary Debulking Surgery and Interval Debulking Surgery for Advanced Ovarian Cancer. The Oncologist 2016;21(6):745–54.

44. Margul D, Coleman RL, Herzog TJ. The current status of secondary cytoreduction in ovarian cancer: a systematic review. Clin Adv Hematol Oncol HO 2020;18(6):332–43.

45. Walther MM, Patel B, Choyke PL, et al. Hypercalcemia in patients with metastatic renal cell carcinoma: effect of nephrectomy and metabolic evaluation. J Urol 1997;158(3 Pt 1):733–9.

46. Garfield DH, Kennedy BJ. Regression of metastatic renal cell carcinoma following nephrectomy. Cancer 1972;30(1):190–6.

47. Marcus SG, Choyke PL, Reiter R, et al. Regression of metastatic renal cell carcinoma after cytoreductive nephrectomy. J Urol 1993;150(2 Pt 1):463–6.

48. Gershman B, Moreira DM, Boorjian SA, et al. Comprehensive Characterization of the Perioperative Morbidity of Cytoreductive Nephrectomy. Eur Urol 2016;69(1):84–91.

49. Roussel E, Campi R, Larcher A, et al. Rates and Predictors of Perioperative Complications in Cytoreductive Nephrectomy: Analysis of the Registry for Metastatic Renal Cell Carcinoma. Eur Urol Oncol 2020;3(4):523–9.

50. Flanigan RC, Salmon SE, Blumenstein BA, et al. Nephrectomy followed by interferon alfa-2b compared with interferon alfa-2b alone for metastatic renal-cell cancer. N Engl J Med 2001;345(23):1655–9.

51. Mickisch GH, Garin A, van Poppel H, et al, European Organisation for Research and Treatment of Cancer

(EORTC) Genitourinary Group. Radical nephrectomy plus interferon-alfa-based immunotherapy compared with interferon alfa alone in metastatic renal-cell carcinoma: a randomised trial. Lancet Lond Engl 2001;358(9286):966–70.

52. Flanigan RC, Mickisch G, Sylvester R, et al. Cytoreductive nephrectomy in patients with metastatic renal cancer: a combined analysis. J Urol 2004; 171(3):1071–6.

53. Hanna N, Sun M, Meyer CP, et al. Survival Analyses of Patients With Metastatic Renal Cancer Treated With Targeted Therapy With or Without Cytoreductive Nephrectomy: A National Cancer Data Base Study. J Clin Oncol Off J Am Soc Clin Oncol 2016; 34(27):3267–75.

54. Conti SL, Thomas IC, Hagedorn JC, et al. Utilization of cytoreductive nephrectomy and patient survival in the targeted therapy era. Int J Cancer 2014;134(9): 2245–52.

55. Mathieu R, Pignot G, Ingles A, et al. Nephrectomy improves overall survival in patients with metastatic renal cell carcinoma in cases of favorable MSKCC or ECOG prognostic features. Urol Oncol 2015; 33(8). 339.e9-15.

56. Alhalabi O, Karam JA, Tannir NM. Evolving role of cytoreductive nephrectomy in metastatic renal cell carcinoma of variant histology. Curr Opin Urol 2019;29(5):521–5.

57. Heng DYC, Wells JC, Rini BI, et al. Cytoreductive nephrectomy in patients with synchronous metastases from renal cell carcinoma: results from the International Metastatic Renal Cell Carcinoma Database Consortium. Eur Urol 2014;66(4):704–10.

58. Bhindi B, Abel EJ, Albiges L, et al. Systematic Review of the Role of Cytoreductive Nephrectomy in the Targeted Therapy Era and Beyond: An Individualized Approach to Metastatic Renal Cell Carcinoma. Eur Urol 2019;75(1):111–28.

59. Petrelli F, Coinu A, Vavassori I, et al. Cytoreductive Nephrectomy in Metastatic Renal Cell Carcinoma Treated With Targeted Therapies: A Systematic Review With a Meta-Analysis. Clin Genitourin Cancer 2016;14(6):465–72.

60. Méjean A, Ravaud A, Thezenas S, et al. Sunitinib Alone or after Nephrectomy in Metastatic Renal-Cell Carcinoma. N Engl J Med 2018;379(5):417–27.

61. Bex A, Mulders P, Jewett M, et al. Comparison of Immediate vs Deferred Cytoreductive Nephrectomy in Patients With Synchronous Metastatic Renal Cell Carcinoma Receiving Sunitinib: The SURTIME Randomized Clinical Trial. JAMA Oncol 2019;5(2):164–70.

62. Mejean A, Thezenas S, Chevreau C, et al. Cytoreductive nephrectomy (CN) in metastatic renal cancer (mRCC): Update on Carmena trial with focus on intermediate IMDC-risk population. J Clin Oncol 2019;37(15_suppl):4508.

63. Abu-Ghanem Y, van Thienen JV, Blank C, et al. Cytoreductive nephrectomy and exposure to sunitinib – a post hoc analysis of the Immediate Surgery or Surgery After Sunitinib Malate in Treating Patients With Metastatic Kidney Cancer (SURTIME) trial. BJU Int 2022;130(1):68–75.

64. Gross EE, Li M, Yin M, et al. A multicenter study assessing survival in patients with metastatic renal cell carcinoma receiving immune checkpoint inhibitor therapy with and without cytoreductive nephrectomy. Urol Oncol Semin Orig Investig 2022. https:// doi.org/10.1016/j.urolonc.2022.08.013.

65. Bakouny Z, El Zarif T, Dudani S, et al. Upfront Cytoreductive Nephrectomy for Metastatic Renal Cell Carcinoma Treated with Immune Checkpoint Inhibitors or Targeted Therapy: An Observational Study from the International Metastatic Renal Cell Carcinoma Database Consortium. Eur Urol 2022. https:// doi.org/10.1016/j.eururo.2022.10.004.

66. Fristrup N. Multicenter Randomized Trial of Deferred Cytoreductive Nephrectomy in Synchronous Metastatic Renal Cell Carcinoma Receiving Checkpoint Inhibitors: A DaRenCa and NoRenCa Trial Evaluating the Impact of Surgery or No Surgery. The NORDIC-SUN-Trial. clinicaltrials.gov. 2022. Available at: https://clinicaltrials.gov/ct2/show/ NCT03977571. Accessed September 25, 2022.

67. Southwest Oncology Group. Phase III Trial of Immunotherapy-Based Combination Therapy With or Without Cytoreductive Nephrectomy for Metastatic Renal Cell Carcinoma (PROBE Trial). clinicaltrials.gov. 2021. Available at: https://clinicaltrials. gov/ct2/show/NCT04510597. Accessed September 25, 2022.

68. Stein M. Cyto-KIK; TRIAL (CYTO Reductive Surgery in Kidney Cancer Plus Immunotherapy (Nivolumab) and Targeted Kinase Inhibition (Cabozantinib). clinicaltrials.gov. 2022. Available at: https://clinicaltrials. gov/ct2/show/NCT04322955. Accessed September 25, 2022.

69. Alt AL, Boorjian SA, Lohse CM, et al. Survival after complete surgical resection of multiple metastases from renal cell carcinoma. Cancer 2011;117(13):2873–82.

70. Dragomir A, Nazha S, Wood LA, et al. Outcomes of complete metastasectomy in metastatic renal cell carcinoma patients: The Canadian Kidney Cancer information system experience. Urol Oncol 2020; 38(10):799.e1–10.

71. Wu K, Liu Z, Shao Y, et al. Nomogram Predicting Survival to Assist Decision-Making of Metastasectomy in Patients With Metastatic Renal Cell Carcinoma. Front Oncol 2020;10:592243.

72. Piltz S, Meimarakis G, Wichmann MW, et al. Long-term results after pulmonary resection of renal cell carcinoma metastases. Ann Thorac Surg 2002; 73(4):1082–7.

73. Kim SH, Park WS, Park B, et al. A Retrospective Analysis of the Impact of Metastasectomy on Prognostic Survival According to Metastatic Organs in Patients With Metastatic Renal Cell Carcinoma. Front Oncol 2019;9:413.

74. Sun M, Meyer CP, Karam JA, et al. Predictors, utilization patterns, and overall survival of patients undergoing metastasectomy for metastatic renal cell carcinoma in the era of targeted therapy. Eur J Surg Oncol J Eur Soc Surg Oncol Br Assoc Surg Oncol 2018;44(9):1439–45.

75. Kudelin N, Bölükbas S, Eberlein M, et al. Metastasectomy with standardized lymph node dissection for metastatic renal cell carcinoma: an 11-year single-center experience. Ann Thorac Surg 2013; 96(1):265–70 [discussion: 270-271].

76. Mikhail M, Chua KJ, Khizir L, et al. Role of metastasectomy in the management of renal cell carcinoma. Front Surg 2022;9:943604.

77. Powles T, Tomczak P, Park SH, et al. Pembrolizumab versus placebo as post-nephrectomy adjuvant therapy for clear cell renal cell carcinoma (KEYNOTE-564): 30-month follow-up analysis of a multicentre, randomised, double-blind, placebo-controlled, phase 3 trial. Lancet Oncol 2022;23(9):1133–44.

78. Appleman LJ, Puligandla M, Pal SK, et al. Randomized, double-blind phase III study of pazopanib versus placebo in patients with metastatic renal cell carcinoma who have no evidence of disease following metastasectomy: a trial of the ECOG-ACRIN cancer research group (E2810). J Clin Oncol 2019;37(15_suppl):4502.

Radiation Therapy in the Treatment of Localized and Advanced Renal Cancer

Kendrick Yim, MD[a], Jonathan E. Leeman, MD[b],*

KEYWORDS

- Renal cell carcinoma • Radiotherapy • Immunotherapy • Stereotactic body radiation therapy
- Radiosensitivity • Oligometastatic disease

KEY POINTS

- Emerging data suggest that stereotactic body radiotherapy (SBRT) is safe and well tolerated in localized renal cell carcinoma (RCC) for nonsurgical candidates. Long-term oncologic, renal functional, and safety outcomes are promising.
- Initial experiences with SBRT for oligometastatic RCC show excellent local control and a favorable toxicity profile.
- Results from ongoing clinical trials will define the oncologic benefit derived from SBRT to sites of metastatic disease in the context of multidisciplinary management of metastatic RCC.

TREATMENT PARADIGMS FOR RENAL CELL CARCINOMA

In the United States alone, an estimated 79,000 new cases of kidney cancer will be diagnosed in 2022, with approximately 14,000 cancer related deaths.[1] Renal cell carcinoma (RCC), which originates from the renal cortex comprises 80% to 85% of primary renal neoplasms. Benign entities such as parenchymal epithelial tumors (oncocytoma) and mesenchymal tumors (angiomyolipomas) make up approximately 15% to 20% of renal masses less than 7 cm in size.[2] Urothelial carcinoma of the renal pelvis, renal sarcomas, lymphomas, and collecting duct tumors are rare. This article will be focusing primarily on RCC, rather than these other rare etiologies. Classically, patients with RCC typically present with the triad of flank pain, abdominal/flank mass, and gross hematuria. However, given the increase in use of cross-sectional imaging, RCC is often now discovered incidentally. At time of diagnosis, 66% of tumors are localized to the kidney, 16% have spread to regional lymph nodes, blood vessels or perinephric tissue (locally advanced), and 15% have metastasized to distant sites.[3]

The standard of care (SOC) for management of localized RCC includes surgical extirpation whether it be partial or radical nephrectomy (RN). For those patients who are nonsurgical candidates, cryoablation (CA) and radiofrequency ablation (RFA) are alternative therapies. However, these treatments are limited by tumor size, tumor location, and anticoagulation status. Stereotactic body radiotherapy (SBRT) is an emerging modality for treatment of localized RCC which, as a noninvasive option, overcomes many of these limitations and can have a role in management for nonsurgical candidates. For patients with metastatic disease, systemic therapy with immunotherapy and/or vascular endothelial growth factor (VEGF)-targeted agents is typically initiated. Initially explored in oligometastatic disease with encouraging results, SBRT has increasingly been investigated as a noninvasive treatment option for patients with localized and metastatic RCC.

[a] Division of Urology, Brigham and Women's Hospital, 45 Francis Street, Boston, MA 02215, USA;
[b] Department of Radiation Oncology, Dana Farber Cancer Institute/ Brigham and Women's Hospital, Boston, MA, USA
* Corresponding author. Brigham and Women's Hospital, 75 Francis Street, Boston, MA 02115.
E-mail address: JONATHANE_LEEMAN@dfci.harvard.edu

Urol Clin N Am 50 (2023) 325–334
https://doi.org/10.1016/j.ucl.2023.01.008

Radiobiology of Renal Cell Carcinoma

Historically, RCC has been considered a radioresistant tumor histology due to preclinical studies performed *in vitro* and initial experience with conventional radiotherapy. In a study by Deschavanne and colleagues,[4] the authors compared the radiosensitivity of approximately 700 cell lines and found that RCC cells were amongst the most resistant to conventionally fractionated radiation therapy (defined as doses per fraction of $\leq$ 2 Gy). These findings were confirmed in several early human investigations. In a study by van der Werf-Messing and colleagues[5] compared RN alone to neoadjuvant conventional radiotherapy followed by RN and found no statistically significant difference in 5-year overall-survival rates. Similarly, multiple studies have found that adjuvant conventional radiotherapy did not improve overall survival but did predispose patients to irradiation-induced gastrointestinal complications (stomach, duodenum, liver), and even death.[6,7] A meta-analysis of seven studies found that postoperative radiation for RCC conducted from 1975 to 1999, typically delivered to adjuvant doses (50 to 60 Gy) with simple techniques such as parallel opposed fields showed an improvement in locoregional failure rates but no significant impact on disease-free survival (DFS) or overall survival.[8]

With technological advances in precision of radiation techniques, there has been improvement in dose delivery, particularly with SBRT. Traditionally, conventionally fractionated radiation consists of lower doses (1 to 2 Gy) delivered daily over a period of weeks, whereas SBRT uses higher dose per fraction (6+ Gy per fraction) delivered in fewer fractions (5 or less) with increased precision and narrower treatment margins. Recent studies have shown that RCC may be characterized by a sensitivity to high dose per fraction radiation as is used in SBRT.[9] In a mouse model of human xenograft RCC, Walsh and colleagues[10] showed that using an ablative, hypo-fractionated dose of 48 Gy over 3 fractions, tumor size decreased to less than 30% of initial volume. At these higher doses, ceramide-induced apoptosis via the sphingomyelinase pathway may drive tumor cell death which has been shown both in vivo and in human studies.[11,12] At high dose per fraction radiation, the vascular injury and endothelial cell response and death may play an active role,[13] which may be particularly relevant for RCC which are typically highly vascularized. These findings led to the hypothesis that the historically observed "radioresistance" of RCC may be overcome by high dose hypofractionated radiotherapy as can be delivered with SBRT.

In addition, developments in cross-sectional imaging, treatment planning, target localization and organ motion control systems such as vacuum stabilization systems and abdominal compression devices have allowed for safe SBRT treatments. Owing to potential off-target effects on kidney, small bowel, liver, pancreas, spleen, and stomach, precise delivery of radiation is imperative. Fiducial markers can be implanted into the renal capsule to allow for improved accuracy of targeting. However, kidney position can vary significantly during the normal respiratory cycle, which needs to be accounted for in treatment planning and delivery. In a study by Sonier and colleagues,[14] the authors evaluated kidney motion in immobilized patients during SBRT to the kidney or adrenal gland. They showed that between inhale and exhale, there was a 1.51 mm, 8.10 mm, and 3.08 mm change in position in left-right, superior-inferior, and anterior-posterior directions, respectively. By using organ motion control systems, respiratory-gated delivery, or abdominal pressure belts, the gross target volume to internal target volume may be reduced.[15] Because of these newfound improvements in SBRT technology, higher doses are able to be more precisely focused to a target of interest.

Radiotherapy Mechanisms of Action and Synergy with Immunotherapy

Immune checkpoint inhibitors have revolutionized the treatment of metastatic RCC. Systemic agents such as nivolumab, pembrolizumab, ipilimumab function to restore the immune response against tumor cells by inhibiting immune-checkpoint receptor/ligand binding. Several randomized trials including CheckMate-025, CheckMate-214, and Keynote-426 have shown improved survival in patients with metastatic RCC compared with previous first line vascular endothelial growth factor receptor (VEGFR) inhibitors.[16–18]

Although radiotherapy has classically been thought to exert its effects on tumor cells by irreversible DNA damage, there is increasing evidence that SBRT also stimulates the immune system. Multiple studies have shown that SBRT mediated cell death upregulates expression of MHC class I molecules, increases dendritic cell presentation of tumor antigens, and promotes CD8+ lymphocyte infiltration of tumor tissue.[19–21] These mechanisms may lead to abscopal effects, or the regression of nonirradiated metastatic deposits distant from the site of irradiation.[22]

Given these immunomodulatory properties, there has been tremendous interest in understanding the interplay between immunotherapy, which is increasingly used in metastatic RCC, and radiotherapy. In a mouse model, Deng and colleagues[23] showed that RT and IO may have synergistic effects. After irradiating each tumor, the investigators found increased levels programmed death-ligand 1 (PD-L1) which may facilitate tumor relapse. Concomitant administration of an anti-PD-L1 therapeutic was able to alter the tumor immune microenvironment and enhanced the effect of radiation via a T-cell-dependent mechanism. In addition, a study by Park and colleagues[24] found that PD-1 blockade in combination with SBRT in a mouse model led to near complete regression of the irradiated primary tumor and elicited a 66% reduction in the size of nonirradiated secondary tumors.

Because of these robust preclinical findings, there are currently several clinical trials investigating combination SBRT and immunotherapy. In a phase II trial of metastatic non-small-cell lung cancer, adding radiation therapy to pembrolizumab significantly increased rates of response, progression-free survival, and overall survival. In a phase II trial of 69 patients receiving SBRT in combination with nivolumab for patients with metastatic RCC who progressed after antiangiogenic therapy, the authors found that delivering SBRT to a metastatic site improved objective response rates (ORR) of irradiated lesions, which was 29% compared with 12% for nonirradiated lesions. Although overall results were less encouraging than previous trials evaluating nivolumab alone, there was a significant proportion of non-clear cell histology patients included in this study, which carries a worse prognosis. Reassuringly, SBRT was well tolerated and did not increase adverse events or lead to treatment delays.[25] In another phase I/II trial of SBRT and short course pembrolizumab of ccRC, authors found that of 30 patients treated (median follow-up 28 months), freedom from local progression at 2 years was 92% and ORR was 63%, and disease control rate was 83% at 2 years. This combination therapy was well tolerated with 13% of patients experiencing grade 3 adverse events, likely related to the pembrolizumab.[26] In addition to these published results, there are several trials in progress including NCT03065179 (SBRT with nivolumab and ipilimumab in patients with metastatic RCC), NCT02599779 (SBRT with pembrolizumab in tyrosine kinase inhibitor (TKI)-resistant metastatic RCC), NCT05327686 (NRG-GU0012, Randomized Phase II Stereotactic Ablative Radiation Therapy (SABR) for Metastatic Unresected Renal Cell Carcinoma (RCC) Receiving Immunotherapy (SAMURAI), IO ± SBRT to renal primary). Although preclinical studies and case reports have characterized abscopal effects occurring following the addition of SBRT to immunotherapy, other randomized trials have been negative[27] and the abscopal effect has not been robustly shown yet in controlled studies.

Stereotactic Body Radiotherapy for Management of Localized Renal Cell Carcinoma

The SOC for localized RCC is surgical extirpation, whether it be partial nephrectomy (PN) or RN.[28,29] PN, also known as nephron sparing surgery involves complete removal of the tumor while preserving normal renal parenchyma. It is the primary treatment strategy for cT1a (<4 cm) renal masses and for select T1b (<7 cm)/cT2 renal masses (≥7 cm, localized to kidney) as it has comparable oncologic outcomes to RN with the benefit of improved renal preservation.[30–33] PN should be prioritized in patients with solitary kidney, bilateral kidney tumors, preexisting chronic kidney disease (CKD), or known familial RCC. Otherwise, for larger localized renal masses or if PN is not technically feasible, RN is the SOC. Concurrent lymphadenectomy, has not shown improved oncologic or overall survival but does provide improved staging.[34,35]

For patients with small renal masses (<4 cm) who are not surgical candidates or those who prefer more conservative therapy, RFA or CA may be possible. However, there are important limitations, including tumor size, tumor location, and anticoagulation status. Although no randomized trials have been developed to compare RFA or CA to other modalities, multiple studies have shown that these procedures are well tolerated, but may have higher rates of tumor recurrence compared with surgical extirpation.[36–40]

For locally advanced RCC which includes tumor spread to regional lymph nodes, renal vein/inferior vena cava, or perinephric tissue, RN is preferred. 10% of patients with RCC will have venous thrombus that will require renal vein or inferior vena cava (IVC) thrombectomy.[41] Several clinical trials have investigated adjuvant therapies for high-risk localized RCC, including VEGF/mTOR inhibitors (sorafenib in ASSURE, sunitinib in S-TRAC, pazopanib in PROTECT) with no to minimal improvement in DFS.[42–44] More recently, adjuvant immune check point inhibitors (pembrolizumab in KEYNOTE-564) have been investigated with a significantly longer DFS in patients when compared with placebo.[45]

Although surgery and ablation have well defined roles in major urologic and oncology guidelines, SBRT has been increasingly investigated and has several advantages.[28,29,46] First, SBRT is noninvasive and can be used in comorbid patients that cannot tolerate surgery/ablation. Second, for patients undergoing CA or RFA, tumors must be < 4 cm or else the risk of incomplete treatment is unacceptably high. Third, tumors that are centrally located have two major issues: (1) nearby renal vessels can act as a heat sink for ablative technologies and decrease treatment efficacy (2) there is an increased risk of major complications such hemorrhage, renal vascular injury, ureteral injury/urine leak, and bowel injury.[47–49] Although there is limited long term data with regards to adverse effects of SBRT, risk of severe toxicity appears very low.[50] Fourth, patients who cannot stop anticoagulation medication have no contraindication to SBRT unlike surgery and ablation. Fifth, patients with multiple tumors or with CKD are at high risk of requiring postoperative dialysis with surgical extirpation. Although difficult to directly compare, SBRT seems to preserve nearby kidney parenchyma in the short term and has been shown to have a modest impact on kidney function.[51] Lastly, SBRT appears to be more cost-effective when compared with RFA for localized RCC. Donovan and colleagues found that over 5 years, SBRT cost $16,097 Canadian dollars (CAD) to gain 4.1 quality-adjusted life years, whereas RFA cost $18,324 to gain 3.6 quality adjusted life years. In addition, for tumors >4 cm, SBRT was $22094 CAD less than RFA per quality adjusted life year. One disadvantage of SBRT is that there is no tissue diagnosis. Unlike a nephrectomy specimen which provides tumor histology and grade, or a core biopsy prior/during time of ablation, patients undergoing SBRT will not have a tissue diagnosis unless biopsy is performed before treatment.

Initial experiences with SBRT for localized kidney cancer have shown encouraging results in several retrospective and prospective studies (**Table 1**).[50,52–58] In a multi-national prospective study (International Radiosurgery Oncology Consortium for Kidney-IROCK) of stereotactic ablative radiotherapy for 223 patients with primary RCC (mean size 2.64 cm) with median follow-up 2.6 years, rates of local control, cancer-specific survival, and progression-free survival were 98.8%, 95.7%, and 77.74% and were similar at 4 years. Importantly, in this cohort with either single-fraction or multi-fraction SBRT, the procedure was well tolerated with 35.6% of patients experiencing grade 1 to 2 toxicities and 1.3% experiencing grade 3 to 4 toxicities. Interestingly, tumors treated with multi-fraction SBRT had poorer progression-free and cancer-specific survival compared with patients treated with single fraction SBRT (hazard ratio of 1.13, $P = .02$, and 1.33, $P = .01$, respectively).[54] Possible reasons for this include, higher biologically effective dose delivered with single fraction SBRT or

alternative mechanisms of cell death when single fraction treatment is delivered. As this study was not randomized, there may also be an element of selection bias whereby patients with more favorable tumors were treated with single fraction SBRT. In this same consortium, the authors performed another analysis in 95 patients with clinical T1b tumors (>4 cm) with a mean tumor size of 4.9 cm and median follow-up of 2.7 years. Cancer-specific survival, overall-survival, and progression-free survival was 96.1%, 83.7%, and 81% at 2 years. At 4 years, rates of local, distant, and any failure was 2.9%, 11.1%, and 12.1%. Despite treating larger tumors, treatment was still well tolerated with 40% of patients had grade 1 to 2 toxicities and there were no grade 3 to 5 toxicities.[59] Lastly, a 5-year follow-up of 190 patients receiving SBRT for localized RCC as part of the IROCK consortium was recently published. The authors found that with a median tumor size of 4 cm, local failure remained low at 5.5%, median eGFR decreased by 14.2 mL/min/1.73 m^2 and only 1 patient who experience grade 4 AE for duodenal ulcer and gastritis.[50] Taken together, these results are encouraging and as the field continues to mature, the longer term oncologic, renal functional, and safety of SBRT will be elucidated. Interestingly, it was also found that single fraction high dose regimens were associated with lower rates of local failure compared with multifraction regimens.

Given these promising findings, there are several ongoing phase II clinical trials evaluating SBRT for primary renal cancer, which are awaiting accrual/publication: (NCT02141919: SBRT for patients with primary renal cancer, NCT01890590: A phase II study for cyberknife radiosurgery for RCC, and NCT02613819: Focal ablative stereotactic radiosurgery for cancers of the kidney [FASTRACK II]).

Effects of Local Therapy on Renal Function

One of the chief concerns of treating of kidney cancer whether it be with surgery, ablation, or radiation is effect on nearby healthy renal parenchyma. Patients with multiple tumors, with functional or solitary kidney, or with CKD are particularly at risk for long-term dialysis which carries significant morbidity, mortality risk and impact on quality of life.

In a review investigating the decline in renal function after PN, Mir and colleagues[52] found that PN led to a 20% decrease in eGFR, likely secondary to ischemic insult or nephron loss during surgery. Moreover, in a multi-institutional study of 665 patients undergoing PN (median tumor size 3 cm) and 715 undergoing RN (median tumor size 7.5 cm) for RCC, Mason and colleagues[53]

Table 1
Published reports of stereotactic body radiotherapy for primary renal tumors

Study	Type	Patients	Tumor Diameter or Volume (Mean)	Dose/Fractions	Median Follow-up	Oncologic Control	AE	Change in Renal Function (mL/min/1.73 m^2)
Ponsky et al,[68] 2015	Prospective (Phase I)	19	57.9 cm^3	24 to 48 Gy/4	13.7 mo	20% PR 80% SD	11% Grade 2 22% Grade 3 to 4	NR
Staehler et al,[72] 2015	Prospective (case control)	40	33.7 to 42 cm^2	25 Gy/1	28.1 mo	98% LC at 9 mo	15% Grade I	−6.5
Chang et al,[73] 2016	Retrospective	16	4cm	30 to 40 Gy/5	19 mo	100% LC	6% Grade I 12% Grade 4	−14.4%
Siva et al,[54] 2017	Prospective (Phase I)	37	4.92 cm	26 Gy/1, 14 Gy/3	24 mo	100% at 24 mo	78% Grade 1 to 2 3% Grade 3	−11
Correa et al,[74] 2018	Retrospective	11	9.5 cm	25 to 40 Gy/5	46.8 mo	71%SD 14% PR 14% PD	45% Grade 1 20% Grade 2 to 3	−2.4
Kasuya et al,[75] 2018	Retrospective	19	3.6 cm	66 to 80 Gy/12 to 16	79.2 mo	94.1% LC at 60 mo	16% Grade 2 5% Grade 4	−6.1
Kasuya et al,[76] 2019	Prospective	8	4.3 cm	66 to 72 Gy/12	43.1 mo	100%LC	No Grade 2 to 4	−10.8
Senger et al,[77] 2019	Retrospective	10	2.8 cm	24 to 51 Gy/3		92.3% LC	20% Grade 1 No Grade 2 to 4	−0.3
Tetar et al,[58] 2020	Prospective	51 (36 primary RCC)	5.6 cm	40 Gy/5	16.4 mo	95.2% LC	2% Grade 2 AE No Grade 3 to 4	−6.0
Yamamoto et al,[15] 2021	Retrospective	29	2.6 cm	50 to 70 Gy/10	57 mo	94% LC	No Grade 3 to 4	−5.4
Siva et al,[50] 2022	Meta-analysis (prospective/ retrospective)	190	4 cm	22 to 26 Gy/1 35 to 48 Gy/ 2 to 10	60 mo	94.5% LC	No Grade 3 1% Grade 4	−14.2

Abbreviations: Gy, Gray; LC, local control; NR, not reported; PD, progressive disease; PR, partial response; SD, stable disease.

showed that at 3-, 12-, and 24- months, patients undergoing RN had a lower eGFR [(35.8 mL/min/1.73 m^2 vs 42.8 mL/min/1.73 m,^{2} $P < .001$), (34.9 mL/min/1.73 m^2 vs 51.7 mL/min/1.73 m,^{2} $P < .001$) and (42.6 mL/min/1.73 m^2 vs 63.2 mL/min/1.73 m,^{2} $P < .001$). In addition, patients undergoing RN had an increase in CKD stage in 76% of patients compared with 41% of patients undergoing PN.

For patients undergoing RFA for cT1a masses (<4 cm) Lucas and colleagues[55] found that there was a mean decrease in eGFR of 1.7 mL/min/1.73 m^2 at 22 months in their cohort of 86 patients. In another study of 200 patients with median tumor size 2.9 cm undergoing RFA, there was a mean decrease in eGFR of 2.0 mL/min/1.73 m,^{2} with only 4 patients developing significant renal function deterioration (>25% decline in eGFR).[55,56] In a study of 102 patients undergoing CA for RCC (median size 2.6 cm) in a solitary kidney, Sriprasand and colleagues[57] reported a mean decrease in eGFR of 3.1 mL/min/1.73 m^2 at 3 months (mean baseline eGFR of 55 mL/min/1.73 m^2). In another study of 41 patients undergoing CA for T1a renal masses (mean tumor size 2.5 cm for both cohorts), Klatte and colleagues[40] found that there was a mean decrease in eGFR of 7.8 mL/min/1.73 m^2 compared with a mean decrease of 9.8 mL/min/1.73 m^2 in patients receiving PN.

In comparison to surgery and ablation, SBRT has a similar modest impact on renal function. In a large study of 223 patients undergoing either single -fraction or multi-fraction SBRT, Siva and colleagues[59] found that with a mean tumor size of 4.36 cm, eGFR decreased by 5.5 mL/min/1.73 m^2 on average at last follow-up (from mean baseline of 55 mL/min/1.73 m^2). The same group also examined 95 patients with ≥T1b renal tumors with an median tumor size of 4.9 cm, and found that average decrease in eGFR was 7.9 mL/min/1.73 m^2 (from mean baseline of 57.2 mL/min/1.73 m^2), after single-fraction SBRT.[54] Of note, these irradiated tumors were on average, 1.5 to 2x the size of those patients undergoing RFA or CA. In a series examining MRI guided SBRT, Tetar and colleagues[58] reported a mean decrease of 6.0 mL/min/1.73 m^2 with a mean starting eGFR of 55.8 mL/min/1.73 m^2 and median follow-up of 16.4 in cohort of 36 patients with an average tumor diameter of 5.6 cm. These results are promising and MR-Linac technology may hold potential for delivering kidney SBRT with decreased renal toxicity and better preservation of kidney parenchyma.

MR-Linac platforms, which combine MRI scanners with radiotherapy delivery systems, are in some ways optimally suited to delivering high dose kidney SBRT using three advantages: superior onboard imaging capabilities, real time MR based tracking of the target to control and account for respiratory motion, and online adaptive planning that involves alteration of the radiation plan in real time to account for daily anatomic changes in tumor or adjacent organs. Tetar and colleagues[58] reported on their experience using a 0.35 T MR-linac for treatment of 36 patients with RCC to a dose of 40 Gy in 5 fractions. Local control was 95% and toxicity rates were low. The phase I experience at Dana-Farber Brigham Cancer Center has similarly found high rates of local control (100%) and very low toxicity rates including minimal impact on kidney function in a cohort of 20 patients.[60]

RCC patients with IVC tumor thrombus represent a particular subset of cases with unique considerations. These cases are typically treated with extirpative surgery that is associated with high rates of morbidity and mortality. Many patients are not surgical candidates or decide to decline surgery given poor prognosis. Consequently, alternative options are critical and SBRT may be increasingly used. In a retrospective study of 15 RCC patients with IVC tumor thrombus (50% level III or level IV) undergoing SBRT to the tumor thrombus, Freifeld and colleagues[61] showed that 58% had tumor regression, 25% had stable disease, and 16% had enlargement. Median overall survival was favorable at 34 months compared with 5 months reported in historical data. Patients tolerated SBRT well with only Grade 1 to 2 adverse events.

Evaluating tumor response after kidney SBRT is an important area of future investigation. Mechanisms of cell death following ionizing radiation include mitotic catastrophe and consequently cell death may not occur instantaneously.[62] This is in contrast to RFA and cryotherapy where cell death occurs at the time of treatment and viable tumor cells should not persist. Consequently, routine biopsy post SBRT to evaluate for oncologic control is not recommended. Evaluating radiographic response has its limitations as well. For CA and RFA, residual enhancement on computed tomography (CT) or MRI within the treatment zone likely denote treatment failure with viable tumor.[63–65] In addition, there may be an immediate increase in size secondary to edema, hemorrhage, and inflammation cause by ablation. However, subsequent to this, there is a strong decrease in size with some studies reporting as high as 20% undetectable rates on follow-up imaging.[66,67] For SBRT, previous studies have shown that contrast enhancement on CT or MRI may persist long after treatment and that decrease in tumor size may not be as robust as previously mentioned ablative techniques.[68] Consequently, "absence of progression" based on radiographic tumor size is commonly used rather than the traditional definitions of treatment response. Abdominal imaging is recommended within the first 6 months following SBRT and then every 6 to 12 months thereafter depending on response and the clinical scenario. Chest imaging should be regularly performed as well.

Stereotactic Body Radiotherapy for Management of Metastatic Renal Cell Carcinoma

In recent years, evidence supporting the role of SBRT in management of oligometastatic disease, commonly defined as 1 to 5 metastatic lesions, has expanded. In a study by Franzese and colleagues[69] of 58 patients with metastatic RCC with 1 to 3 metastatic deposits treated with SBRT, the authors found that local control rates at 12 and 18 months were both 90.2%, suggesting effective local control of oligometastatic RCC. Prospective studies have started to validate these preliminary studies. In a prospective randomized trial of 99 patients with metastatic solid tumors that included a variety of histologies (1 to 5 metastatic lesions) comparing palliative SOC versus SOC + SBRT to metastatic deposits, the authors found that overall survival at 5 years was significantly higher in the SBRT group (42.3% vs 17.7%, P = .006), without any difference in quality of life (QOL) or difference in grade $\geq$2 adverse events.[70] Reassuringly, as new metastatic deposits presented themselves, patients were able to receive salvage treatment with repeat SBRT. In fact, 30% of patients living greater than 5 years after initial treatment received repeat SBRT. This suggests that although SBRT may not eliminate all micro-metastatic disease, it may be used to provide local control and extend overall survival.

For patients with metastatic RCC, a subset of which have indolently growing disease, there may be a role for SBRT to address sites of metastatic disease. In addition, although the role of systemic therapies and immunotherapies have advanced, patients may experience oligorecurrence or oligoprogression of isolated sites that are not responsive. Instead of switching systemic therapy regimens, SBRT to progressive sites can be undertaken with the goal of keeping the patient on an otherwise active systemic treatment. Tang and colleagues undertook a single arm phase II study of SBRT to sites of metastatic disease in patients with metastatic RCC limited to 1 to 5 sites and found a median progression-free survival of

22.7 months. Ten percent of patients experienced grade 3 or higher toxicity events.[71]

Importantly, many intrabdominal organs that are common destinations of metastasis from RCC are also some of the most challenging to treat with high dose radiation, such as pancreatic lesions and abdominal lymph nodes which can be adjacent to bowel and are subject to respiratory motion and organ motion. There may be a particular role for MR guided adaptive radiotherapy, which can account for motion and organ uncertainties, in treatment of these lesions with SBRT to maximize local control and minimize toxicity risks.

FUTURE DIRECTIONS

There are several important future directions and avenues of ongoing research which will help to better characterize the role of SBRT in the multidisciplinary management of RCC patients and improve clinical outcomes. In particular, additional randomized evidence is needed in the settings of both localized and oligo- or poly-metastatic RCC to establish outcomes associated with kidney SBRT or the addition of SBRT to sites of metastasis compared with current standards of care. An important example of such studies is the newly activated NRG-GU 012 SAMURAI trial which randomizes patients with metastatic RCC to either SOC immunotherapy versus immunotherapy + SBRT to the primary kidney tumor with a primary endpoint of nephrectomy and radiographic progression-free survival. Novel studies such as this will help to clarify how SBRT can most effectively be integrated into the modern multi-disciplinary management of RCC.

CLINICS CARE POINTS

- Stereotactic body radiotherapy (SBRT) is a promising treatment modality for localized RCC in non-surgical candidates with respect to oncologic, renal functional, and safety outcomes.

- New data has demonstrated favorable outcomes when using SBRT to address sites of metastatic disease in oligometastatic RCC.

- Technological advancements in radiation technology (such as MRI-guided SBRT) and combinatorial treatment paradigms with immunotherapy are currently under investigation and there is a need for continued prospective clinical trial development to better characterize clinical benefit.

DISCLOSURE

K. Yim has no relevant financial or nonfinancial relationships to disclose. J. Leeman reports research funding from Viewray and NH TherAguix and speaker's honoraria from Viewray.

REFERENCES

1. Siegel RL, Miller KD, Fuchs HE, et al. Cancer statistics, 2022. CA A Cancer J Clin 2022;72(1):7–33.

2. Akdogan B, Gudeloglu A, Inci K, et al. Prevalence and predictors of benign lesions in renal masses smaller than 7 cm presumed to be renal cell carcinoma. Clin Genitourin Cancer 2012;10(2):121–5.

3. Cancer of the Kidney and Renal Pelvis - Cancer Stat Facts. SEER. Available at: https://seer.cancer.gov/statfacts/html/kidrp.html. Accessed September 17, 2022.

4. Deschavanne PJ, Fertil B. A review of human cell radiosensitivity in vitro. Int J Radiat Oncol Biol Phys 1996;34(1):251–66.

5. van der Werf-Messing B. Proceedings: Carcinoma of the kidney. Cancer 1973;32(5):1056–61.

6. Finney R. The Value of Radiotherapy in the Treatment of Hypernephroma-a Clinical Trial. Br J Urol 1973;45(3):258–69.

7. Kjaer M, Iversen P, Hvidt V, et al. A Randomized Trial of Postoperative Radiotherapy Versus Observation in Stage II and III Renal Adenocarcinoma. Scand J Urol Nephrol 1987;21(4):285–9.

8. Tunio MA, Hashmi A, Rafi M. Need for a new trial to evaluate postoperative radiotherapy in renal cell carcinoma: a meta-analysis of randomized controlled trials. Ann Oncol 2010;21(9):1839–45.

9. Ning S, Trisler K, Wessels BW, et al. Radiobiologic studies of radioimmunotherapy and external beam radiotherapy in vitro and in vivo in human renal cell carcinoma xenografts. Cancer 1997;80(12 Suppl): 2519–28.

10. Walsh L, Stanfield JL, Cho LC, et al. Efficacy of ablative high-dose-per-fraction radiation for implanted human renal cell cancer in a nude mouse model. Eur Urol 2006;50(4):795–800. ; discussion 800.

11. Garcia-Barros M, Paris F, Cordon-Cardo C, et al. Tumor response to radiotherapy regulated by endothelial cell apoptosis. Science 2003;300(5622):1155–9.

12. Marathe S, Schissel SL, Yellin MJ, et al. Human vascular endothelial cells are a rich and regulatable source of secretory sphingomyelinase. Implications for early atherogenesis and ceramide-mediated cell signaling. J Biol Chem 1998;273(7):4081–8.

13. Song CW, Glatstein E, Marks LB, et al. Biological Principles of Stereotactic Body Radiation Therapy (SBRT) and Stereotactic Radiation Surgery (SRS): Indirect Cell Death. Int J Radiat Oncol Biol Phys 2021;110(1):21–34.

14. Sonier M, Chu W, Lalani N, et al. Evaluation of kidney motion and target localization in abdominal SBRT patients. J Appl Clin Med Phys 2016;17(6): 429–33.

15. Yamamoto T, Kawasaki Y, Umezawa R, et al. Stereotactic body radiotherapy for kidney cancer: a 10-year experience from a single institute. J Radiat Res 2021;62(3):533–9.

16. Motzer RJ, Escudier B, McDermott DF, et al. Nivolumab versus Everolimus in Advanced Renal-Cell Carcinoma. N Engl J Med 2015;373(19):1803–13.

17. Motzer RJ, Tannir NM, McDermott DF, et al. Nivolumab plus Ipilimumab versus Sunitinib in Advanced Renal-Cell Carcinoma. N Engl J Med 2018;378(14): 1277–90.

18. Rini BI, Plimack ER, Stus V, et al. Pembrolizumab plus Axitinib versus Sunitinib for Advanced Renal-Cell Carcinoma. N Engl J Med 2019;380(12): 1116–27.

19. Garnett CT, Palena C, Chakraborty M, et al. Sublethal irradiation of human tumor cells modulates phenotype resulting in enhanced killing by cytotoxic T lymphocytes. Cancer Res 2004;64(21):7985–94.

20. Kachikwu EL, Iwamoto KS, Liao YP, et al. Radiation Enhances Regulatory T Cell Representation. Int J Radiat Oncol Biol Phys 2011;81(4):1128–35.

21. Teitz-Tennenbaum S, Li Q, Okuyama R, et al. Mechanisms involved in radiation enhancement of intratumoral dendritic cell therapy. J Immunother 2008; 31(4):345–58.

22. Wersäll PJ, Blomgren H, Pisa P, et al. Regression of nonirradiated metastases after extracranial stereotactic radiotherapy in metastatic renal cell carcinoma. Acta Oncol 2006;45(4):493–7.

23. Deng L, Liang H, Burnette B, et al. Irradiation and anti–PD-L1 treatment synergistically promote antitumor immunity in mice. J Clin Invest 2014;124(2): 687–95.

24. Park SS, Dong H, Liu X, et al. PD-1 Restrains Radiotherapy-Induced Abscopal Effect. Cancer Immunol Res 2015;3(6):610–9.

25. Masini C, Iotti C, De Giorgi U, et al. Nivolumab in Combination with Stereotactic Body Radiotherapy in Pretreated Patients with Metastatic Renal Cell Carcinoma. Results of the Phase II NIVES Study. Eur Urol 2022;81(3):274–82.

26. Siva S, Bressel M, Wood ST, et al. Stereotactic Radiotherapy and Short-course Pembrolizumab for Oligometastatic Renal Cell Carcinoma-The RAPPORT Trial. Eur Urol 2022;81(4):364–72.

27. McBride S, Sherman E, Tsai CJ, et al. Randomized Phase II Trial of Nivolumab With Stereotactic Body Radiotherapy Versus Nivolumab Alone in Metastatic Head and Neck Squamous Cell Carcinoma. J Clin Oncol 2021;39(1):30–7.

28. Ljungberg B, Albiges L, Abu-Ghanem Y, et al. European Association of Urology Guidelines on Renal

Cell Carcinoma: The 2022 Update. Eur Urol 2022; 82(4):399–410.

29. Campbell SC, Clark PE, Chang SS, et al. Renal Mass and Localized Renal Cancer: Evaluation, Management, and Follow-Up: AUA Guideline: Part I. J Urol 2021;206(2):199–208.

30. Leibovich BC, Blute ML, Cheville JC, et al. Nephron sparing surgery for appropriately selected renal cell carcinoma between 4 and 7 cm results in outcome similar to radical nephrectomy. J Urol 2004;171(3): 1066–70.

31. Van Poppel H, Da Pozzo L, Albrecht W, et al. A prospective, randomised EORTC intergroup phase 3 study comparing the oncologic outcome of elective nephron-sparing surgery and radical nephrectomy for low-stage renal cell carcinoma. Eur Urol 2011;59(4):543–52.

32. Huang WC, Levey AS, Serio AM, et al. Chronic kidney disease after nephrectomy in patients with renal cortical tumours: a retrospective cohort study. Lancet Oncol 2006;7(9):735–40.

33. Kopp RP, Mehrazin R, Palazzi KL, et al. Survival outcomes after radical and partial nephrectomy for clinical T2 renal tumours categorised by R.E.N.A.L. nephrometry score. BJU Int 2014;114(5):708–18.

34. Crispen PL, Breau RH, Allmer C, et al. Lymph node dissection at the time of radical nephrectomy for high-risk clear cell renal cell carcinoma: indications and recommendations for surgical templates. Eur Urol 2011;59(1):18–23.

35. Blom JHM, van Poppel H, Maréchal JM, et al. Radical nephrectomy with and without lymph-node dissection: final results of European Organization for Research and Treatment of Cancer (EORTC) randomized phase 3 trial 30881. Eur Urol 2009;55(1):28–34.

36. Gore JL, Kim HL, Schulam P. Initial experience with laparoscopically assisted percutaneous cryotherapy of renal tumors. J Endourol 2005;19(4):480–3.

37. Clark TWI, Malkowicz B, Stavropoulos SW, et al. Radiofrequency ablation of small renal cell carcinomas using multitined expandable electrodes: preliminary experience. J Vasc Interv Radiol 2006;17(3):513–9.

38. Bandi G, Wen CC, Hedican SP, et al. Cryoablation of small renal masses: assessment of the outcome at one institution. BJU Int 2007;100(4):798–801.

39. Zagoria RJ, Traver MA, Werle DM, et al. Oncologic efficacy of CT-guided percutaneous radiofrequency ablation of renal cell carcinomas. AJR Am J Roentgenol 2007;189(2):429–36.

40. Klatte T, Mauermann J, Heinz-Peer G, et al. Perioperative, Oncologic, and Functional Outcomes of Laparoscopic Renal Cryoablation and Open Partial Nephrectomy: A Matched Pair Analysis. J Endourol 2011;25(6):991–7.

41. Kirkali Z, Van Poppel H. A critical analysis of surgery for kidney cancer with vena cava invasion. Eur Urol 2007;52(3):658–62.

42. Haas NB, Manola J, Uzzo RG, et al. Adjuvant sunitinib or sorafenib for high-risk, non-metastatic renal-cell carcinoma (ECOG-ACRIN E2805): a double-blind, placebo-controlled, randomised, phase 3 trial. Lancet 2016;387(10032):2008–16.

43. Ravaud A, Motzer RJ, Pandha HS, et al. Adjuvant Sunitinib in High-Risk Renal-Cell Carcinoma after Nephrectomy. N Engl J Med 2016;375(23):2246–54.

44. Motzer RJ, Haas NB, Donskov F, et al. Randomized Phase III Trial of Adjuvant Pazopanib Versus Placebo After Nephrectomy in Patients With Localized or Locally Advanced Renal Cell Carcinoma. J Clin Oncol 2017;35(35):3916–23.

45. Choueiri TK, Tomczak P, Park SH, et al. Adjuvant Pembrolizumab after Nephrectomy in Renal-Cell Carcinoma. N Engl J Med 2021;385(8):683–94.

46. Motzer RJ, Jonasch E, Agarwal N, et al. Kidney Cancer, Version 3.2022, NCCN Clinical Practice Guidelines in Oncology. J Natl Compr Cancer Netw 2022;20(1):71–90.

47. Park BK, Kim CK. Complications of image-guided radiofrequency ablation of renal cell carcinoma: causes, imaging features and prevention methods. Eur Radiol 2009;19(9):2180–90.

48. Hegarty NJ, Gill IS, Desai MM, et al. Probe-ablative nephron-sparing surgery: Cryoablation versus radiofrequency ablation. Urology 2006;68(1 Supplement): 7–13.

49. Atwell TD, Carter RE, Schmit GD, et al. Complications following 573 Percutaneous Renal Radiofrequency and Cryoablation Procedures. J Vasc Interv Radiol 2012;23(1):48–54.

50. Siva S, Ali M, Correa RJM, et al. 5-year outcomes after stereotactic ablative body radiotherapy for primary renal cell carcinoma: an individual patient data meta-analysis from IROCK (the International Radiosurgery Consortium of the Kidney). Lancet Oncol 2022;23(12):1508–16.

51. Correa RJM, Louie AV, Zaorsky NG, et al. The Emerging Role of Stereotactic Ablative Radiotherapy for Primary Renal Cell Carcinoma: A Systematic Review and Meta-Analysis. European Urology Focus 2019;5(6):958–69.

52. Mir MC, Ercole C, Takagi T, et al. Decline in Renal Function after Partial Nephrectomy: Etiology and Prevention. J Urol 2015;193(6):1889–98.

53. Mason R, Kapoor A, Liu Z, et al. The natural history of renal function after surgical management of renal cell carcinoma: Results from the Canadian Kidney Cancer Information System. Urol Oncol 2016; 34(11):486.e1–7.

54. Siva S, Pham D, Kron T, et al. Stereotactic ablative body radiotherapy for inoperable primary kidney cancer: a prospective clinical trial. BJU Int 2017; 120(5):623–30.

55. Lucas SM, Stern JM, Adibi M, et al. Renal function outcomes in patients treated for renal masses

smaller than 4 cm by ablative and extirpative techniques. J Urol 2008;179(1):75–9. ; discussion 79-80.

56. Wah TM, Irving HC, Gregory W, et al. Radiofrequency ablation (RFA) of renal cell carcinoma (RCC): experience in 200 tumours. BJU Int 2014; 113(3):416–28.

57. Sriprasad S, Aldiwani M, Pandian S, et al. Renal Function Loss After Cryoablation of Small Renal Masses in Solitary Kidneys: European Registry for Renal Cryoablation Multi-Institutional Study. J Endourol 2020;34(2):233–9.

58. Tetar SU, Bohoudi O, Senan S, et al. The Role of Daily Adaptive Stereotactic MR-Guided Radiotherapy for Renal Cell Cancer. Cancers 2020; 12(10):2763.

59. Siva S, Louie AV, Warner A, et al. Pooled analysis of stereotactic ablative radiotherapy for primary renal cell carcinoma: A report from the International Radiosurgery Oncology Consortium for Kidney (IROCK). Cancer 2018;124(5):934–42.

60. Yim K, Cagney DN, Mak RH, et al. Safety and Efficacy of Stereotactic MRI-Guided Adaptive Radiation Therapy for Localized Kidney Cancer. Int J Radiat Oncol Biol Phys 2022;114(3):e207.

61. Freifeld Y, Pedrosa I, Mclaughlin M, et al. Stereotactic ablative radiation therapy for renal cell carcinoma with inferior vena cava tumor thrombus. Urol Oncol 2022;40(4):166.e9.

62. Sia J, Szmyd R, Hau E, et al. Molecular Mechanisms of Radiation-Induced Cancer Cell Death: A Primer. Front Cell Dev Biol 2020;8. Available at: https://www.frontiersin.org/articles/10.3389/fcell.2020.00041. Accessed October 7, 2022.

63. Wile GE, Leyendecker JR, Krehbiel KA, et al. CT and MR imaging after imaging-guided thermal ablation of renal neoplasms. Radiographics 2007;27(2): 325–39. ; discussion 339-340.

64. Weight CJ, Kaouk JH, Hegarty NJ, et al. Correlation of radiographic imaging and histopathology following cryoablation and radio frequency ablation for renal tumors. J Urol 2008;179(4):1277–81. ; discussion 1281-1283.

65. Raman JD, Stern JM, Zeltser I, et al. Absence of viable renal carcinoma in biopsies performed more than 1 year following radio frequency ablation confirms reliability of axial imaging. J Urol 2008;179(6): 2142–5.

66. Nadler RB, Kim SC, Rubenstein JN, et al. Laparoscopic renal cryosurgery: the Northwestern experience. J Urol 2003;170(4 Pt 1):1121–5.

67. Gill IS, Novick AC, Meraney AM, et al. Laparoscopic renal cryoablation in 32 patients. Urology 2000; 56(5):748–53.

68. Ponsky L, Lo SS, Zhang Y, et al. Phase I dose-escalation study of stereotactic body radiotherapy (SBRT) for poor surgical candidates with localized renal cell carcinoma. Radiother Oncol 2015;117(1): 183–7.

69. Franzese C, Franceschini D, Di Brina L, et al. Role of Stereotactic Body Radiation Therapy for the Management of Oligometastatic Renal Cell Carcinoma. J Urol 2019;201(1):70–6.

70. Palma DA, Olson R, Harrow S, et al. Stereotactic Ablative Radiotherapy for the Comprehensive Treatment of Oligometastatic Cancers: Long-Term Results of the SABR-COMET Phase II Randomized Trial. J Clin Oncol 2020;38(25):2830–8.

71. Tang C, Msaouel P, Hara K, et al. Definitive radiotherapy in lieu of systemic therapy for oligometastatic renal cell carcinoma: a single-arm, single-centre, feasibility, phase 2 trial. Lancet Oncol 2021;22(12): 1732–9.

72. Staehler M, Bader M, Schlenker B, et al. Single Fraction Radiosurgery for the Treatment of Renal Tumors. J Urol 2015;193(3):771–5.

73. Chang JH, Cheung P, Erler D, et al. Stereotactic Ablative Body Radiotherapy for Primary Renal Cell Carcinoma in Non-surgical Candidates: Initial Clinical Experience. Clin Oncol 2016;28(9):e109–14.

74. Correa RJM, Rodrigues GB, Chen H, et al. Stereotactic Ablative Radiotherapy (SABR) for Large Renal Tumors: A Retrospective Case Series Evaluating Clinical Outcomes, Toxicity, and Technical Considerations. Am J Clin Oncol 2018;41(6):568–75.

75. Kasuya G, Tsuji H, Nomiya T, et al. Updated long-term outcomes after carbon-ion radiotherapy for primary renal cell carcinoma. Cancer Sci 2018;109(9): 2873–80.

76. Kasuya G, Tsuji H, Nomiya T, et al. Prospective clinical trial of 12-fraction carbon-ion radiotherapy for primary renal cell carcinoma. Oncotarget 2019; 10(1):76–81.

77. Senger C, Conti A, Kluge A, et al. Robotic stereotactic ablative radiotherapy for renal cell carcinoma in patients with impaired renal function. BMC Urol 2019;19(1):96.

The Changing Landscape of Immunotherapy for Advanced Renal Cancer

Soki Kashima, MD, PhD[a,b], David A. Braun, MD, PhD[a,*]

KEYWORDS

- Renal cell carcinoma • Kidney cancer • Immunotherapy • Immune checkpoint inhibitor
- Molecularly targeted therapy • Combination therapy

KEY POINTS

- Clear cell renal cell carcinoma (RCC) is an immunogenic tumor, historically in the cytokine era (with interleukin-2 and interferon-α), and contemporarily in the immune checkpoint inhibitor (ICI) era.
- ICI, particularly with antibodies targeting the PD-1–PD-L1 pathway, form the foundation of systemic therapy for advanced clear cell RCC. Since the approval of nivolumab plus ipilimumab in 2018, ICI-based combination therapies are now the recommended first-line strategy for most patients with advanced RCC.
- Pembrolizumab is the first FDA-approved adjuvant immunotherapy for RCC, although other adjuvant ICI therapies have not demonstrated clear benefit. The decision to initiate adjuvant therapy should be individualized for each patient.
- Although biomarkers in other solid tumors do not predict ICI efficacy in RCC (eg, total mutation burden, T-cell infiltration), sarcomatoid dedifferentiation is associated with improved response to ICIs.

INTRODUCTION

Conventional immune therapies, such as interleukin-2 (IL-2) and interferon-α, have historically played an important role in the treatment of metastatic renal cell carcinoma (RCC).[1,2] Since 2005, molecularly targeted therapies, such as anti-angiogenic therapy and mammalian target of rapamycin inhibitors (mTORi) were placed in the center of advanced RCC management.[3–7] More recently, immune checkpoint inhibitors (ICIs) have demonstrated greatly improved therapeutic efficacy across many solid tumors, including RCC.[8,9] Currently, combination therapies including ICI are the mainstay in RCC therapy.[10] In this review, we look back on the historical changes in systemic therapy for advanced RCC, and we focus on the characteristic mechanisms of ICI efficacy by examining the crosstalk of immune cells within the tumor microenvironment in RCC. Finally, we discuss the possibility of developing biomarkers of ICI efficacy and novel immunotherapeutic strategies for this disease.

HISTORY

Cytokine Therapy Era

In 1976, RCC was reported to be the most frequent spontaneously regressing of human cancers.[11] This provided early support for RCC becoming known as an immunogenic solid tumor. Classic immunotherapies have been applied against RCC, such as the systemic administration of IL-2 and interferon-α as a standard therapy (**Fig. 1**).[12,13] In addition to

^a Center of Molecular and Cellular Oncology, Yale Cancer Center, Yale School of Medicine, 300 George Street, Suite 6400, New Haven, CT, USA; ^b Department of Urology, Akita University, Graduate School of Medicine, Akita, Japan
* Corresponding author. Department of Medical Oncology, Yale School of Medicine, 300 George Street, Suite 6400, New Haven, CT 06511.
E-mail address: david.braun@yale.edu

Urol Clin N Am 50 (2023) 335–349
https://doi.org/10.1016/j.ucl.2023.01.012

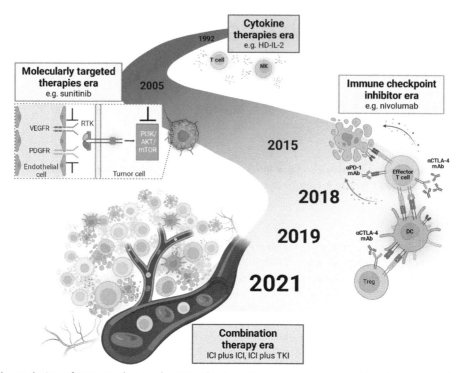

Fig. 1. The evolution of systemic therapy for RCC. This trajectory demonstrates the historical changes in the treatment of RCC, with conventional cytokine therapies, such as interleukin-2 and interferon-α since 1992, molecularly targeted therapies as antiangiogenic therapy and mTORi since 2005, and ICIs since 2015. Currently, combination therapies including ICI plus molecularly targeted therapies are the mainstay in RCC therapy. αCTLA-4 mAb, anticytotoxic T-lymphocyte antigen-4 monoclonal antibody; αPD-1 mAb, antiprogrammed cell death protein 1 monoclonal antibody; AKT, protein kinase B; DC, dendritic cell; HD-IL-2, high-dose interleukin-2; PDGFR, platelet-derived growth factor receptor; PI3K, phosphoinositide 3-kinase; RTK, receptor tyrosine kinase; TKI, tyrosine kinase inhibitor; Treg, regulatory T cell; VEGFR, vascular endothelial growth factor receptor. (Created with BioRender.com.)

these standard therapies, clinical researchers have investigated early cellular immunotherapies, including autologous lymphokine-activated killer cells therapy,[14–16] or nonmyeloablative allogeneic stem cell transplantation.[17,18]

BACKGROUND
Immune Checkpoint Inhibitor Rationale/ Mechanism

To understand the mechanism of ICIs, it is critical to first review the normal mechanism of tolerance in human immunity. The immune system has natural mechanisms to suppress an overactive response against self-targets, which is broadly known as self-tolerance.[19] Self-tolerance in T cells has two primary mechanisms: central tolerance by negative selection in the thymus and peripheral tolerance.[19,20] Peripheral tolerance consists of three major mechanisms: anergy, regulatory T cells (Treg), and the immune checkpoint system.[20,21] In cancer specifically, tumor cells escape from immune attack by T cells through multiple mechanisms, including

the recruitment of Tregs and the exploitation of immune checkpoint systems.[22]

Generally, T-cell activation requires the combination of an antigen-specific signal through T-cell receptor (TCR) and CD3 (signal 1), and costimulatory signal through several costimulatory molecules, including CD28 as a primary molecule (signal 2).[23–25] The molecule of cytotoxic T-lymphocyte antigen 4 (CTLA-4) binds more strongly to CD80/86 (ligands of CD28) on dendritic cells than CD28 as a costimulatory molecule on T cells binds to it, thereby preventing signal 2 and inhibiting proper T-cell activation.[26–28]

Activated T cells express inhibitory receptors, such as programmed cell death 1 (PD-1).[29,30] When PD-1 on T cells bind PD-1 ligands on myeloid or tumors cells, downstream signaling of TCR, such as the CD3 ζ-subunit and ZAP70, and CD28 signaling are inhibited,[30–32] inducing a state of T-cell dysfunction called "exhaustion." Cancer cells use these peripheral tolerance mechanisms of CTLA-4/CD80/86 or PD-1/PD-1 ligand axes to escape from T-cell cytotoxicity.[31,33,34]

MODERN IMMUNOTHERAPY

CTLA-4 was cloned as a new molecule on activated T cells by Golstein and colleagues in 1987.[26] About 10 years later, it was discovered that CTLA-4 has a suppressive mechanism by Allison and colleagues and Bluestone and colleagues.[35,36] Shortly thereafter, Allison and colleagues demonstrated that anti-CTLA-4 antibody treatment could suppress cancer growth in mouse models.[33] This was the first demonstration of ICI efficacy against cancer. In the first of human therapeutic studies, it was reported that ipilimumab, an anti-CTLA-4 antibody, improved survival in patients with metastatic melanoma.[37] Based on the trial, ipilimumab was approved for advanced melanoma in the United States in 2011.

PD-1 was cloned by Honjo and colleagues in 1992,[38] and it was shown that PD-1 regulates the immune system through T-cell suppression.[39] Later, it was reported that anti-PD-L1 antibody and anti-PD-1 antibody treatments had efficacy against cancer in mouse models.[31,40,41] Furthermore, it was demonstrated that PD-1 was selectively upregulated by the exhausted T cells in mice chronically infected with lymphocytic choriomeningitis virus, and anti-PD-L1 antibody was able to restore their ability to kill infected cells.[42] In 2012, nivolumab as an anti-PD-1 antibody proved efficacy in several types of cancers including melanoma and RCC.[43] In 2013, an anti-PD-1 antibody was approved for metastatic melanoma first in Japan, and it was approved for the disease next year in the United States.

Immune-Related Adverse Events

Toxicities caused by ICIs are commonly referred to as "immune-related adverse events (irAE)," because they differ from ones caused by other therapies. Because blockade of immune checkpoints interferes with peripheral tolerance system, autoreactive T cells may attack various organs in the body, causing autoimmune diseases against skin, digestive, endocrine, or nervous systems.[44] These diseases often have an acute onset, can occur after drug discontinuation, and have the potential to cause lifelong and even life-threatening complications. Common irAEs are rash, colitis, endocrinopathies (including hypothyroidism, and less commonly hypophysitis or autoimmune diabetes), and pneumonitis. Rare but potentially fatal irAEs can also occur, including myocarditis, encephalitis, gastrointestinal perforation associated with colitis, and fulminant type 1 diabetes.[9,45–47] Of note, endocrine disorders are typically permanent, and therefore lifelong hormone replacement is required in these cases. The most important

consideration in the management of irAEs is early detection, including self-monitoring, family cooperation, and physician vigilance.[48] If irAEs are suspected, ICI should be generally discontinued and, for higher grade toxicities, organ-specific symptomatic therapy should be initiated. Steroids are commonly administered in situations where the initial symptoms are severe (ie, high grade) or do not improve after treatment discontinuation and symptomatic treatment. In steroid-refractory cases, additional immunosuppressants may be used, with specific agents being used for different toxicities (eg, infliximab for colitis, mycophenolate mofetil or azathioprine for liver disorder),[48] and it is typically advised to refer the patient for subspecialty consultation. Overall, given the role of ICIs in treating advanced RCC, physicians should be aware of common and potentially serious irAEs.

Immune Checkpoint Inhibitor for Tyrosine Kinase Inhibitor–Refractory Renal Cell Carcinoma

In more than 80% of ccRCC, there is an abnormality of von Hippel–Lindau tumor suppressor (VHL) protein, typically through chromosomal loss of regions of 3p and somatic mutation of the *VHL* gene (or, less commonly, through germline mutation of *VHL* or methylation of its promoter region).[49–52] In normal oxygen conditions, VHL mediates repression of the hypoxia-inducible factors (including HIF-2α) transcriptional activity through ubiquitination and targeting for degradation. When VHL is inactive (as is the case in RCC), HIF-2α is not ubiquitinated, and as a result the HIF complex is activated even in normoxia.[53] HIF-2α activates expression of proangiogenesis factors (eg, vascular endothelial growth factor [VEGF]), prosurvival and proliferation factors (eg, cyclin D1), and metabolism (eg, GLUT1).[54,55] In addition, VHL-associated ccRCC frequently has loss-of-function mutations in genes encoding molecules associated with mTOR pathway (eg, *TSC1*, *PTEN*, and *PIK3CA*).[52] The mTOR kinase consists of complexes mTORC1 and mTORC2, and the mTORC2 signaling has the function to stabilize HIF2α.[56,57] Therefore, either VEGF receptor tyrosine kinase inhibitors (VEGFR TKIs), the anti-VEGF-A antibody, or mTOR inhibitors have been used to inhibit the VEGF signaling pathway and mTOR signaling pathway in RCC (see **Fig. 1**). These molecularly targeted therapies were at the center of RCC therapy for a decade; however, essentially all tumors ultimately develop resistance against these therapies.[58] The CheckMate 025 trial was the first phase III trial that demonstrated a clinical benefit of nivolumab (anti-PD-1 antibody) therapy compared with everolimus (mTORi) in patients with advanced RCC previously treated with VEGFR TKIs in 2015 (see **Fig. 1**).[9] The results with long-term follow-up (minimum of 64 months; median of 72 months) showed significantly improved overall survival (OS) (25.8 vs 19.7 months; hazard ratio, 0.73), objective response rate (ORR) (23 vs 4%; $P < .001$), progression-free survival (PFS) (hazard ratio, 0.84; $P = .0331$), and quality of life.[45]

First-Line Therapy (Immune Checkpoint Inhibitor Plus Immune Checkpoint Inhibitor)

The initial approval of nivolumab in the refractory setting set the stage for investigating ICI-based strategies for the front-line treatment of advanced RCC. In 2018, the CheckMate 214 trial demonstrated that the combination therapy of ipilimumab (anti-CTLA-4 antibody) plus nivolumab significantly improved ORR, PFS, and OS compared with sunitinib (VEGFR TKI) among patients with previously untreated ccRCC and International Metastatic RCC Database Consortium intermediate- and poor-risk disease (see **Fig. 1**).[46] The results with long-term follow-up (minimum of 60 months, median of 67.7 months) showed significantly improved PFS (median, 11.6 vs 8.3 months; hazard ratio, 0.73) and OS (median, 47.0 vs 26.6 months; hazard ratio, 0.68) in patients with intermediate- and poor-risk disease.[47] Also, there is a clear plateau in the PFS curve at around 25% to 30%, representing long-term response. The introduction of ICI-based therapies into the front-line treatment of RCC has substantially improved survival in this disease.

First-Line Therapy (Immune Checkpoint Inhibitor Plus Tyrosine Kinase Inhibitor)

Along with the development of ICI plus ICI combination therapy, investigators have also sought to combine ICI with other therapeutic agents with different mechanisms of action and demonstrated efficacy in advanced RCC. One potential mechanism of immune escape in cancer involves dysfunction in the DC compartment, inhibiting DC maturation and antigen presentation.[59–62] Additionally, VEGF activity in the tumor may prevent infiltration of functional immune cells into the microenvironment.[63,64] Therefore, VEGF blockade may impact DC maturation from immature precursor cells,[62,65] normalize the tumor vessels, and promote immune cell infiltration into the tumor.[64,66,67] Furthermore, VEGF inhibitors also suppress the activation of myeloid-derived suppressor cells and thereby enhance antitumor immunity.[63,68] These lines of evidence support a role for antiangiogenic agents in improving the immunosuppressive tumor microenvironment, and have served as a rationale for the combination therapy for ICI plus VEGF/VEGFR targeted drugs.

The first of these ICI plus TKI trials in advanced RCC were the KEYNOTE-426 and JAVELIN Renal 101 trials. The KEYNOTE-426 trial demonstrated superiority of pembrolizumab (anti-PD-1 antibody) and axitinib (VEGFR TKI) over sunitinib (VEGFR TKI) with respect to OS (median not reached vs 35.7 months; hazard ratio, 0.68; $P < .0003$), PFS (median, 15.1 vs 11.1 months; hazard ratio, 0.71; $P < .0001$), and ORR (59.3% vs 35.7%, respectively; $P < .0001$).[69,70] However, the JAVELIN Renal 101 trial demonstrated superiority of avelumab (anti-PD-L1 antibody) and axitinib over sunitinib with respect to PFS (median, 13.8 vs 7.0 months; hazard ratio, 0.62; $P < .0001$) in patients with PD-L1-positive tumors (OS data as the coprimary end point were immature).[71,72] These new regimens were approved by US Food and Drug Administration (FDA) in 2019. Two years later, the results of the CLEAR trial and the CheckMate 9ER trial were also published. The CLEAR trial demonstrated superiority of pembrolizumab (anti-PD-1 antibody) and lenvatinib (VEGFR TKI) over sunitinib with respect to PFS (median, 23.9 vs 9.2 months; hazard ratio, 0.39; $P < .001$), OS (hazard ratio, 0.66; $P = .005$), and ORR (67.3% vs 35.0%).[73] The CheckMate 9ER trial demonstrated superiority of nivolumab (anti-PD-1 antibody) and cabozantinib (multikinase inhibitor) over sunitinib with respect to PFS (median, 16.6 vs 8.3 months; hazard ratio, 0.51; $P < .001$), OS (hazard ratio, 0.60; $P = .001$), and ORR (55.7% vs 27.1%; $P < .001$).[74,75] These two treatment regimens (pembrolizumab plus lenvatinib, and nivolumab plus cabozantinib) were approved in 2021, and therefore there are now four innovative ICI plus TKI regimens available for first-line treatment of advanced RCC since 2019 (see **Fig. 1**, **Table 1**). In contrast, the IMmotion151 trial demonstrated superiority of atezolizumab (anti-PD-L1 antibody) and bevacizumab (anti-VEGF antibody) over sunitinib with respect to PFS in patients with PD-L1-positive tumors (median, 11.2 vs 7.7 months; hazard ratio, 0.74; $P < .0217$)[76]; however, it was not able to demonstrate superiority with respect to OS in the intention-to-treat population as coprimary end point (median, 36.1 vs 35.3 months; hazard ratio, 0.91; $P = .27$).[77]

Although one cannot directly compare these therapies because of different patient populations, there are some notable trends. The latest two regimens (pembrolizumab plus lenvatinib and nivolumab plus cabozantinib) demonstrated the lowest progression of disease (PD) rates (5.4% and

Table 1
Review of randomized phase III trials of approved regimens investigating ICI efficacy for patients with advanced RCC

PDA Approved	Study	Intervention	Control	Patients (n)	Primary End Point	Outcomes (Intervention vs Control) (month)	P Value	Reference
2015	CheckMate 025	Nivolumab	Everolimus	821	OS	25.8 vs 19.7	<.0001	9,45
2018	CheckMate 214	Ipilimumab plus nivolumab	Sunitinib	1096	OS, PFS, ORR in inter/poor risk	OS, 47.0 vs 26.6 PFS, 11.6 vs 8.3 DOR, NR vs 19.7	<.0001 .0004 <.0001	46,47
2019	KEYNOTE-426	Pembrolizumab plus axitinib	Sunitinib	861	OS, PFS	OS, NR vs 35.7 PFS, 15.4 vs 11.1	<.0003 .0001	69,70
2019	JAVELIN Renal 101	Avelumab plus axitinib	Sunitinib	886	OS, PFS in PD-L1+ (TICs)	OS, NR vs 28.6 PFS, 13.8 vs 7.0	<.1301 .0001	71,72
2021	CLEAR	Pembrolizumab plus lenvatinib	Sunitinib	1069	PFS	23.9 vs 9.2	<.001	73
2021	CheckMate 9ER	Nivolumab plus cabozantinib	Sunitinib	651	PFS	16.6 vs 8.3	<.0001	74,75

Abbreviations: DOR, duration of response; FDA, Food and Drug Administration; ICI, immune checkpoint inhibitor; NR, not reached; ORR, objective response rate; OS, overall survival; PFS, progression-free survival; RCC, renal cell carcinoma; TICs, tumor-infiltrating immune cells.

5.6%, respectively).[78] Furthermore, pembrolizumab plus lenvatinib demonstrated the highest complete response (CR) rate compared with other therapies (16.1% vs 3.8%–10%), whereas grade 3 or higher adverse event rate was the highest compared with other therapies (82.4% vs 65.0%–71.2%).[73] Although nivolumab plus cabozantinib demonstrated higher grade 3 or higher adverse event rate than sunitinib (71.2% vs 53.8%), quality of life (as measured by the 19-item Functional Assessment of Cancer Therapy-Kidney Symptom Index) was improved lower in nivolumab plus cabozantinib compared with the sunitinib group (hazard ratio, 0.63; P = .0001).[79]

Although large randomized trials have not been performed in variant RCC histology (ie, nonclear cell), numerous regimens have demonstrated efficacy in multiple histologic subtypes, including atezolizumab plus bevacizumab, nivolumab plus cabozantinib, and pembrolizumab plus lenvatinib.[80–82] However, a consistent exception is the lower efficacy of ICI-based treatment regimens in chromophobe RCC,[81] highlighting an area of unmet clinical need.

Adjuvant Therapy

There is no globally accepted adjuvant therapy for patients with RCC after surgery. In the adjuvant setting, VEGF-targeted therapies, axitinib, pazopanib, and sorafenib did not improve disease-free survival (DFS) in randomized phase III trials.[83–87] Among VEGF-targeted agents, although only sunitinib had controversial data that it demonstrated improved DFS in the S-TRAC trial (sunitinib vs placebo),[88] sunitinib did not significantly impact DFS in the ASSURE trial (sunitinib or sorafenib vs placebo),[83] and had no signal for OS benefit in both of trials.

In contrast, the KEYNOTE-564 trial of adjuvant pembrolizumab demonstrated DFS benefit for select patients with ccRCC after surgery. Patients with ccRCC who were at intermediate-high risk (stage 2 with nuclear grade 4 or sarcomatoid differentiation, tumor stage 3 or higher), high risk (T4 or regional lymph node metastasis), or metastatic (M1) but with no evidence of disease after surgery were randomly assigned to receive either adjuvant pembrolizumab or placebo for approximately 1 year. Pembrolizumab was associated with significantly longer DFS than placebo with a greater proportion of patients free of disease at 30 months (75.2 vs 65.5%; hazard ratio, 0.63). Although OS data are still immature and not yet significant, the estimated percentage of patients alive at 30 months was numerically higher in those treated with pembrolizumab (95.7% vs 91.4%;

hazard ratio, 0.52).[89,90] However, it is worth noting that other adjuvant or perioperative trials of ICI did not significantly impact DFS (ipilimumab plus nivolumab in CheckMate 914,[91] atezolizumab in IMmotion010,[92] and perioperative nivolumab in PROSPER trial[93]) (**Table 2**). These results suggested that trial eligibility (ie, including higher risk patients) and the choice of ICI agent (and associated toxicity and treatment discontinuation rates) are important considerations for patients with RCC after surgery.

With approval of pembrolizumab as the first adjuvant therapy, we have to carefully consider which patients benefit most. The absolute DFS benefit at 2 years in the KEYNOTE-564 trial was approximately a 10% increase, and although OS data are trending in an encouraging way it is not yet statistically positive.[90] Furthermore, although uncommon with single-agent use, ICIs can cause severe adverse events, including life-altering toxicities, such as type I diabetes or adrenal insufficiency. Therefore, the decision to proceed with this adjuvant therapy should be made jointly with the patient after thorough discussion of the risks and benefits.

Future Combinations

With the success of "doublet" therapies (ie, combination of two drugs, at least one of which is an ICI), a current generation of trials is exploring the potential benefit of "triplet" regimens. The COSMIC-313 trial is a phase III randomized trial of ipilimumab plus nivolumab plus cabozantinib or placebo among patients with previously untreated ccRCC and International Metastatic RCC Database Consortium intermediate- and poor-risk disease (NCT03937219). The trial demonstrated superiority of the triplet over doublet with respect to PFS (median not reached vs 11.3 months; hazard ratio, 0.73; P = .013) without available OS data.[94] Notably, the triplet therapies had higher rates of grade 3 to 4 adverse events over the doublet (73% vs 41%), therefore there were potentially early discontinuation of ipilimumab and more frequent use of steroids.[95] Another triplet trial, the MK-6482-012 trial, is investigating the combination of pembrolizumab, belzutifan (HIF-2α inhibitor), and lenvatinib, or pembrolizumab, quavonlimab (anti-CTLA-4 antibody), and lenvatinib, compared with the standard-of-care doublet combination therapy of pembrolizumab and lenvatinib for patients with previously untreated ccRCC (NCT04736706) (**Table 3**).

These cutting-edge trials may indicate that the "triplet regimen era" is just around the corner. One needs to carefully consider the fine line

Table 2
Review of randomized phase III trials of regimens investigating perioperative ICI efficacy for patients with RCC

Study	Intervention	Control	Patients (n)	Primary End Point	Outcome (Intervention vs Control)	P Value	Reference
Perioperative							
PROSPER RCC	Nivolumab	Surgery alone	819	RFS	NA	.43	93
Adjuvant							
KEYNOTE-564	Pembrolizumab	Placebo	994	DFS at 24 mo	77.3% vs 68.1%	.002	89,90
IMmotion010	Atezolizumab	Placebo	778	DFS	57.2 vs 49.5 mo	.50	92
CheckMate 914	1. Ipilimumab plus nivolumab 2. Nivolumab	Placebo	NA	DFS	NA	NA (fail to meet)	91

Abbreviations: DFS, disease-free survival; ICI, immune checkpoint inhibitor; NA, not available; RCC, renal cell carcinoma; RFS, recurrence-free survival.

between a benefits and risks. In COSMIC-313, the addition of cabozantinib to ipilimumab plus nivolumab may overcome some of the challenges with ICI plus ICI therapy, the higher primary PD rate. Although ipilimumab plus nivolumab has already demonstrated the most robust evidence for durability in combination therapies, there are 19% patients with primary progressive disease that may limit the use of this regimen in some patients with rapidly progressing disease.[47] Therefore, these triplet regimens probably may "derisk" ICI therapy; it may allow clinicals to prescribe ICI plus ICI therapy to all patients, without risking rapid progression.

In that context, one can also consider the schedule of when to start an additional agent. The PDIGREE trial is a phase III trial for patients with metastatic untreated RCC and intermediate and poor risk. Patients with CR after completing ipilimumab plus nivolumab undergo maintenance nivolumab, patients with PD switch to cabozantinib, and patients with non-CR/non-PD are randomized to continue nivolumab alone (current standard) versus nivolumab plus the addition of cabozantinib (NCT03793166). This schedule of an additional TKI for patients with suboptimal responses may minimize adverse effects by triplet agents and to select the patients who are most likely to receive benefit from a third agent.

DISCUSSION

Through the development of modern immunotherapies, the prognosis for patients with RCC has

Table 3
Review of randomized phase III trials of ongoing regimens investigating ICI efficacy for patients with previously untreated advanced RCC

Study	Intervention	Control	Primary End Point	Clinical Trial ID
COSMIC-313	Cabozantinib, ipilimumab, and nivolumab	Placebo, ipilimumab, and nivolumab	PFS	NCT03937219
MK-6482-012	1. Pembrolizumab, lenvatinib, and belzutifan 2. Pembrolizumab, lenvatinib, and quavonlimab	Pembrolizumab and lenvatinib	PFS, OS	NCT04736706

Abbreviations: ICI, immune checkpoint inhibitor; OS, overall survival; PFS, progression-free survival; RCC, renal cell carcinoma.

greatly improved over the past 5 years. Furthermore, trials including new mechanisms of action, such as HIF-2α inhibition, are certainly promising. However, with the plethora of therapeutic options, it is more important than ever to advocate for the development of personalized medicine approaches based on validated biomarkers. To address some of these challenges and to understand the underlying mechanisms of therapeutic response of ICIs, many studies of other solid tumors have investigated predictive biomarkers of ICI response, including tumor mutation burdens, the presence of microsatellite instability from defects in DNA mismatch repair mechanisms, and CD8 infiltration within the tumor microenvironment.[96–99] However, these biomarkers do not seem to be associated with ICI efficacy in RCC.[100] RCC has a modest tumor mutation burden, and higher mutation burden is not associated with improved ICI response in this disease.[101–103] Furthermore, CD8+ T-cell infiltration is not associated with improved response or survival with ICI across multiple trials.[100,104] Although these results suggest that the underlying RCC immunobiology is likely different from other ICI-responsive solid tumors,[105] the RCC-specific mechanisms of effective antitumor immunity have not been fully elucidated. One consistent histologic biomarker that has emerged is the presence of sarcomatoid differentiation being associated with substantially improved ORR (and CR rate) compared with TKIs in RCC.[106,107] One possible mechanisms of ICI efficacy in sarcomatoid RCC is high expression of PD-1 ligands in tumor cells,[106] although there are certainly other mechanisms at play. Similarly, it was reported that sarcomatoid RCC had higher PD-L1 expression and higher CD8+PD-1+ T-cell density than ccRCC in an immunohistochemical analysis of 210 clinical samples.[108] These results suggest a need to further dissect the immunobiology of ccRCC to fully understand effective antitumor immunity with ICI in this histology.

Future Directions

ICI-based therapies have improved the outcomes of patients with advanced RCC, and for some patients, have even led to durable responses or even cure. Although these cases prove the concept that immunotherapies can lead to long-term survival in patients with advanced RCC, primary and acquired resistance to these therapies remains a fundamental unsolved issue for most patients. Moving forward, a new generation of therapies to overcome these challenges is required. To rationally design next-generation immunotherapies, it will be critical to understand RCC-specific biology underlying effective antitumor immunity.[105] Previous reports have demonstrated that multiple immunosuppressive mechanisms are at work in advanced RCC, including other inhibitory immune checkpoint molecules[109,110]; tumor-associated macrophages[111,112]; Tregs[113]; and an immunologically unfavorable cytokine milieu, including higher levels of IL-8.[114,115]

Among these targets, numerous clinical trials of antibodies targeting other inhibitory immune checkpoints, including lymphocyte-activation gene 3 (LAG-3),[116] T-cell immunoglobulin and ITIM domain (TIGIT),[117,118] and T-cell immunoglobulin and mucin-domain containing-3 (TIM-3),[119] are ongoing in RCC and in other solid tumors (**Fig. 2**). For example, a coformulation of nivolumab and the anti-LAG-3 antibody relatlimab were FDA-approved in 2022 for patients with advanced melanoma, and early trials are exploring this combination in RCC (NCT02996110; FRACTION-RCC, NCT05148546, NCT03849469, NCT02465060).[105]

Beyond targeting the T-cell compartment, it is clear now that the myeloid compartment plays a key immunosuppressive role in RCC and should be therapeutically targeted as well.[109] IL-8 (also known as CXCL8), is one of ligands of CXCR2 that requires tumor-associated macrophages,[120] myeloid-derived suppressor cells,[121,122] or neutrophils,[123] which are all associated with immune suppression within the tumor microenvironment. High plasma levels of IL-8 were reported to correlate with poor ICI efficacy in patients with advanced RCC treated by atezolizumab in the phase II IMmotion150 trial.[114] A combination trial with anti-IL-8 antibody (BMS-986253) is ongoing now (NCT03400332) (see **Fig. 2**).

Beyond conventional immunotherapies, we are also witnessing the development of novel antigen-specific therapies for ccRCC, including vaccination therapy and adoptive cellular therapies. Vaccination against cancer-specific antigens is a classical method steering the immune system toward tumor epitopes, and clinical trials of shared antigen-specific vaccination were performed, such as targeting CAIX,[124] VEGF-R1,[125] HIG2,[126] mutant VHL,[127] MUC1,[128] or WT-1.[129] Although these studies showed an increase in antigen-specific T cells and/or release of cytotoxic cytokines, objective antitumor effects were not significantly impacted.[130,131] To increase antigen priming and vaccine-induced T-cell responses, trials with multiepitope vaccines have been developed, including a peptide-based personalized neoantigen vaccination (with or without ipilimumab; NCT04024878), and an mRNA-based personalized neoantigen multiepitope vaccine

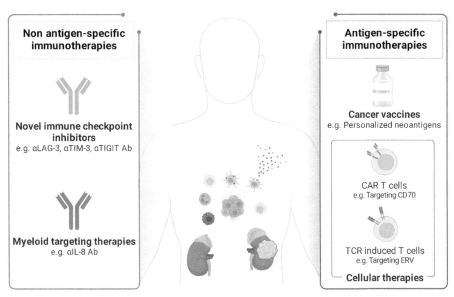

Fig. 2. Emerging immunotherapies in RCC. These are promising nonantigen-specific immunotherapies in ongoing clinical trials, targeting immunosuppressive mechanisms at work in advanced RCC, including other inhibitory immune checkpoint molecules, the myeloid cell compartment, and the immunologically unfavorable cytokine milieu, such as IL-8. Numerous clinical trials of antibodies targeting other ICIs are underway, including LAG-3, TIM-3, and TIGIT. Furthermore, IL-8 is one of the ligands of CXCR2 that recruits immunosuppressive TAMs, MDSCs, and neutrophils. A combination trial with anti-IL-8 antibody targeting these immunosuppressive cells is ongoing now. Novel antigen-specific therapies also have investigated for ccRCC, including vaccination therapy (including personalized neoantigen vaccines) and adoptive cellular therapies, such as CAR T-cell therapy, and ERV-specific TCR T-cell therapy. (Created with BioRender.com.)

combined with the anti-PD-L1 antibody (NCT03289962) (see **Fig. 2**).

Vaccination therapy indirectly activates antigen-specific T cells through antigen-presenting cells, whereas adoptive T-cell therapy directly transfers antigen-specific effector cells into patients.[130] Building on recent success of chimeric antigen receptor (CAR) T-cell therapies in hematologic malignancies, trials are now being developed for solid tumors.[132] Among patients with advanced RCC, the most promising surface target for CAR T therapy is the CD70 antigen, which is currently being investigated in multiple active trials (NCT02830724; NCT04438083; NCT04696731) (see **Fig. 2**).[133,134]

Beyond targeting surface epitopes (ie, antigens found on the surface of tumor cells), genetically modified T-cell therapies expressing antigen-specific TCRs have also been investigated.[135] The most significant difference between CAR and TCR-induced therapy is whether the treatment targets the surface antigen or the complex of HLA and peptide (which can derive from an intracellular protein). Therefore, engineered TCR-based T-cell therapies could target endogenous antigens, including overexpressed proteins more than normal tissue, cancer-testis antigens,

neoantigens derived from nonsynonymous somatic mutations, or aberrant expression of human endogenous retroviruses.[105] It is worth noting that re-expression of normally quiescent endogenous retroviruses sequence might occur with epigenetic dysregulation preferentially in RCC more than other tumors.[130,136,137] It was reported that retroviral epitopes are widely shared among patients,[138] and engineered TCR therapy targeting a specific endogenous retrovirus is ongoing (NCT03354390) (see **Fig. 2**). Most adoptive T-cell therapies use autologous T cells; however, this approach is costly, time consuming, and depends on the quality of the patient's T cells. To resolve these issues, more recent trials are exploring allogeneic products, "off-the-shelf" therapeutic T cells modified to prevent clearance and graft-versus-host disease, or derived from pluripotent stem cells.[139,140] These promising studies may herald the beginning of precision immunotherapy for RCC.

SUMMARY

With the introduction of ICIs, the treatment of RCC has experienced a true paradigm shift. Between 2018 and 2021, five combination therapies (one

ICI plus ICI, and four ICI plus TKI regimens) were added to first-line therapeutic armamentarium for patients with advanced RCC. In 2021 pembrolizumab was also approved by the FDA as adjuvant therapy for patients with RCC at high risk for recurrence after nephrectomy. These treatments have dramatically improved outcomes for patients with RCC, and the next generation of immunotherapies may further improve the lives of patients living with this disease.

CLINICS CARE POINTS

- Although the choice of therapy should always be individualized, ICI-based combination therapies should be considered for all patients with previously untreated advanced clear cell RCC.

- The choice between ICI plus ICI therapy or ICI plus TKI therapy should be individualized; considerations include durability of response, need for immediate response, and toxicity.

- Pembrolizumab is approved as adjuvant therapy in patients with clear cell RCC and patients with high risk for recurrence after nephrectomy.

- A new generation of immunotherapies targeting novel immune checkpoints, inhibiting the myeloid compartment, and providing antigen-specific immune targeting offers hope that therapy for advanced RCC will continue to improve.

DISCLOSURE

D.A. Braun reports nonfinancial support from Bristol Myers Squibb; honoraria from LM Education/Exchange Services; advisory board fees from Exelixis and AVEO; personal fees from Charles River Associates, Schlesinger Associates, Imprint Science, Insight Strategy, Trinity Group, Cancer Expert Now, Adnovate Strategies, MDedge, CancerNetwork, Catenion, OncLive, Cello Health Bio-Consulting, PWW Consulting, Haymarket Medical Network, Aptitude Health, ASCO Post/Harborside, Targeted Oncology, and AbbVie; and research support from Exelixis, outside of the submitted work.

REFERENCES

1. Bukowski RM. Natural history and therapy of metastatic renal cell carcinoma: the role of interleukin-2. Cancer 1997;80(7):1198–220.

2. Interferon-alpha and survival in metastatic renal carcinoma: early results of a randomised controlled trial. Medical Research Council Renal Cancer Collaborators. Lancet 1999;353(9146):14–7.

3. Motzer RJ, Hutson TE, Tomczak P, et al. Sunitinib versus interferon alfa in metastatic renal-cell carcinoma. N Engl J Med 2007;356(2):115–24.

4. Hudes G, Carducci M, Tomczak P, et al. Temsirolimus, interferon alfa, or both for advanced renal-cell carcinoma. N Engl J Med 2007;356(22):2271–81.

5. Motzer RJ, Escudier B, Oudard S, et al. Efficacy of everolimus in advanced renal cell carcinoma: a double-blind, randomised, placebo-controlled phase III trial. Lancet 2008;372(9637):449–56.

6. Sternberg CN, Davis ID, Mardiak J, et al. Pazopanib in locally advanced or metastatic renal cell carcinoma: results of a randomized phase III trial. J Clin Oncol 2010;28(6):1061–8.

7. Rini BI, Escudier B, Tomczak P, et al. Comparative effectiveness of axitinib versus sorafenib in advanced renal cell carcinoma (AXIS): a randomised phase 3 trial. Lancet 2011;378(9807):1931–9.

8. Postow MA, Callahan MK, Wolchok JD. Immune checkpoint blockade in cancer therapy. J Clin Oncol 2015;33(17):1974–82.

9. Motzer RJ, Escudier B, McDermott DF, et al. Nivolumab versus everolimus in advanced renal-cell carcinoma. N Engl J Med 2015;373(19):1803–13.

10. Motzer RJ, Jonasch E, Agarwal N, et al. Kidney cancer, Version 3.2022, NCCN Clinical Practice Guidelines in Oncology. J Natl Compr Canc Netw 2022;20(1):71–90.

11. Cole WH. Spontaneous regression of cancer and the importance of finding its cause. Natl Cancer Inst Monogr 1976;44:5–9.

12. Motzer RJ, Bander NH, Nanus DM. Renal-cell carcinoma. N Engl J Med 1996;335(12):865–75.

13. Klapper JA, Downey SG, Smith FO, et al. High-dose interleukin-2 for the treatment of metastatic renal cell carcinoma: a retrospective analysis of response and survival in patients treated in the surgery branch at the National Cancer Institute between 1986 and 2006. Cancer 2008;113(2):293–301.

14. Rosenberg SA, Lotze MT, Muul LM, et al. A progress report on the treatment of 157 patients with advanced cancer using lymphokine-activated killer cells and interleukin-2 or high-dose interleukin-2 alone. N Engl J Med 1987;316(15):889–97.

15. Fisher RI, Coltman CA Jr, Doroshow JH, et al. Metastatic renal cancer treated with interleukin-2 and lymphokine-activated killer cells. A phase II clinical trial. Ann Intern Med 1988;108(4):518–23.

16. Negrier S, Philip T, Stoter G, et al. Interleukin-2 with or without LAK cells in metastatic renal cell

carcinoma: a report of a European multicentre study. Eur J Cancer Clin Oncol 1989;25(Suppl 3): S21–8.

17. Childs RW, Clave E, Tisdale J, et al. Successful treatment of metastatic renal cell carcinoma with a nonmyeloablative allogeneic peripheral-blood progenitor-cell transplant: evidence for a graft-versus-tumor effect. J Clin Oncol 1999;17(7): 2044–9.

18. Childs RW. Nonmyeloablative allogeneic peripheral blood stem-cell transplantation as immunotherapy for malignant diseases. Cancer J May-Jun 2000; 6(3):179–87.

19. Grossman Z, Paul WE. Self-tolerance: context dependent tuning of T cell antigen recognition. Semin Immunol 2000;12(3):197–203. ; discussion 257-344.

20. Goodnow CC, Sprent J, Fazekas de St Groth B, et al. Cellular and genetic mechanisms of self tolerance and autoimmunity. Nature 2005;435(7042): 590–7.

21. Sakaguchi S. Regulatory T cells: key controllers of immunologic self-tolerance. Cell 2000;101(5): 455–8.

22. Wherry EJ, Kurachi M. Molecular and cellular insights into T cell exhaustion. Nat Rev Immunol 2015;15(8):486–99.

23. Lafferty KJ, Misko IS, Cooley MA. Allogeneic stimulation modulates the in vitro response of T cells to transplantation antigen. Nature 1974;249(454): 275–6.

24. Riley JL, Mao M, Kobayashi S, et al. Modulation of TCR-induced transcriptional profiles by ligation of CD28, ICOS, and CTLA-4 receptors. Proc Natl Acad Sci U S A 2002;99(18):11790–5.

25. Diehn M, Alizadeh AA, Rando OJ, et al. Genomic expression programs and the integration of the CD28 costimulatory signal in T cell activation. Proc Natl Acad Sci U S A 2002;99(18):11796–801.

26. Brunet JF, Denizot F, Luciani MF, et al. A new member of the immunoglobulin superfamily–CTLA-4. Nature 1987;328(6127):267–70.

27. Dariavach P, Mattéi MG, Golstein P, et al. Human Ig superfamily CTLA-4 gene: chromosomal localization and identity of protein sequence between murine and human CTLA-4 cytoplasmic domains. Eur J Immunol 1988;18(12):1901–5.

28. Linsley PS, Greene JL, Brady W, et al. Human B7-1 (CD80) and B7-2 (CD86) bind with similar avidities but distinct kinetics to CD28 and CTLA-4 receptors. Immunity 1994;1(9):793–801.

29. Parry RV, Chemnitz JM, Frauwirth KA, et al. CTLA-4 and PD-1 receptors inhibit T-cell activation by distinct mechanisms. Mol Cell Biol 2005;25(21): 9543–53.

30. Freeman GJ, Long AJ, Iwai Y, et al. Engagement of the PD-1 immunoinhibitory receptor by a novel B7 family member leads to negative regulation of lymphocyte activation. J Exp Med 2000;192(7): 1027–34.

31. Iwai Y, Ishida M, Tanaka Y, et al. Involvement of PD-L1 on tumor cells in the escape from host immune system and tumor immunotherapy by PD-L1 blockade. Proc Natl Acad Sci U S A 2002;99(19): 12293–7.

32. Hui E, Cheung J, Zhu J, et al. T cell costimulatory receptor CD28 is a primary target for PD-1-mediated inhibition. Science 2017;355(6332):1428–33.

33. Leach DR, Krummel MF, Allison JP. Enhancement of antitumor immunity by CTLA-4 blockade. Science 1996;271(5256):1734–6.

34. Waldman AD, Fritz JM, Lenardo MJ. A guide to cancer immunotherapy: from T cell basic science to clinical practice. Nat Rev Immunol 2020;20(11): 651–68.

35. Krummel MF, Allison JP. CD28 and CTLA-4 have opposing effects on the response of T cells to stimulation. J Exp Med 1995;182(2):459–65.

36. Tivol EA, Borriello F, Schweitzer AN, et al. Loss of CTLA-4 leads to massive lymphoproliferation and fatal multiorgan tissue destruction, revealing a critical negative regulatory role of CTLA-4. Immunity 1995;3(5):541–7.

37. Hodi FS, O'Day SJ, McDermott DF, et al. Improved survival with ipilimumab in patients with metastatic melanoma. N Engl J Med Aug 19 2010;363(8): 711–23.

38. Ishida Y, Agata Y, Shibahara K, et al. Induced expression of PD-1, a novel member of the immunoglobulin gene superfamily, upon programmed cell death. Embo J 1992;11(11):3887–95.

39. Nishimura H, Nose M, Hiai H, et al. Development of lupus-like autoimmune diseases by disruption of the PD-1 gene encoding an ITIM motif-carrying immunoreceptor. Immunity 1999;11(2):141–51.

40. Iwai Y, Terawaki S, Honjo T. PD-1 blockade inhibits hematogenous spread of poorly immunogenic tumor cells by enhanced recruitment of effector T cells. Int Immunol 2005;17(2):133–44.

41. Hirano F, Kaneko K, Tamura H, et al. Blockade of B7-H1 and PD-1 by monoclonal antibodies potentiates cancer therapeutic immunity. Cancer Res 2005;65(3):1089–96.

42. Barber DL, Wherry EJ, Masopust D, et al. Restoring function in exhausted CD8 T cells during chronic viral infection. Nature 2006;439(7077):682–7.

43. Topalian SL, Hodi FS, Brahmer JR, et al. Safety, activity, and immune correlates of anti-PD-1 antibody in cancer. N Engl J Med Jun 28 2012;366(26): 2443–54.

44. Michot JM, Bigenwald C, Champiat S, et al. Immune-related adverse events with immune checkpoint blockade: a comprehensive review. Eur J Cancer 2016;54:139–48.

45. Motzer RJ, Escudier B, George S, et al. Nivolumab versus everolimus in patients with advanced renal cell carcinoma: updated results with long-term follow-up of the randomized, open-label, phase 3 CheckMate 025 trial. Cancer 2020;126(18): 4156–67.

46. Motzer RJ, Tannir NM, McDermott DF, et al. Nivolumab plus ipilimumab versus sunitinib in advanced renal-cell carcinoma. N Engl J Med 2018;378(14): 1277–90.

47. Motzer RJ, McDermott DF, Escudier B, et al. Conditional survival and long-term efficacy with nivolumab plus ipilimumab versus sunitinib in patients with advanced renal cell carcinoma. Cancer 2022;128(11):2085–97.

48. Brahmer JR, Lacchetti C, Schneider BJ, et al. Management of immune-related adverse events in patients treated with immune checkpoint inhibitor therapy: American Society of Clinical Oncology Clinical Practice Guideline. J Clin Oncol Jun 10 2018;36(17):1714–68.

49. Kaelin WG. Von Hippel-Lindau disease. Annu Rev Pathol 2007;2:145–73.

50. Sgambati MT, Stolle C, Choyke PL, et al. Mosaicism in von Hippel-Lindau disease: lessons from kindreds with germline mutations identified in offspring with mosaic parents. Am J Hum Genet 2000;66(1):84–91.

51. Latif F, Tory K, Gnarra J, et al. Identification of the von Hippel-Lindau disease tumor suppressor gene. Science May 28 1993;260(5112):1317–20.

52. Comprehensive molecular characterization of clear cell renal cell carcinoma. Nature Jul 4 2013; 499(7456):43–9.

53. Bratslavsky G, Sudarshan S, Neckers L, et al. Pseudohypoxic pathways in renal cell carcinoma. Clin Cancer Res Aug 15 2007;13(16):4667–71.

54. Kaelin WG Jr. The von Hippel-Lindau tumour suppressor protein: O2 sensing and cancer. Nat Rev Cancer 2008;8(11):865–73.

55. Choueiri TK, Kaelin WG Jr. Targeting the HIF2-VEGF axis in renal cell carcinoma. Nat Med Oct 2020;26(10):1519–30. https://doi.org/10.1038/s41591-020-1093-z.

56. Saxton RA, Sabatini DM. mTOR signaling in growth, metabolism, and disease. Cell 2017; 168(6):960–76.

57. Toschi A, Lee E, Gadir N, et al. Differential dependence of hypoxia-inducible factors 1 alpha and 2 alpha on mTORC1 and mTORC2. J Biol Chem 2008;283(50):34495–9.

58. van Beijnum JR, Nowak-Sliwinska P, Huijbers EJ, et al. The great escape; the hallmarks of resistance to antiangiogenic therapy. Pharmacol Rev 2015; 67(2):441–61.

59. Gabrilovich DI, Ciernik IF, Carbone DP. Dendritic cells in antitumor immune responses. I. Defective antigen presentation in tumor-bearing hosts. Cell Immunol 1996;170(1):101–10.

60. Chaux P, Favre N, Martin M, et al. Tumor-infiltrating dendritic cells are defective in their antigen-presenting function and inducible B7 expression in rats. Int J Cancer 1997;72(4):619–24.

61. Gabrilovich DI, Corak J, Ciernik IF, et al. Decreased antigen presentation by dendritic cells in patients with breast cancer. Clin Cancer Res 1997;3(3): 483–90.

62. Gabrilovich D, Ishida T, Oyama T, et al. Vascular endothelial growth factor inhibits the development of dendritic cells and dramatically affects the differentiation of multiple hematopoietic lineages in vivo. Blood Dec 1 1998;92(11):4150–66.

63. Hegde PS, Wallin JJ, Mancao C. Predictive markers of anti-VEGF and emerging role of angiogenesis inhibitors as immunotherapeutics. Semin Cancer Biol Oct 2018;52(Pt 2):117–24.

64. Fukumura D, Kloepper J, Amoozgar Z, et al. Enhancing cancer immunotherapy using antiangiogenics: opportunities and challenges. Nat Rev Clin Oncol May 2018;15(5):325–40.

65. Gabrilovich DI, Chen HL, Girgis KR, et al. Production of vascular endothelial growth factor by human tumors inhibits the functional maturation of dendritic cells. Nat Med Oct 1996;2(10):1096–103.

66. Wallin JJ, Bendell JC, Funke R, et al. Atezolizumab in combination with bevacizumab enhances antigen-specific T-cell migration in metastatic renal cell carcinoma. Nat Commun Aug 30 2016;7: 12624.

67. Jain RK. Normalizing tumor vasculature with anti-angiogenic therapy: a new paradigm for combination therapy. Nat Med 2001;7(9):987–9.

68. Yuan H, Cai P, Li Q, et al. Axitinib augments anti-tumor activity in renal cell carcinoma via STAT3-dependent reversal of myeloid-derived suppressor cell accumulation. Biomed Pharmacother Jul 2014; 68(6):751–6.

69. Rini BI, Plimack ER, Stus V, et al. Pembrolizumab plus axitinib versus sunitinib for advanced renal-cell carcinoma. N Engl J Med 2019;380(12): 1116–27.

70. Powles T, Plimack ER, Soulières D, et al. Pembrolizumab plus axitinib versus sunitinib monotherapy as first-line treatment of advanced renal cell carcinoma (KEYNOTE-426): extended follow-up from a randomised, open-label, phase 3 trial. Lancet Oncol Dec 2020;21(12):1563–73.

71. Motzer RJ, Penkov K, Haanen J, et al. Avelumab plus axitinib versus sunitinib for advanced renal-cell carcinoma. N Engl J Med 2019;380(12): 1103–15.

72. Choueiri TK, Motzer RJ, Rini BI, et al. Updated efficacy results from the JAVELIN Renal 101 trial: first-line avelumab plus axitinib versus sunitinib in

patients with advanced renal cell carcinoma. Ann Oncol Aug 2020;31(8):1030–9.

73. Motzer R, Alekseev B, Rha SY, et al. Lenvatinib plus pembrolizumab or everolimus for advanced renal cell carcinoma. N Engl J Med Apr 8 2021; 384(14):1289–300.

74. Choueiri TK, Powles T, Burotto M, et al. Nivolumab plus cabozantinib versus sunitinib for advanced renal-cell carcinoma. N Engl J Med 2021;384(9): 829–41.

75. Motzer RJ, Powles T, Burotto M, et al. Nivolumab plus cabozantinib versus sunitinib in first-line treatment for advanced renal cell carcinoma (Check-Mate 9ER): long-term follow-up results from an open-label, randomised, phase 3 trial. Lancet Oncol 2022;23(7):888–98.

76. Rini BI, Powles T, Atkins MB, et al. Atezolizumab plus bevacizumab versus sunitinib in patients with previously untreated metastatic renal cell carcinoma (IMmotion151): a multicentre, open-label, phase 3, randomised controlled trial. Lancet 2019;393(10189):2404–15.

77. Motzer RJ, Powles T, Atkins MB, et al. Final overall survival and molecular analysis in IMmotion151, a phase 3 trial comparing atezolizumab plus bevacizumab vs sunitinib in patients with previously untreated metastatic renal cell carcinoma. JAMA Oncol 2022;8(2):275–80.

78. Hahn AW, Msaouel P, Tannir NM. CLEAR Trial: is lenvatinib plus pembrolizumab the best first-line immunotherapy doublet in metastatic renal cell carcinoma? In: The ASCO Post. Available at: https://ascopost.com/issues/april-25-2021/clear-trial-is-lenvatinib-plus-pembrolizumab-the-best-first-line-immunotherapy-doublet-in-metastatic-renal-cell-carcinoma/. Accessed September 23, 2022.

79. Cella D, Motzer RJ, Suarez C, et al. Patient-reported outcomes with first-line nivolumab plus cabozantinib versus sunitinib in patients with advanced renal cell carcinoma treated in Check-Mate 9ER: an open-label, randomised, phase 3 trial. Lancet Oncol 2022;23(2):292–303.

80. McGregor BA, McKay RR, Braun DA, et al. Results of a multicenter phase II study of atezolizumab and bevacizumab for patients with metastatic renal cell carcinoma with variant histology and/or sarcomatoid features. J Clin Oncol 2020;38(1): 63–70.

81. Lee CH, Voss MH, Carlo MI, et al. Phase II trial of cabozantinib plus nivolumab in patients with non-clear-cell renal cell carcinoma and genomic correlates. J Clin Oncol 20 2022;40(21):2333–41.

82. Lee C-H, Li C, Perini RF, et al. KEYNOTE-B61: open-label phase 2 study of pembrolizumab in combination with lenvatinib as first-line treatment for non-clear cell renal cell carcinoma (nccRCC). J Clin Oncol 2021;39.

83. Haas NB, Manola J, Uzzo RG, et al. Adjuvant sunitinib or sorafenib for high-risk, non-metastatic renal-cell carcinoma (ECOG-ACRIN E2805): a double-blind, placebo-controlled, randomised, phase 3 trial. Lancet May 14 2016;387(10032): 2008–16.

84. Haas NB, Manola J, Dutcher JP, et al. Adjuvant treatment for high-risk clear cell renal cancer: updated results of a high-risk subset of the ASSURE randomized trial. JAMA Oncol Sep 1 2017;3(9): 1249–52.

85. Motzer RJ, Haas NB, Donskov F, et al. Randomized phase III trial of adjuvant pazopanib versus placebo after nephrectomy in patients with localized or locally advanced renal cell carcinoma. J Clin Oncol Dec 10 2017;35(35):3916–23.

86. Sun M, Marconi L, Eisen T, et al. Adjuvant vascular endothelial growth factor-targeted therapy in renal cell carcinoma: a systematic review and pooled analysis. Eur Urol. Nov 2018;74(5):611–20.

87. Gross-Goupil M, Kwon TG, Eto M, et al. Axitinib versus placebo as an adjuvant treatment of renal cell carcinoma: results from the phase III, randomized ATLAS trial. Ann Oncol Dec 1 2018;29(12): 2371–8.

88. Ravaud A, Motzer RJ, Pandha HS, et al. Adjuvant sunitinib in high-risk renal-cell carcinoma after nephrectomy. N Engl J Med Dec 8 2016;375(23): 2246–54. https://doi.org/10.1056/NEJMoa1611406.

89. Choueiri TK, Tomczak P, Park SH, et al. Adjuvant pembrolizumab after nephrectomy in renal-cell carcinoma. N Engl J Med Aug 19 2021;385(8):683–94.

90. Powles T, Tomczak P, Park SH, et al. Pembrolizumab versus placebo as post-nephrectomy adjuvant therapy for clear cell renal cell carcinoma (KEYNOTE-564): 30-month follow-up analysis of a multicentre, randomised, double-blind, placebo-controlled, phase 3 trial. Lancet Oncol 2022; 23(9):1133–44.

91. Bex A, Russo P, Tomita Y, et al. A phase III, randomized, placebo-controlled trial of nivolumab or nivolumab plus ipilimumab in patients with localized renal cell carcinoma at high-risk of relapse after radical or partial nephrectomy (CheckMate 914). American Society of Clinical Oncology 2020;38(15):suppl.

92. Pal SK, Uzzo R, Karam JA, et al. Adjuvant atezolizumab versus placebo for patients with renal cell carcinoma at increased risk of recurrence following resection (IMmotion010): a multicentre, randomised, double-blind, phase 3 trial. Lancet 2022. https://doi.org/10.1016/s0140-6736(22)01658-0.

93. Haas NB, Puligandla M, Allaf ME, et al. PROSPER: phase III randomized study comparing perioperative nivolumab versus observation in patients with renal cell carcinoma (RCC) undergoing

nephrectomy (ECOG-ACRIN EA8143). American Society of Clinical Oncology 2020;38(15):suppl.

94. Choueiri TK. ESMO 2022: Phase 3 Study of Cabozantinib in Combination With Nivolumab and Ipilimumab in Previously Untreated Advanced Renal Cell Carcinoma of Imdc Intermediate or Poor Risk (COSMIC-313). In: ESMO 2022 Kidney Cancer. Available at: https://www.urotoday.com/conference-highlights/esmo-2022/esmo-2022-kidney-cancer/139513-esmo-2022-lba8-phase-3-study-of-cabozantinib-c-in-combination-with-nivolumab-n-and-ipilimumab-i-in-previously-untreated-advanced-renal-cell-carcinoma-arcc-of-imdc-intermediate-or-poor-risk-cosmic-313.html. Accessed September 23, 2022.

95. Pal SK. ESMO 2022: Invited Discussant: Results of COSMIC-313. In: ESMO 2022 Kidney Cancer. Available at: https://www.urotoday.com/conference-highlights/esmo-2022/esmo-2022-kidney-cancer/139522-esmo-2022-invited-discussant-lba8.html. Accessed September 23, 2022.

96. Cristescu R, Mogg R, Ayers M, et al. Pan-tumor genomic biomarkers for PD-1 checkpoint blockade-based immunotherapy. Science Oct 12 2018;362(6411). https://doi.org/10.1126/science.aar3593.

97. Le DT, Uram JN, Wang H, et al. PD-1 blockade in tumors with mismatch-repair deficiency. N Engl J Med Jun 25 2015;372(26):2509–20.

98. Le DT, Durham JN, Smith KN, et al. Mismatch repair deficiency predicts response of solid tumors to PD-1 blockade. Science Jul 28 2017;357(6349):409–13.

99. Bruni D, Angell HK, Galon J. The immune contexture and Immunoscore in cancer prognosis and therapeutic efficacy. Nat Rev Cancer 2020;20(11):662–80.

100. Braun DA, Hou Y, Bakouny Z, et al. Interplay of somatic alterations and immune infiltration modulates response to PD-1 blockade in advanced clear cell renal cell carcinoma. Nat Med 2020;26(6):909–18.

101. Yarchoan M, Hopkins A, Jaffee EM. Tumor mutational burden and response rate to PD-1 inhibition. N Engl J Med Dec 21 2017;377(25):2500–1.

102. Latham A, Srinivasan P, Kemel Y, et al. Microsatellite instability is associated with the presence of Lynch syndrome pan-cancer. J Clin Oncol Feb 1 2019;37(4):286–95.

103. Mandal R, Samstein RM, Lee KW, et al. Genetic diversity of tumors with mismatch repair deficiency influences anti-PD-1 immunotherapy response. Science May 3 2019;364(6439):485–91.

104. Motzer RJ, Choueiri TK, McDermott DF, et al. Biomarker analysis from CheckMate 214: nivolumab plus ipilimumab versus sunitinib in renal cell carcinoma. J Immunother Cancer. Mar 2022;10(3).

105. Braun DA, Bakouny Z, Hirsch L, et al. Beyond conventional immune-checkpoint inhibition: novel immunotherapies for renal cell carcinoma. Nat Rev Clin Oncol Apr 2021;18(4):199–214.

106. Bakouny Z, Braun DA, Shukla SA, et al. Integrative molecular characterization of sarcomatoid and rhabdoid renal cell carcinoma. Nat Commun Feb 5 2021;12(1):808.

107. Tannir NM, Signoretti S, Choueiri TK, et al. Efficacy and safety of nivolumab plus ipilimumab versus sunitinib in first-line treatment of patients with advanced sarcomatoid renal cell carcinoma. Clin Cancer Res Jan 1 2021;27(1):78–86.

108. Kawakami F, Sircar K, Rodriguez-Canales J, et al. Programmed cell death ligand 1 and tumor-infiltrating lymphocyte status in patients with renal cell carcinoma and sarcomatoid dedifferentiation. Cancer Dec 15 2017;123(24):4823–31.

109. Braun DA, Street K, Burke KP, et al. Progressive immune dysfunction with advancing disease stage in renal cell carcinoma. Cancer Cell May 10 2021;39(5):632–48.e8.

110. Kraehenbuehl L, Weng CH, Eghbali S, et al. Enhancing immunotherapy in cancer by targeting emerging immunomodulatory pathways. Nat Rev Clin Oncol 2022;19(1):37–50.

111. Xu L, Zhu Y, Chen L, et al. Prognostic value of diametrically polarized tumor-associated macrophages in renal cell carcinoma. Ann Surg Oncol Sep 2014;21(9):3142–50.

112. Hakimi AA, Voss MH, Kuo F, et al. Transcriptomic profiling of the tumor microenvironment reveals distinct subgroups of clear cell renal cell cancer: data from a randomized phase III trial. Cancer Discov Apr 2019;9(4):510–25.

113. Davidsson S, Fiorentino M, Giunchi F, et al. Infiltration of M2 macrophages and regulatory T cells plays a role in recurrence of renal cell carcinoma. Eur Urol Open 2020;20:62–71.

114. Yuen KC, Liu LF, Gupta V, et al. High systemic and tumor-associated IL-8 correlates with reduced clinical benefit of PD-L1 blockade. Nat Med 2020;26(5):693–8.

115. Bakouny Z, Choueiri TK. IL-8 and cancer prognosis on immunotherapy. Nat Med 2020;26(5):650–1.

116. Sauer N, Szlasa W, Jonderko L, et al. LAG-3 as a potent target for novel anticancer therapies of a wide range of tumors. Int J Mol Sci 2022;23(17). https://doi.org/10.3390/ijms23179958.

117. Florou V, Garrido-Laguna I. Clinical development of anti-TIGIT antibodies for immunotherapy of cancer. Curr Oncol Rep 2022;24(9):1107–12.

118. Annese T, Tamma R, Ribatti D. Update in TIGIT immune-checkpoint role in cancer. Front Oncol 2022;12:871085.

119. Gomes de Morais AL, Cerdá S, de Miguel M. New checkpoint inhibitors on the road: targeting TIM-3

in solid tumors. Curr Oncol Rep May 2022;24(5): 651–8.

120. Hosono M, Koma YI, Takase N, et al. CXCL8 derived from tumor-associated macrophages and esophageal squamous cell carcinomas contributes to tumor progression by promoting migration and invasion of cancer cells. Oncotarget Dec 1 2017; 8(62):106071–88.

121. Korbecki J, Kupnicka P, Chlubek M, et al. CXCR2 receptor: regulation of expression, signal transduction, and involvement in cancer. Int J Mol Sci 2022; 23(4). https://doi.org/10.3390/ijms23042168.

122. Najjar YG, Rayman P, Jia X, et al. Myeloid-derived suppressor cell subset accumulation in renal cell carcinoma parenchyma is associated with intratumoral expression of IL1β, IL8, CXCL5, and Mip-1α. Clin Cancer Res May 1 2017;23(9):2346–55.

123. Jaillon S, Ponzetta A, Di Mitri D, et al. Neutrophil diversity and plasticity in tumour progression and therapy. Nat Rev Cancer 2020;20(9):485–503.

124. Uemura H, Fujimoto K, Tanaka M, et al. A phase I trial of vaccination of CA9-derived peptides for HLA-A24-positive patients with cytokine-refractory metastatic renal cell carcinoma. Clin Cancer Res 2006;12(6):1768–75.

125. Yoshimura K, Minami T, Nozawa M, et al. Phase I clinical trial of human vascular endothelial growth factor receptor 1 peptide vaccines for patients with metastatic renal cell carcinoma. Br J Cancer Apr 2 2013;108(6):1260–6.

126. Obara W, Karashima T, Takeda K, et al. Effective induction of cytotoxic T cells recognizing an epitope peptide derived from hypoxia-inducible protein 2 (HIG2) in patients with metastatic renal cell carcinoma. Cancer Immunol Immunother Jan 2017; 66(1):17–24.

127. Rahma OE, Ashtar E, Ibrahim R, et al. A pilot clinical trial testing mutant von Hippel-Lindau peptide as a novel immune therapy in metastatic renal cell carcinoma. J Transl Med Jan 28 2010;8:8.

128. Wierecky J, Müller MR, Wirths S, et al. Immunologic and clinical responses after vaccinations with peptide-pulsed dendritic cells in metastatic renal cancer patients. Cancer Res Jun 1 2006;66(11): 5910–8.

129. Iiyama T, Udaka K, Takeda S, et al. WT1 (Wilms' tumor 1) peptide immunotherapy for renal cell carcinoma. Microbiol Immunol 2007;51(5):519–30.

130. Xu Y, Miller CP, Warren EH, et al. Current status of antigen-specific T-cell immunotherapy for advanced renal-cell carcinoma. Hum Vaccin Immunother Jul 3 2021;17(7):1882–96.

131. Rosenberg SA, Restifo NP. Adoptive cell transfer as personalized immunotherapy for human cancer. Science Apr 3 2015;348(6230):62–8.

132. Chen K, Wang S, Qi D, et al. Clinical investigations of CAR-T cell therapy for solid tumors. Front Immunol 2022;13:896685.

133. Wang QJ, Yu Z, Hanada KI, et al. Preclinical evaluation of chimeric antigen receptors targeting CD70-expressing cancers. Clin Cancer Res May 1 2017;23(9):2267–76.

134. Kim TJ, Lee YH, Koo KC. Current and future perspectives on CAR-T cell therapy for renal cell carcinoma: a comprehensive review. Investig Clin Urol 2022;63(5):486–98.

135. Morgan RA, Dudley ME, Wunderlich JR, et al. Cancer regression in patients after transfer of genetically engineered lymphocytes. Science Oct 6 2006;314(5796):126–9.

136. Florl AR, Löwer R, Schmitz-Dräger BJ, et al. DNA methylation and expression of LINE-1 and HERV-K provirus sequences in urothelial and renal cell carcinomas. Br J Cancer Jul 1999;80(9):1312–21.

137. Siebenthall KT, Miller CP, Vierstra JD, et al. Integrated epigenomic profiling reveals endogenous retrovirus reactivation in renal cell carcinoma. EBioMedicine 2019;41:427–42.

138. Smith CC, Selitsky SR, Chai S, et al. Alternative tumour-specific antigens. Nat Rev Cancer 2019; 19(8):465–78.

139. Kashima S, Maeda T, Masuda K, et al. Cytotoxic T lymphocytes regenerated from iPS cells have therapeutic efficacy in a patient-derived xenograft solid tumor model. iScience Apr 24 2020;23(4):100998.

140. Kawamoto H, Masuda K, Nagano S. Regeneration of antigen-specific T cells by using induced pluripotent stem cell (iPSC) technology. Int Immunol 2021;33(12):827–33.

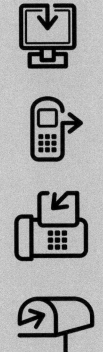